Teaching Mindfulness

Donald McCown · Diane Reibel
Marc S. Micozzi

Teaching Mindfulness

A Practical Guide for Clinicians
and Educators

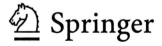 Springer

Donald McCown
School of Health Professions
Thomas Jefferson University
Philadelphia, PA
USA
don.mccown@jefferson.edu

Diane Reibel
Jefferson Medical College
Thomas Jefferson University
Philadelphia, PA
USA
diane.reibel@jefferson.edu

Marc S. Micozzi
School of Medicine
Georgetown University
Washington, DC
USA
marcsmicozzi@aol.com

ISBN 978-0-387-09483-0   e-ISBN 978-0-387-09484-7
DOI 10.1007/978-0-387-09484-7
Springer New York Dordrecht Heidelberg London

Library of Congress Control Number: 2009932118

Printed on acid-free paper

Springer is part of Springer Science+Business Media (www.springer.com)

For the light and love of my life, Gail.
                              Donald McCown

*For my beautiful daughters, Rachel
and Lauren, with love.*
                              Diane Reibel

*For my dear, departed father, Edio,
with gratitude*
                              Marc S. Micozzi

Acknowledgments

We are indebted to Jon Kabat-Zinn, whose vision and dedication in bringing mindfulness to the world has transformed and informed our work and our lives. Our teaching arises from and is grounded in the embodied wisdom of the teachers of the Center for Mindfulness at UMASS Medical School, present and past, and we thank Saki Santorelli for his clarity, compassion, and fire, Melissa Blacker for her limitless love and patience (especially when supervising us!), Florence Meleo-Meyer for her kindness and gentleness, Elana Rosenbaum for the brilliant light she emits, and Ferris Urbanowski for the delight of her loving presence. We are continually nourished and challenged to grow by our noble friends in the Delaware Valley MBSR teacher sangha. Special thanks to our proofing team: Eileen Abrams, Julie Agresta, Carleton Dallery, and Aleeze Moss. We are grateful for the ongoing support of the staff at the Jefferson-Myrna Brind Center of Integrative Medicine. And, after years of teaching, we remain awed and humbled by the incredible courage and unique wisdom of the participants in our classes — they truly are our most powerful teachers.

Donald McCown: I am grateful to those who have shaped my practice, teaching, and way of being in the world: Warren Soule and Chip Prehn for Christian formation and friendship, Larry Kaiden for psychological courage and comfort (and the worst-ever puns), Steve Antinoff for the hard questions about compassion and ethics, Chip Dallery for subtleties of scholarship and social constructionism. Gratitude and bows to Stephen Batchelor and Charles Genoud for bringing Western minds to Eastern thought and teaching in a way that touches my heart and mind, and to Louise Boedeker for connecting me to the transforming power of sensory awareness practice and its lineage. I offer deep appreciation for those who read and commented upon various drafts of the manuscript and important bits and pieces, including Jon Kabat-Zinn, John Dunne, Kenneth Gergen, Jeffrey Brantley, Carleton Dallery, and especially Daniel Siegel — for neuroscience help and encouragement. Given all this wonderful support, any deficiencies and stumbling blocks that have found their way into this book may be laid at the authors' feet. Thanks to the Bryn Mawr College Graduate School of Social Work and Social Research for making space and resources available for research and writing, and to the staff of the Bryn Mawr College library for bearing with all my ILLs, misplaced books, and teetering carts. Finally, much appreciation to Guy Tourangeau, who turned my sketches and scribbles of diagrams into art.

Diane Reibel: Many thanks to my dear friends and colleagues Steven Rosenzweig, MD, and Bud Brainard, PhD, who co-founded the Stress Reduction Program at Jefferson in 1996 at a time when mindfulness was not "hot". They trusted in me to teach MBSR and supported me to develop the program from the ground up (literally, from its start in a dingy basement — a somewhat common theme in MBSR!). Special thanks to Steve, who, at a time when I was uncertain if I had what it takes to teach MBSR, told me, in his infinite wisdom, not to worry: "Your students will be your greatest resource." I share this story with my students till this day, acknowledging that they are indeed my greatest resource. A deep bow to all of my friends from the CFM Teacher Development Intensive 2000. What a blessing to be supported by you and to support you as we continually grow in our own unique way bringing mindfulness to the world! Through the years I have studied with many teachers from different wisdom traditions, each one of you who has enriched my spiritual path beyond measure. I am deeply indebted to Jack Kornfield, Tara Brach, Sylvia Boorstein, Thich Nhat Hanh, Tenzin Wangyal Rinpoche, Tsoknyi Rinpoche, Lama Orgyen Zangpo, Rabbi Zalman Schachter-Shalomi, and Jason Shulman. Deepest gratitude to my dear teacher Rabbi David Cooper for his accessibility, generosity, wisdom, and love. His guidance has been invaluable to me as I navigate the waters of the unknown.

Marc S. Micozzi: I am grateful for having met Don McCown and renewed my contact with Diane Reibel while serving as Executive Director of the Thomas Jefferson University Center for Integrative Medicine (2002–2005). We persisted in our intention to create this book and it will be the lasting legacy of my time there. You might wonder why a university and hospital in Philadelphia are named after Thomas Jefferson of Virginia (my own birth state) given all the distinguished Philadelphians who were also "Founding Fathers." The answer is a long story for another time and something upon which to meditate.

Foreword

What you have in your hands is an important and finely honed work, the first of its kind, as far as I know — a guide for exploring from the inside and making explicit what is involved in teaching mindfulness to adults in mainstream secular settings within mainstream society. This is a pioneering and courageous breaking of new ground, in part because it explicitly brings together different ways of studying and knowing the world of human experience from the perspectives of the scientific, meditative, and philosophical traditions. The authors provide a great deal of context and substance for developing the rich interior space from which all good teaching emerges, as well as the background and history relevant to the emergence of the growing interest in teaching mindfulness among professionals in health care, education, and beyond. They offer a close examination of the range of skill sets required, and the potential positive effects of this pedagogy associated with the cultivation of mindfulness within the community of a classroom. What I hope to contribute to this offering are a range of perspectives and concerns that are essential, in my view at least, to understanding the great responsibility and challenges of teaching mindfulness, and the great benefits that can emerge for others and for oneself if we can keep certain principles and contexts in mind as we engage in this potentially life-transforming work.

Many Streams, One Ocean

In the year 2000, during a meeting in Dharamsala, India, organized by the Mind and Life Institute, in which the Dalai Lama and a group of psychologists, neuroscientists, scholars, and contemplatives explored together the subject of destructive emotions and what might be done to mitigate the enormous personal and societal harm that so often stems from them, the Dalai Lama, amazingly and yet characteristically, challenged the scientists to come up with non-Buddhist, secular methods for working with and transforming the energies of these said emotions.[1] He acknowledged that Buddhism might have a lot to offer, in terms of its elaborate and detailed understanding of what he termed *afflictive emotions*, including a range of meditative practices that have been utilized for centuries and millennia in monastic settings to work with them in skillful ways. At the same time, he was saying that the real hope lay in a non-Buddhist, a truly universal and secular approach that would make use of whatever elements of Buddhist understanding and methods were found to be helpful, but only combined with and integrated into Western culture, its understanding of the psyche, and in particular, its scientific understanding of emotions, emotional expression, and emotion regulation.*

It was truly impressive that the Dalai Lama was encouraging such a secular approach. It affirmed the view that it was only by bringing together the epistemologies and practices of the different cultures represented in the dialogue that whatever might develop would be of any use to people in non-Buddhist countries. Out of that meeting came a very strong and ongoing effort to respond to the Dalai Lama's challenge. It has given rise to a range of new approaches, innovations in teaching methods, books, and studies just now being published in the scientific literature, reporting on major efforts to operationalize this secular challenge and the outcomes of these efforts in terms of brain science, psychology, and medicine.

It was also pointed out at that meeting that there already was an approach that had been doing much of what the Dalai Lama was calling for in clinical settings, primarily hospitals, for twenty-one years at that point, namely mindfulness-based stress reduction (MBSR) and the family of mindfulness-based interventions that have arisen around it. It was also pointed out and discussed in considerable detail that there was a growing base of evidence from scientific studies that MBSR training resulted in profound effects on medical patients and others in terms of relief of pain and suffering, and also in terms of immune response and specific brain changes related to more effective emotion regulation. Of course, it was well known by many of the participants in that meeting that the curriculum of MBSR and other mindfulness-based interventions is deeply rooted in a universal expression of the Buddhadharma[ς]; and that the curriculum features the cultivation of mindfulness of mind states and body states, including in particular, awareness of reactive emotions, as well as how to deploy specific strategies to respond mindfully rather than react reflexively when they are triggered — and even more so if these emotions tend to linger and color one's longer term experience, actions, and relationships, as they so frequently do.

In the emerging of new and compelling fields of inquiry and understanding, in this case the various potential applications of mindfulness in mainstream society, there are usually many different streams of thought and effort that arise more or less simultaneously, sometimes running in parallel, sometimes taking very different directions, but all issuing into the one ocean of what is. All can be said to add value in one way or another to the overall vector of the work because their experience and findings, particularly if the individual efforts have integrity, expand

---

* This would include supporting the development of new research agendas to investigate our understanding of emotions, including happiness, and those not usually studied in the West, or even seen as emotions, such as kindness and compassion.

[ς] The foundational teachings of the Buddha.

our understanding of what works well under what circumstances, and what doesn't. But, sooner or later, the different streams tend to recognize each other, take stock of each other's virtues and limitations, and finally come together in the emergence of a new and inclusive synthesis, one that does indeed add value to what has come before.

In the context of this book, that synthesis would be the emerging in this era of a new way of understanding the nature of the mind and how it works, grows, and continues learning, its relationship to the new-found plasticity of the brain and to the self-healing body, and, in terms of practical applications, what might be possible in a vast array of different venues in society and its institutions, such as medicine and health care, education, business, sports, economics, and politics, were we to individually and collectively avail ourselves of the depths of these emergent discoveries that shed new light on core dimensions of our true nature as human beings.

Motivation and Integrity

Teaching Mindfulness is a welcome and very timely response to the exponential growth of professional interest in mindfulness and its applications in society, and to the need, now upon us, to scale up the teaching of mindfulness to a much broader level within many of society's institutions, as noted above, in response to the rapidly growing interest and demand. This of course, requires a very large cadre of well-trained and highly competent and skilled mindfulness teachers. One critical challenge that the authors are well aware of is that of maintaining the highest levels of mastery and integrity necessary to insure that there is deep authenticity and fidelity in the teaching of mindfulness. Otherwise, it wouldn't be mindfulness, it wouldn't be dharma, and the effort itself wouldn't be very mindful or tap the vast potential energies that lie at the heart of why people are so drawn to mindfulness in the first place. For mindfulness is not just one more method or technique, akin to other familiar techniques and strategies we may find instrumental and effective in one field or another. It is a way of being, of seeing, of tapping into the full dimensionality of our humanity, and this way has a critical non-instrumental essence inherent in it. From the very first chapter, the authors describe a process and pedagogy that speak to the depths of what the work is, what it asks of those who come to teach it, and what the challenges are for anyone hoping to pursue such a path.

One of those challenges is to examine one's own motivation for embarking on such an unusual path in the first place. Motivation is an ongoing and crucial factor for teaching mindfulness, and even more so, for maintaining, sustaining, and deepening one's practice. It invites continual re-examination and reflection, as motivations can grow and change, and richly mature over time and with experience.

In terms of initial motivations, the authors recognize that the mushrooming professional interest in mindfulness in different arenas carries with it the inevitable risk that for some, becoming a mindfulness teacher is now something of a smart career move. This is not necessarily bad. Actually it is a sign of success that so many young people, graduate students, medical students, new teachers, are wanting to work in this area, sometimes even introducing mindfulness as a field of professional inquiry to their mentors and advisors. So even if mindfulness is a smart career move for some at this point in time, that is still simply a starting off point on an extended journey, a place to begin, and a profound opportunity to follow one's intuition and ambition into something far deeper than one might suspect at first. It is almost inevitable that one will discover that the trajectory one has embarked upon goes way beyond the concept that mindfulness is merely a technique that one can easily pick up at a workshop or professional training and then integrate into one's repertoire of skills. This challenge will become, whether anticipated or not by those drawn to this work, a central feature of one's effectiveness as a teacher.

The early years of MBSR and the development of other mindfulness-based clinical interventions were the province of a small group of people who gave themselves over to practicing and teaching mindfulness basically out of love, out of passion for the practice, knowingly and happily putting their careers and economic well-being at risk because of that love, usually stemming from deep first-person encounters with the dharma and its meditative practices, often through the mediation of Buddhist teachers and acknowledged masters within a number of well-defined traditions and lineages. For better or for worse, the next generations of mindfulness teachers may not have the same opportunities or even interest in studying and practicing with Asian Buddhist teachers, or Asian teachers in other traditions that value the wisdom of mindfulness, such as Sufism, the yogas, and Taoism. Fortunately, there are ample opportunities, for those who wish to pursue them, to study and practice with Asian teachers and with seasoned Western dharma teachers who have themselves practiced in Asia with respected teachers, and to sit long retreats at wonderful Dharma centers in the West. I personally consider sitting long teacher-led retreats periodically to be an absolute necessity in the developing of one's own meditation practice, understanding, and effectiveness as a teacher. But while sitting periodic long retreats may be necessary, it is not in itself sufficient. Mindfulness in everyday life is the ultimate challenge and practice.

The practice of mindfulness is a life-time's engagement. Growth, development, and maturation as a mindfulness practitioner and teacher of mindfulness are a critical part of the process. It is not always painless. Self-awareness can be very humbling, so the motivation to carry on and face what needs facing must mature as well in the process.

Opportunity and Calling

Why is mindfulness so sought after in this moment, and so necessary? In part, I would say, because the world and its institutions and denizens are literally and metaphorically starving for authentic ways to live and to be and to act in the world. We long for some degree of effective balance and wisdom that supports meaningful, embodied, and significant work — the work of making a difference in the world, of adding value and beauty, of individually and collectively waking up to the full range of human intelligences and capacities we share for wisdom, ease of being and kindness. Those capacities and intelligences also include a love of learning, the urge to continue growing into our full potential as beings across the lifespan, into our capacity for healing ourselves and society, into becoming agents of healing out of the response of our compassionate hearts, in a word, an aspiration from deep within our bones and cells and DNA for contributing to the flowering of what is deepest and best in ourselves as human beings, as the species name *homo sapiens sapiens* [the species that knows and knows that it knows] suggests. Without this waking up from the endemic unawareness and self-absorption that we are also subject to, our propensity as a species for ignoring what is most important, coupled with our intellectual and technological precocity and tendency to be blinded by our own volatile emotions and desires, may get us and our now small and crowded planet into even greater trouble than it is already in.

If we were to name some of the emergent streams at the moment that are germane to the subject of *Teaching Mindfulness*, the list would include the domains of mind/body medicine, integrative medicine, mindfulness-based clinical interventions of all kinds in health care, medicine, psychology, and psychotherapy, including mindfulness-based stress reduction (MBSR), mindfulness-based cognitive therapy (MBCT), mindfulness-based relapse prevention for binge drinking (MBRP), mindfulness-based childbirth and parenting (MBCP), mindfulness-based art therapy for cancer patients (MBAT), mindfulness-based eating awareness training (MB-EAT), mindfulness-based trauma therapy (MBTT), mindfulness-based relapse prevention — Women (MBRP-W), mindfulness-based elder care (MBEC), dialectical behavior therapy (DBT), acceptance and commitment therapy (ACT), mindfulness-based psychotherapy, mindfulness-informed psychotherapy, mindfulness-based mind fitness training (MMFT) in the military, the Shamatha Project, the Contemplative Mind in Society, Google's main campus employee program in mindfulness-based emotional intelligence — Search Inside Yourself (SIY), the emerging fields of contemplative neuroscience and neuro-phenomenology, and perhaps the biggest challenge of all in many ways, the emerging stream of bringing mindfulness into education, especially K-12 education, but also higher education. That is a lot of mindfulness-based work. Of course, this trend implies that we will soon require a lot of mindfulness teachers, a lot more than are presently available. And good ones. It is up to us, individually and collectively, to recognize what that might mean.

This remarkable and ambitious book is a uniquely welcome contribution to the flowering of mindfulness in the West in mainstream professional circles. To date, no other book has even attempted to synthesize the various elements of the MBSR model into a coherent and explicit teaching pedagogy that could serve as a foundation for the skillful development of new teachers, and the ongoing deepening development of experienced teachers of mindfulness in this wholly secular idiom, yet which is wholly based on the non-dual universal dharma that the Dharma within Buddhism is and has always pointed to.... a basic lawfulness in the universe, and in the nature of what we call "the mind" and its behavior. In this context, which can sound quite daunting, it is important to keep in mind that the Buddha himself was not a Buddhist, and that even the term *Buddhism* was coined by Westerners only several hundred years ago.[2]

This book has many virtues. One salient example is the explicit emphasis on and fine-structure analysis of the pedagogy of the classroom and the processes of inquiry and dialogue that lie at the heart of good dharma teaching. The emphasis on the group experience is critical, since almost all mindfulness-based approaches work in a class setting with sizable groups of people, whether they be medical patients or children in a kindergarten or high school classroom. The authors address many domains in the field of mindfulness-based interventions that have remained up to this point more implicit than explicit. One is an overview of the historical roots of Western, and particularly North American interest in meditation. Another is the art and the science and the skill set of teaching mindfulness in a professional clinical context.

Every element of the pedagogy offered here, as the authors themselves point out, is potentially subject to debate and reflection, and to be put to the test in practice. What makes a "good enough" mindfulness teacher is something of a lifetime koan[ᴪ], at least I have found it to be so in my own life, and that koan reminds me constantly of how audacious the undertaking is (and how inadequate we all may feel), and yet, how important and priceless it is as well (see section 8).

Fidelity and Innovation in Any Curriculum

One characteristic of the MBSR curriculum that the authors explicitly point out is that it has what they refer to as "integrity." Where MBSR itself is concerned, and other clinical interventions modeled on it, this integrity needs to be protected, especially in the face of the inevitable impulse on the part of new teachers to improve the curriculum, or add new "modules" to it, or put in their favorite pedagogical material to enrich the program to make it there own. These are all understandable and in some cases, admirable and creative impulses. And in some instances, they work and work well, and are a necessary element of making the teaching your own.

At the same time, because the foundation lies in mindfulness, it also lies in silence, stillness, and spaciousness. For that reason, we need to guard against the

---

[ᴪ]a koan is a Zen teaching device, like a puzzle in the form of a question or statement or dialogue one attempts to hold in mind during meditation and understand and respond to without responding with the discursive thinking mind, since no response coming out of thought will be authentic and adequate to the circumstances of the moment. An example would be "What am I?" or "Does a dog have Buddha nature" or "What is Buddha?" Almost any life circumstance could be seen as a koan. You could think of it as "What is this?" or even, "What now?" In every moment, the response might be different. The only requirement is that it be authentic and appropriate, and not come out of dualistic thinking. Responses can be non-verbal.

impulse we might have, especially if we feel uncomfortable with extended silences or uncertain that the participants in the class are "getting" what we want them to "get," to fill all the empty space in MBSR with extra "stuff." The emptiness, the "sparseness" of the curriculum is that way for a reason. Without the silence, the stillness, the spaciousness of the non-conceptual, it would merely become a cognitive exercise, no longer speaking to or cultivating the heart of mindfulness, which is practice.

Several MBSR teachers have shared with me over the years that they have tried at times to change the curriculum in one way or another, to add things, or take things out, even the core practices themselves. In the end, they came back to the core structure of MBSR, having found that their changes didn't work as well as they had thought. One of the reasons they returned to the core curriculum was discovering that, without meaning for it to happen, all the space and feelings of openness and silence had been filled up.

So when teaching MBSR, it is important that it be MBSR and not simply whatever one wants to put in or take out or modify according to one's liking or feelings of inadequacy under that umbrella. This means that if you don't feel competent to teach mindful yoga, then you develop that competency through study and practice with good yoga teachers. You don't bring a yoga expert in to do the yoga, any more than you would bring a breathing expert in to teach the breathing. You don't throw out the body scan because you think it is too slow, or too threatening to some, but you learn to work skillfully with the body scan in various ways, realizing that it does have the potential to trigger reactions in people with histories of abuse, etc.

One lesson that scientists have learned from evolution is that certain molecular structures within our cells have been conserved and relatively or even highly invariant over time, and across species. An example would be the structure of actin and myosin molecules, which work together to form muscle that is capable of contracting when it needs to contract, and releasing when it needs to release. Another even more elemental example would be the structure of ribosomes and other cellular organelles. Having refined a process and a structure that functioned effectively over unthinkable amounts of time, almost any change in the structure is bound to lead to a diminishment of function. People have said that MBSR may be similar in some ways. It is important to be innovative, and pull on everything the teacher knows and loves, as appropriate. There is a great deal of latitude and space built into the MBSR curriculum for the teacher to bring in himself or herself in critical ways, including, where appropriate, new information and practices. That latitude in creativity is essential for the curriculum to come alive. But at the same time, there is little room in the 8-week MBSR curriculum for putting in more stuff, however interesting or relevant, without sacrificing something perhaps more important.

It is usually more space that is needed, rather than more information or methods or learning modules. What is important is that the structure reflects the depths of the opportunity that mindfulness offers both each individual and the class as a whole. For the teachers, all that comes out of throwing oneself into the practice itself, and trusting the practice and life to be the real teacher.

Thus, the emergence of the pedagogy elaborated in this book will be, as the authors hope and suggest, an ongoing contemplation in its own right regarding what the teaching of mindfulness is all about. While the 8-week format and curriculum of MBSR in the clinical setting may have its own inner logic for conserving the format and not introducing all sorts of extraneous concepts because of the teacher's pet interests, other forms of mindfulness teaching in other contexts will *require* and *demand* just this kind of spontaneous creativity. When developing new and innovative mindfulness programs for new venues, whether it be at Google headquarters, or in stressful workplaces, prisons, the inner city, sports teams, or for bringing mindfulness into elementary and middle schools, it is important to keep in mind that modifications and innovation are absolutely necessary. At the same time, you wouldn't want to lose the essence. In order not to, you have to live inside that essence yourself, and know who you are working with, what the dominant culture and idiom are, what the specific needs of the culture and its community of constituents might be, in a word, the full spectrum of what each teaching opportunity presents you with. Just dealing with the fact that in many venues a high proportion of participants may have known or unknown histories of trauma requires a degree of sensitivity and flexibility that may change how the curriculum is unfolded, both qualitatively and quantitatively. Of course, you may never know the culture you are entering all that well, so a lot of your capacity to innovate effectively will rely, once again, on trust, on your intuition and sensitivity, as well as on your own good will and clarity, and of course, on your practice.

Languaging and Reification

In my own teaching and practice, I try to bring a highly refined ear to the possible uses of the language so that the languaging itself recognizes and points to and embodies the non-dual. Without opening to this dimension of experience, there is no reason for teaching mindfulness, nor for practicing it. Thus the valuable gift of present participles in the English language, what the Buddhist scholar, John Dunne termed, in observing how much care is given to it in MBSR, "the secret heart of the English gerund." It's virtue is that it transcends duality. That is not the case in all languages, but in English, we are blessed with this part of speech, and it can be very effective in the teaching of mindfulness and dharma. For one thing, it can help us to avoid unwittingly falling into the imperative verb form in guiding meditations, as in "breathe in" or "breathe out," which posits an authority (me), telling someone, namely *you*, who I expect to obey this command, what to do. But by saying "breathing in," you the teacher are no longer giving an order, privileging your position over the student's. We are in this together, and the breathing takes care of itself. The only question is, can we be here for it? Is there any awareness of it? For it is never the objects of attention that are the key to mindfulness practice. It is the *attending* itself. In the attending, there need not be any subject reified who is "doing the attending," or "doing the meditating," for that matter.

With a modicum of awareness, we do not need to fall into what amounts to a very strong habit, built right into the language, of identifying ourselves as the seer, the listener, the smeller, the taster, the toucher, the doer, the knower, absolutely separate and distinct from what is seen, heard, smelled, tasted, touched, done, or known, as opposed to a more co-creative and co-arising, relational unity. At first, it might seem artificial in the extreme, and certainly the use of present participles can be overdone or mindlessly abused, just like anything else. But, as pointed to over and over again by the authors, there is a profound opportunity in every moment to rest in awareness without falling into separation and a reification of self or other, and disregarding the relationality and interconnectedness that is so fundamental to experience. So, while there is observing, for instance, we do not have to create, or reify, an "observer;" while breathing a "breather;" while thinking a "thinker;" or while meditating, a "meditator."

Needless to say, from a relative point of view, of course it is *we* who are breathing. It is not somebody else's breath coming out of our body. It is not somebody else's checking account that has your name on the checks. We certainly are seeing, we are hearing, etc. But the mystery lies in who we think that "we" or "I" or "me" is. The mystery lies in the personal pronouns, and how much we identify with them without awareness of the reciprocity of relationality, of interconnectedness, and what Thich Nhat Hanh calls *interbeing*. That may be why the Buddha once said that all of his years of teaching could be encapsulated into the one sentence: "Nothing is to be clung to as I, me, or mine."[3,4]

One valuable use of the present participle in the English language is that it can leave subject and object indeterminate, unvoiced. This is a new (and very old) kind of experiencing, underneath thought itself, in the domain of being, the domain of the timeless, of knowing without a knower, of pure awareness. This understanding lies at the heart of the pedagogy presented here.

Trust

Donald McCown and Diane Reibel are experienced teachers of mindfulness in various contexts, particularly MBSR and its applications in heath care and business. They are very clear to point out that the pedagogy presented here is a beginning, a means rather than an end. It is meant to be exploratory, tentative, and invitational, clay on the wheel, shaped by their own experience and backgrounds, and aimed at getting us as readers and teachers or possible teachers of mindfulness in secular settings to think and talk together about how we see and work with the challenges of bringing mindfulness in various ways into different contexts and settings. The invitation is to enter into a conversation, to share approaches and perspectives, to reflect together on skillful means for igniting passionate engagement in people, whatever the context, for being more present in their own lives, and for understanding the value of consistent practice and cultivation of embodied mindfulness. They are explicit about this being a collective inquiry, dialogue, and investigation within the community of mindfulness teachers, as well as an occasion to reflect deeply within oneself as to one's motivation for doing this work or for being drawn to it as a professional, one's relationship to one's own practice of mindfulness and the never-ending learning curve it entails, and to situate one's own understanding within a much broader historical and social perspective that we sometimes shy away from or frankly ignore. It also asks us to reflect on the synergies of practicing and teaching mindfulness in the context of a gathering of people, specifically in a classroom, where the potential for maximizing attunement within oneself and among the group, what the authors term "intersubjective resonance," based on the work of Ed Tronick, Daniel Siegel, and others in attachment theory and interpersonal neurobiology[5], is profound and enormously valuable.

Importantly, such resonances are not something one attempts to bring into being. That would be a tantamount to forcing or seeking a particular effect, and thus, an attachment to a particular outcome. The desire to bring about an effect is a trap that, if one falls into it, belies one's understanding of mindfulness and the work in the first place, and potentially betrays it as well as yourself and your students, at least for that moment. Of course, we all have fallen into that trap at one moment or another, and hopefully, we learn from such moments as we grow into becoming good-enough teachers. But if we can anticipate and appreciate the potential of such impulses arising, notice them when they do, and resist filling the space with one's own thoughts, anxiety, and agenda-driven aims, that noticing itself allows for the ultimately mysterious emerging of such intra- and inter-subjective resonances within the container of stillness, silence, and awareness in the room.

For this to have even a chance to unfold, trust is paramount. Trust in the practice, trust in the silence, in the spaciousness of awareness that does not have to be filled with anything, trust in a moment that does not have to give rise to anything else, or be described, trust in the beauty of each person in the room as they are. This is one of the many many reasons why we frequently say, as a sort of short-hand, that, when it comes right down to it, *the teaching has to come out of one's practice.* There is simply no other way. Therefore, exquisite intimacy with one's own mind states, including those invariable impulses that *do* want to fill any empty space, that *are* very much attached to preconceived outcomes that are favorable to one's aims and philosophy or ego, is essential.

And you who take on this challenge, or will, or have, will know or come to know that you are probably the greatest beneficiary of your own teaching, practice, and study, more than anybody you teach no matter how much they benefit from it. And you will realize that your students, whoever they are, whatever the context, what-ever the chosen mindfulness-based vehicle you are working within, are teaching you at least as much as you are teaching them, until you come to realize that it is life itself that is the only teacher of any note here, life itself that is both the curriculum, the path, and the end of any path, right here, in the present moment, in the circumstances and context we have chosen to walk into and stand within, wherever and however that might be.

Lineage

To stand within such human potential for learning, growing, connecting, healing, transformation, realization, liberation, however you want to frame it, usually requires some sense of lineage. How did you arrive at this spot, in this moment, carrying the message of awareness, of mindfulness, of presence, allowing yourself to be a catalyst in its dissemination to others? Chances are, it wasn't totally by yourself. In all likelihood it has resulted from a journey, perhaps an inner one, perhaps since childhood, perhaps it has come as a transmission from someone else, a gift of sorts, a structure, a curriculum, or the opportunity and necessity to craft a curriculum of your own out of sometimes very trying and often unfamiliar circumstances. Here is another place where your recognition of your personal journey, your path, your teachers, what Yeats called "the unknown instructors," is so essential. Sometimes, you have to answer, when the question is posed: "What tradition do you teach in?"

It happened to me in an unanticipated moment, in Shenzhen, China in 2004, when I was visiting a Chan temple along with some friends, Helen Ma and Rosalie Kwong, who teach MBSR in Hong Kong.

Venerable Ben Huan, a sparkling-eyed 98 year-old Chinese Chan master, after MBSR had been explained to him by one of his senior monks and Dharma successors [the Venerable Hin Hung, who had read and studied the literature on mindfulness-based applications in medicine and health care and was bringing similar principles into both psychotherapy and the education of children, and so was equipped to explain it accurately], commented: "There are an infinite number of ways in which people suffer; therefore there must be an infinite number of ways in which the Dharma is made available to them."

He said this looking straight at me. When it was translated by Hin Hung, I realized that this old Chan Master was giving me and the other teachers in the room a tremendous gift by saying such a thing, by according such a profound recognition and acceptance to another dharma vehicle, potentially suspect, of course, from halfway round the world, that he could easily have felt might be inauthentic.

Then, totally unexpectedly, in his very next utterance, he asked, "What tradition do you teach in?" He clearly wanted to push this foreigner a bit and in a friendly way, "test his understanding," as is the way of Chan and Zen, by probing with a bit of dialogue, with what is sometimes called *dharma combat*. In such exchanges, it is not so much the specific response to a question in words that is critical, but *how* one responds to the challenge it throws out.

I responded, "I teach in the tradition of the Buddha and of Hui Neng*." It was an attempt to be authentic while at the same time, giving him a reference frame that he would recognize and understand. He came right back with "What's the primary point?" I smiled and replied, "Why non-attachment, of course," at which point he

---

* The sixth Patriarch of Chinese Chan Buddhism (638-713 AD).

said, "Would you like to become my student?" I smiled again, leaned in close to him, and said, "I thought I already was your student." He laughed and said, "Let's go eat lunch."

All this is to say that you cannot worry about being "enlightened" or "a realized being" if you aspire to be an MBSR teacher, or an MBCT teacher, or any other kind of mindfulness-based instructor. But what you very much do need to take care of — and not worry about — is tending to, deepening, and nurturing in every possible way, many of which may be unconventional and untraditional, your own meditation practice. This might include exposure to and studying with great teachers in the various Buddhist traditions and lineages: *Theravada*, *Mahayana*, and *Vajrayana* to whatever degree possible. Because if mindfulness-based interventions have anything profound, healing, and transformational to offer the world, it is only because they are firmly grounded in the Dharma — not so much as expressed in the particular cultural and religious forms of the Buddhadharma — but as *universal dharma*, which it is up to us to understand, realize for ourselves (clearly a life-time's engagement), find ways to language, and share authentically with others without idealizing any of it. Matter-of-fact is the way to go.

I answered Ben Huan as I did in that moment. In another place, or at another time, or under different circumstances, I might have answered very differently. The answer itself is not important, but one's open awareness of the question and where it is coming from *is* very important. There is never one right answer, just as there is no one right way to practice. This is one small way in which we have to shoulder responsibility for our own work, situating it honestly within our own practice, our own understanding, our own lineage, learning from everything that arises for us in our lives, in our searching for right livelihood, in our professional calling and fields of expertise, and certainly in our desire to be a mindfulness teacher. Not knowing is preferable to too much knowing. But when we are on the spot, any spot, we will need to respond, and respond authentically. Our students require it. The curriculum requires it. Your very integrity requires it.

At the same time, the dharma is very forgiving. If you make a mis-take, as we all have done countless times, if you regret something you did, or said, or forgot to do, or didn't say, the very next moment, or week, provides amply opportunities for correcting, adjusting, apologizing, whatever feels appropriate. This work is not about being perfect, whatever that might mean. It is very much about being human, and about learning as we, like everybody else, get caught by our own unawareness, our own fears, our own feelings of inadequacy, whatever it might be in a particular moment when we feel we do not measure up to our own standards and expectations, or those of others we admire. These too, are opportunities, precious ones: for mindfulness, for practicing what we may too often be preaching as good for others, forgetting that we will always be the greatest beneficiary of our own teaching, and experience, because it really isn't *ours*, it just is what it is. It is hard not to take things personally, especially when we feel we have made a serious mistake, but taking personally what is not personal might be the biggest, and the most recalcitrant mis-take of all.

The koan of "What is good-enough teaching."

No one ever said it was easy to be a mindfulness teacher, or practitioner. In many ways, it is the hardest work in the world, just to be present for a moment, and open-hearted. That is why it might just be worthy of our energy and commitment. We need to be grounded in our own practice and trust that it will be adequate when we most need it, and have to act out of it *without thinking* but with that other core capacity we have, the only one capable of containing and taming thoughts and emotions, namely *awareness*.

Competency in teaching mindfulness within secular mindfulness-based frameworks is a combination of knowing and not knowing. It helps to know from the inside, through your bones and skin, the general framework of the Dharma, including the Four Noble (Ennobling) Truths, the Eight-Fold Noble Path, something of the Abhidharma, stories of certain teachers and teaching stories, and perhaps the teaching lineage of at least one Buddhist tradition. But *not* for the purpose of teaching any of it, or to tell any of those stories. Only to use it in a wordless way, to inform yourself, remind yourself about the meaning of practice, and of key elements embedded in our experience, such as anicca, anatta, dukkha, the kelesas, the four foundations of mindfulness, the four immeasurables (Brama Viharas — loving kindness, compassion, empathic joy, and equanimity), etc.

Also, it might be essential for you to participate in various professional training programs in mindfulness and its myriad applications, offered by a number of centers in various parts of the world. These are listed in the Appendix of this book. All are the product of an intensive commitment to the practice on the part of the founders and staff, coupled with unique perspectives on professionalism and skillful means for training people to do the work of teaching mindfulness in different professional settings and fields. The one I know best is the one offered by the Oasis Institute for Mindfulness-Based Professional Education and Innovation of The Center for Mindfulness in Medicine, Health Care, and Society (CFM) at the University of Massachusetts Medical School, where MBSR originated. Oasis offers teacher certification in MBSR, and a range of professional training programs in mindfulness and divers specific applications throughout the world.[6]

Hopefully you will become intimate over time with classroom moments of not knowing what to do, what to say, who your students are, and what or who you are, and yet be willing to sit/stand/be/move in the not-knowing and reside in the present moment in full awareness — with an agenda (since you are the teacher) and with *no* agenda (since you are the teacher), and no attachment to any outcome, yet with the intention to be of service and the aspiration that everybody's suffering in the room will be honored and held in awareness, without any attempt to fix anything that you think might be broken. The invitation for yourself is that you are, together with all the classroom participants (who are equally as wise and beautiful and worthy as yourself), co-creating or "enacting" or "allowing" the mindfulness-based curriculum to emerge, and trusting in that emergence moment by moment as you rest in awareness — an awareness that is intrinsically boundless, spacious, luminous, empty, and kind.

So a question we might address to ourselves, and which *Teaching Mindfulness* will help us in exploring, comes down to "What is good enough?" What is good enough in terms of preparation for teaching, beyond all the essential planning and thought that may need to go into a class? What is good enough in terms of the quality of one's own mindfulness practice? What is good enough in terms of the teachers you have trained with, and the books you have or haven't read, or the retreats you have or haven't sat? What is good enough in terms of your presence in the classroom? In terms of your comfort with silence and stillness? Or lack thereof?

Here are a few offerings from my experience, although the only authentic responses will be those of your own heart:

It is "good enough" *for now* if you don't contribute to or exacerbate the harm and suffering others are experiencing, or become aware that you are and alter your approach and even apologize when you inadvertently do.

It is "good enough" *for now* if you know you don't really know what you are doing but somehow find a way to be real within the container of the MBSR curriculum or other curriculum you are facilitating in support of mindfulness, and bring it to life in the face of life unfolding and expressing itself in the human beings you are working with, and in yourself, of course.

It is "good enough" *for now* if you carefully drink in what is being offered in this book and take it to heart as you develop your own unique strengths and skills and questions as a meditation teacher and mindfulness instructor.

It is "good enough" *for now* if you keep in mind at all times that life is the real meditation teacher, and life is the real meditation practice.

It is "good enough" if you can remember from time to time, especially when you forget, that nothing you think is personal is personal, so it is best not to take things personally, including your own performance, since it is not a performance but an exchange, a gift, a love affair.

Then you just might make a very big and beneficial difference in some people's lives, and in your own.

Jon Kabat-Zinn
September 18, 2009

Endnotes

1. Goleman, Daniel *Destructive Emotions: How Can We Overcome Them?*, Bantam Books, NY, 2003.
2. Batchelor, Stephen *The Awakening of the West: The Encounter of Buddhism and Western Culture*, Parallax Press, Berkeley CA, 1994, Chapter 14.
3. Buddhadasa Bhikkhu *The Heartwood of the Bodhi Tree: The Buddha's Teachings on Voidness*, Wisdom, Boston, 1994, pp 15–17.
4. Goldstein, Joseph *One Dharma: The Emerging Western Buddhism*, HarperSanFrancisco, 2002, pg 134.
5. Siegel, Daniel *The Mindful Brain: Reflection and Attunement in the Cultivation of Well-Being*, WW Norton, NY, 2007.
6. See http://www.umassmed.edu/cfm/oasis/index.aspx

Preface

Why We Wrote this Book

It would be simple and easy to say that this book is about passing on the gift of mindfulness. But that would be a bit glib, and would miss a subtle and vital point. Mindfulness, the capacity to be with and in the constant flow of awareness, is an inherent ability that we all share: It's not so much a gift as a given. The real gift, then, is the teaching of mindfulness, the act of pointing out and tending to the development of what is already given in the other.

This gift of teaching mindfulness flows in two directions. There is the possibility of mutual transformation. The one who is taught is enriched beyond measure as the practice of mindfulness helps reveal and realize her unique, authentic being, and she participates more deeply and with greater freedom in her own inner life and life with others. The one who teaches receives powerful instruction through this process. In finding ways to reach the other in her difference, a teacher is continually brought up short, pressed in each moment to question, adjust, even overturn, her own understandings and assumptions of the practice, her teaching, and herself. The value of such destabilization — and the attendant opportunities for growth — is limitless.

This book is our contribution to keep the gift of teaching mindfulness in circulation. It is rooted in gratitude for the grace of the practice, the generosity of our own teachers through the years, and the power of the challenges posed by the uniqueness and authenticity of those we have taught — and those we have been teaching to teach.

Who Should Read this Book

If the practice of mindfulness has transformed your life in huge or tiny ways (or both!), this book is for you. You can most fully express gratitude for the teaching you've received by sharing it with others. However large or small an undertaking that may become for you, you'll find hints and help here.

We're writing from a frame of reference defined by a complex of influences, the most salient of which are many years of teaching within the Mindfulness-Based Stress Reduction curriculum, the requirements of working within hospital and academic settings, and the demands of training professionals from across a range of disciplines. As a result, the book may seem at first glance to be most accessible to clinicians, such as physicians, psychologists, social workers, marriage and family therapists, professional counselors, nurses, occupational therapists, physical therapists, and others, as well as to clergy and educators.

Yet, the accessibility is ultimately much wider. If you have experienced the benefits of mindfulness practice, the material here can help you better understand your own practice, reveal ways that you can deepen it, and bring clarity to how you speak about mindfulness practice with others in your life.

How to Use this Book

The three-part structure of this book gives you several points of entry. If you're coming with just a little background to investigate the possibilities of teaching mindfulness, Part I (Chapters 1, 2, and 3) may be the place to start. Chapter 1 provides an overview of the contemporary mindfulness-based interventions in medicine and mental healthcare. Chapter 2 places those interventions in the wider historical and cultural context of the meeting of East and West in Western, particularly North American culture, suggesting the ripple effects and the expanding openness to contemplative practices in general and mindfulness in particular. Chapter 3 attempts to offer a pragmatic definition and felt understanding of mindfulness that will be useful for a teacher when inquiring about her practice or the practice of those she is teaching.

For those who have ongoing personal practices of mindfulness meditation and are currently teaching or considering stepping out in that way, Part II (Chapters 4 and 5) may make a sensible beginning. Chapter 4 will help you towards a realization of what is required of you in the process of teaching, and what you might wish to explore or develop further in your practice and teaching. Chapter 5 outlines the skills of teaching, explaining how and when they come into play, and offering vignettes of the skills in use with participants.

Part III (Chapters 6, 7, and 8) is the most pragmatic way in, for those concerned primarily with curricular and pedagogical questions. The final three chapters focus on the unfolding of the pedagogy of mindfulness (as we understand it at this moment) and its concrete expressions in curricula and guided practice. Chapter 6 provides a schematic of the process of teaching and learning within mindfulness-based interventions, whether with groups or individuals. Chapter 7 is our identification and description of a series of "gestures" of the process of teaching and learning, illustrated with interchanges between teachers and participants. Chapter 8 is meant as a resource for teaching, with scripts for audio recordings and step-by-step descriptions of activities and practices that can be used as jumping off points for development of any teacher's own presentations.

Wherever you are in your development as a teacher, wherever you start in this book, we trust that you'll find something you can use immediately, something that challenges your assumptions, and something that brings you right to the breath in the present moment – an inspiration to share the gift of teaching mindfulness.

Contents

Part I
Clinical and Cultural Context

Chapter 1
Getting Grounded (In Our Own Instability)

The applications and use of mindfulness-based interventions (MBIs) in medicine and mental healthcare have been expanding as rapidly as the empirical evidence base that is validating and recommending them. This growth has created a powerful demand for professionals who can effectively deliver these interventions and for training new professionals who can enter the fold.

The very idea of teaching mindfulness as a professional creates a conundrum. Questions of *why*, and *who*, and *how* arise immediately to send us into a spiral of alternating definitions and possible doubts. The terrain of our cultural moment is unstable ground on which those of us who choose to do this work must stand.

One answer to *why* one should teach mindfulness as a professional, then, is simple and cold: because of market demand. A simultaneous and likewise simple answer adds some warmth: because mindfulness really seems to help relieve suffering.

Next, the *who* question sidles up to lean on the *why* answers, and the spiral begins. The person of the teacher of mindfulness is little considered and loosely defined in the scientific literature. Depending on the intervention, the "mindfulness professional" may be placed anywhere along a continuum that extends from a workshop-trained instructor who provides introductions to some useful techniques, all the way to an accomplished meditator with decades of intensive practice and study with traditional masters, who embody to a large degree mindfulness as a way of being.

So, at this point, the *how* question gives a push, and the spiral speeds up and spins. The art, or craft, or science of teaching mindfulness is too rarely discussed in public forums. Many mindfulness teachers work in relative isolation, following their pedagogical whims and intuitions into success in one direction, frustration in another, and uncertainty at every turn. Even where local communities of practice have sprung up, sharing and development of pedagogical theory and best practices are more sought after than found.

Perhaps the first step in resolving the conundrum presented by teaching mindfulness as a professional is to become more solidly grounded in our own instability, to look more closely at the questions of *why* and *who* and *how*. Let's take them in order.

D. McCown et al., *Teaching Mindfulness: A Practical Guide
for Clinicians and Educators*, DOI 10.1007/978-0-387-09484-7_1,
© Springer Science+Business Media, LLC 2010

Why? Responding to the Demand

Certainly, implicit and explicit practices that can be identified as "mindfulness" have long been a part of medicine and mental healthcare in the West. Influences from the philosophies and spiritualities of both Eastern and Western cultures have helped to shape professional practice in important ways since the middle of the nineteenth century and especially since the middle of the twentieth. Such influences are evident in the course of development of what are now called complementary and alternative medicine (CAM) and integrative medicine (IM), and in both the psychodynamic and humanistic traditions of psychotherapy — and related approaches — since their inceptions. We will discuss this history in more depth in Chapter 2.

The current demand for professionals who can teach mindfulness is much more recent. According to commentators, the year 1990 was a watershed, after which "mindfulness" as a discrete term began to take hold in the discourse of academic medicine and psychology (Dryden and Still, 2006). That's the publication date of Jon Kabat-Zinn's *Full Catastrophe Living*, describing the mindfulness-based stress reduction (MBSR) program that he developed in 1979 at the University of Massachusetts Medical Center. The book made the concepts and content of the program and the benefits of mindfulness accessible to a general audience. The enterprise quickly got a boost when Bill Moyers featured Kabat-Zinn and the MBSR program on his *Healing and the Mind* public television series in 1993. Interest by medical and mental healthcare professionals as well as healthcare consumers grew dramatically from that point onward. In a count taken five years after the Moyers series, there were MBSR programs in more than 240 hospitals and clinics in the Unites States and in other countries (Salmon et al. 1998). Ten years after the series, meditation and mindfulness were featured in cover stories in both *Time* and *Newsweek* (Kalb, 2003; Stein, 2003). The professional and public acceptance of MBSR epitomized a wider cultural change, as contemplative philosophies and practices — such as yoga, Tai Chi, meditation, and prayer — came into the mainstream not merely of medicine and academia, but of church basements and shopping malls, daytime talk shows, and primetime sitcoms.

As Dryden and Still (2006) suggest, the epochal growth and influence of MBSR have arisen from its position at the confluence of certain social and institutional factors. Perhaps most important is its emerging status as an "evidence-based treatment," creating a theoretical appeal to academic, government, and public sector funding sources and service providers. From the beginning, MBSR has been the focus of outcome studies with specific medical or psychiatric conditions and populations, as well as with the general population. Although early studies often lacked methodological rigor, as interest and evidence have mounted, resources and funding have become available for randomized, controlled clinical trials, which have continued to provide support for the efficacy of MBSR and other mindfulness-based and informed interventions. As we are writing this, clinical trials have been funded or are underway to study the efficacy of mindfulness-based interventions in asthma, bone marrow transplant, breast cancer, chronic pain, chronic obstructive pulmonary disease (COPD), fibromyalgia, human immunodeficiency virus/acquired immunodeficiency syndrome (HIV/AIDS), hot flashes, hypertension, immune response to human papillomavirus, irritable bowel syndrome, lupus, myocardial ischemia, obesity, prostate cancer, rheumatoid arthritis, solid organ transplant, type-2 diabetes, and other medical conditions, as well as psychiatric disorders, including anxiety disorders, delusional disorder, depression, drug abuse and dependence, eating disorders, personality disorders, post-traumatic stress disorder, schizophrenia, suicidality, and others (Clinical Trials, 2008). It would seem that MBSR and other mindfulness-based interventions are filling an aching need within academic medicine and psychology for new avenues of research. For example, at this writing, in one of the academic psychology programs with which we are familiar, 11 of 12 approved doctoral dissertation topics concern mindfulness.

Mindfulness-based interventions and health benefits: Meta-analyses

The two meta-analyses abstracted in the tables below act as a snapshot of the state of the empirical research at a moment when interest in MBSR and other MBIs began to surge. Strict criteria were set in both meta-analyses for selection of the studies to be analyzed. Conclusions may be characterized by this statement from Grossman et al. (2004), "Thus far, the literature seems to clearly slant toward support for basic hypotheses concerning the effects of mindfulness on mental and physical well-being".

Baer (2003)

Variable	N	Mean effect size[a]
By research design		
Pre–post	8	0.71
Between group	10	0.69
By population		
Chronic pain	4	0.37
Axis 1 (anxiety, depression)	4	0.96
Medical (fibromyalgia, cancer, psoriasis)	4	0.55
Nonclinical (medical students, healthy volunteers)	4	0.92
By outcome measure		
Pain	17	0.31
Anxiety	8	0.70
Depression	5	0.86
Medical symptoms (self-report)	11	0.44
Global psychological[b]	18	0.64
Medical symptoms (objective)[c]	2	0.80

[a]At post treatment.
[b]POMS — total mood disturbance; SCL-90 R global severity index.
[c]Urine and skin.
N = Number of studies included in the meta-analysis. Of the studies included in the analysis, two employed MBCT as the intervention, one employed listening to mindfulness tapes, and the remaining used MBSR or a variant of MBSR as the treatment intervention.

Grossman et al. (2004)

Variables	N	Mean effect size[a]
Mental health variables		
Pre–post	18	0.50
Between groups	10	0.54
Physical health variables		
Pre-post	9	0.42
Between groups	5	0.53

[a]At post treatment.
N = Number of Studies included in the meta-analysis.
Between Groups (controlled studies) include both wait list controls (WLC) and active controls (AC). No difference in mean effect size noted between WLC and AC.

There is also a human dimension, an affective and relational set of factors in the success of MBSR. The personal energy and charisma of Jon Kabat-Zinn must be reckoned into the equation. The sheer drive and *chutzpah* with which he argues the case for mindfulness has been on display across a range of venues: a continually growing presence in the professional literature of both research and commentary; an expanding catalog of best selling books, including *Full Catastrophe Living* (1990), *Wherever You Go There You Are* (1994), and *Coming to Our Senses* (2005), plus popular audio and video recordings; exposure in the public media, alone and in association with other bellwether cultural figures such as the Dalai Lama, author Daniel Goleman, and integrative physician Andrew Weil; ongoing speaking engagements, workshops, and retreats; and training of professionals who may choose to teach MBSR or other MBIs. At last count, Kabat-Zinn and colleagues at the University of Massachusetts Medical School's Center for Mindfulness (CFM) had helped more than 9,000 mindfulness researchers and teachers expand their understanding of the MBSR curriculum and pedagogical theory. What also must be mentioned here is Kabat-Zinn's thoroughly welcoming stance to those who would contribute to moving mindfulness into the mainstream. His gift of enthusiasm and encouragement is best described by the statement of the freedom granted to those who choose to teach MBSR: "Rather than 'clone' or 'franchise' one cookie cutter approach, mindfulness ultimately requires effective use of the present moment as the core indicator of the appropriateness of particular choices" (Kabat-Zinn, 1996).

Beyond Kabat-Zinn's personal magnetism, there is a powerful attraction in the intervention itself. MBSR is multifaceted, yet it may be epitomized by three distinctive characteristics. It is secular, non-pathologizing, and transformational for teachers and participants alike.

Kabat-Zinn is direct and unapologetic about the Buddhist roots of the mindfulness practices in MBSR, yet he also goes to great lengths to assure his audiences that there is nothing exclusively Eastern, or Buddhist, or even generically religious about mindfulness. Paying attention to what is arising in the present moment is a universal human capacity. That means, of course, that the MBSR program itself can be seen as purely secular, carrying no denominational charge or baggage. This secular identity, coupled with many participants' intuitive recognition that mindfulness practice does indeed mesh with their own spiritual traditions or lack thereof, increases MBSR's appeal and reduces barriers to participation.

MBSR is inherently non-pathologizing. It is designed for a heterogeneous population from all walks of life, with almost any medical and/or psychological diagnosis — or none at all. No one needs to carry her specific diagnosis into the class; in effect, all participants share the same one, the "stress" or suffering of the human condition. Perhaps the clearest non-pathologizing statement is Kabat-Zinn's (1990, p. 2) insistence that "...as long as you are breathing, there is more right with you than there is wrong...." Further, MBSR is not positioned as a clinical intervention at all, but rather as an educational program. It is not about training to remove something unwanted from your experience, but rather about learning to open up to all that you are from moment to moment, to live life to the fullest.

Within the secular and non-pathologizing environment of an MBSR class, then, there is a democracy of participants and teachers. There is no hierarchy. In the emerging present moment, no one (or everyone!) is special. Participants and teachers practice mindfulness *together* from the very start. They explore their own experiences and, at times, share inquiry into those experiences. New insights and understandings become available to touch and transform anyone and everyone. This sense of shared possibilities, of a community of growth and healing, accounts for much of MBSR's appeal, we believe. Further, this sense is renewed for the teacher in each new class, and reinforces us in our choice of vocation.

The power of the evidence base, the charisma of the leadership, and the humanity of the MBSR program itself combine to suggest an answer to *why* there is such a need — and desire — for professionals to teach mindfulness. The MBSR curriculum and pedagogical approach to mindfulness have become a framework, an armature on which programs are being built to reach out to and serve particular populations. The list of such interventions is growing continuously. As just a few examples, mindfulness-based art therapy (MBAT) adds an expressive dimension in an approach to medical patients, particularly those with cancer (Monti et al., 2006); mindfulness-based relationship enhancement (MBRE) adds interpersonal practices for couples (Carson et al., 2004); and mindfulness-based eating awareness training (MB-EAT) adds elements of cognitive behavioral therapy and specific practices around eating and body image for patients with eating disorders (Kristeller and Hallett, 1999). In addition, of course, other approaches to bringing the benefits of mindfulness to various populations grew up in the early 1990s. Many have their roots in the evidence-based world of cognitive and behavioral approaches to psychotherapy. These interventions have added considerably to the evidence base for mindfulness, and to the legitimization of mindfulness-based interventions in the eyes of the public and of other professionals.

Perhaps a quick overview of the most influential streams of MBIs will be valuable. This would include, of course, MBSR, which needs but little further description; mindfulness-based cognitive therapy (MBCT), an integration of MBSR and cognitive therapy developed to prevent relapse in depression; dialectical behavior therapy (DBT), developed independently of MBSR and integrating mindfulness skills among others for treatment of borderline personality disorder; acceptance and commitment therapy (ACT), developed independently as a "third wave" within the cognitive-behavioral

tradition, and applied across a wide range of conditions; and, within the psychodynamic and humanistic traditions of psychotherapy, the ongoing engagement of the
world's contemplative traditions for use in the therapeutic encounter. By understanding the parallels and crosscurrents of these approaches, both the need for and the
complexity of teaching mindfulness as a professional may become more clear.

Mindfulness-Based Stress Reduction

The structure of the MBSR program developed and modeled by Kabat-Zinn (1990)
and colleagues at the Stress Reduction Clinic at the University of Massachusetts
Medical Center is a group-based, 8-week, 9-session course that is educational and
experiential. Participants attend 2½ hour sessions once a week for eight weeks, with
a full-day (7-hour) class between the sixth and seventh sessions. Class time, apart
from a very few didactic presentations on stress by the teacher, is divided between
formal meditation practice, small and large group discussions, and inquiry with
individuals into their present-moment experiences.

Formal mindfulness practices include body scan, sitting meditation (with focus
on the breath), mindful Hatha yoga, sitting meditation (moving from focus on the
breath to an expanded awareness of other objects of attention, i.e., body sensations,
hearing, thoughts, emotions, and ending with an open awareness of all that is
arising in the present moment), walking meditation, and eating meditation. Class
discussions focus on group members' experiences in the formal meditation
practices and the application of mindfulness in day-to-day life. Home practice is an
integral part of MBSR. Participants are asked to commit to formal practice, supported by audio recordings that guide the meditations, once a day, six days a week.

Mindfulness-Based Cognitive Therapy

Segal et al. (2002) used the 8-week structure and the core mindfulness practices of the
MBSR curriculum as an armature on which to mount an integration of cognitive
therapy to help people with histories of major depressive episodes to avoid relapse.
Their intervention is based on the parallel between the actions of cognitive therapy in
helping patients to *decenter* or *distance* from their negative thoughts and emotions and
the work of mindfulness practice in cultivating nonjudgmental awareness and acceptance of all experience — including thoughts. Following on a distinction in Full
Catstrophe living pertaining to MBSR, MBCT contrasts two modes of mind: *doing*
and *being*. In doing mode, one compares the wished-for with the actual (compara-
tively unsatisfactory) situation and struggle or suffering begins. In being mode, one
settles into the actual situation and allows it to be a focus of exploration, revealing its
impermanent nature. By cultivating the capacity for being, MBCT gives participants the
opportunity to encounter their triggers for depressive relapse in a way that provides
the extra time and affective distance to make skillful choices. MBCT is a shift away
from the more traditional cognitive therapy conceptualizations, because thoughts are
allowed rather than evaluated, disputed, and (in theory) changed.

MBCT varies from MBSR in several significant ways that characterize and set precedents for other integrations of cognitive/behavioral therapies and mindfulness training. First, it narrows the focus to a particular population. This allows the incorporation of very specific didactic materials and fine-tuning of the practices and guidance to bring out the most germane experiences and potential knowledge. Second, it manualizes the curriculum. This provides greater support for beginning teachers and, of course, ensures the reproducibility of the intervention in research studies. These two features set the pattern for the elaboration of MBCT-based curricula for a very quickly growing list of populations and disorders, including children, the elderly, stroke survivors, bipolar affective disorder, conversion disorder, eating disorders, generalized anxiety disorder, suicidal behavior, and co-occurring addictive and mood disorders.

Dialectical Behavior Therapy

Linehan (1993a,b) developed DBT originally to treat chronically suicidal patients who have the symptoms of borderline personality disorder. It synthesizes strategies for change from the cognitive-behavioral therapy tradition and strategies for acceptance from Eastern and Western contemplative traditions. It is a yearlong, multimodal program that incorporates weekly individual therapy and group-based skills training sessions, plus individual skills coaching by telephone when needed. The key is mindfulness: "it is both the practice of the therapist and the core skill taught to clients" (Robins et al., 2004, p. 37).

The client population has difficulties complying with extended formal mindfulness practices, so mindfulness in DBT is instead taught as an interlocking set of skills through structured exercises. The first of the skills is *wise mind,* which is the result of integrating two more commonly accessed states of mind, *emotion mind* and *reasonable mind.* In emotion mind, the client feels controlled by emotional reactivity, while in reasonable mind, the client can apply logic and critical thinking. Wise mind arises, then, when clients know what they feel and can think clearly about it — a capacity that DBT trusts is inherent in everyone. There are six other skills, which amount to a practical definition of mindfulness. The three "what" skills are what one does to be mindful. *Observing*: sensing and attending to the experience of the present moment without being caught up in it, or attempting to change or escape it. *Describing*: labeling present-moment experience very simply with words; identifying thoughts, emotions, urges — without acting on them. *Participating*: becoming completely involved in the unfolding of the present-moment experience; acting spontaneously and un-self-consciously. The three "how" skills are how the "what" skills are done. *Nonjudgmentally*: does not imply approval of an experience; rather, it means accepting both the experience and any judgment that arises as ultimately neither good nor bad. *One-Mindfully*: attending to one thing at a time; single-tasking in sequence, rather than multitasking. *Effectively*: instead of being caught up in how things *should be*, having the freedom to do what works in the present moment.

The evidence base for DBT's efficacy as a discrete intervention is very strong, and it shares the evidence of the efficacy of mindfulness. DBT was one of the first manualized treatments to place mindfulness at its core. And Linehan's imaginative and effective translation of formal meditation practices into everyday skills significantly broadens the applicability of mindfulness to challenging populations.

Acceptance and Commitment Therapy

Hayes et al. (1999), Hayes and Strosahl (2004) developed ACT originally as a general approach to individual therapy that allows for brief, targeted interventions for specific issues. They defined a theoretical outlook called relational frame theory (RFT), to provide an empirically testable explanatory platform upon which to build and extend ACT. RFT proposes that people suffer because they become embedded in the language of their problems, creating a psychological rigidity. This is manifested in two pathological positions: cognitive fusion and experiential avoidance. In cognitive fusion, a situation and one's thinking about it become inextricably linked through language. For example, the logical construction of the thought "I can't change careers because I need to keep paying the mortgage" blocks counter action. In experiential avoidance, one develops and consistently applies maladaptive strategies to escape inner and outer events that cause distress. For example, one may drink alcohol to suppress painful memories, or isolate oneself to avoid social anxiety.

The goal of ACT therapy, then, is psychological flexibility, defined as the capacity to accept what each situation or moment brings and, when possible, to choose to work towards change in the direction of one's closely held values. The ACT model of therapy has six core processes, which can be evenly divided (with overlaps) between the processes for mindfulness and acceptance, and the processes for commitment and behavioral change. The mindfulness and acceptance processes include *acceptance* and *defusion*, plus *contact with the present moment* and *self as context*. The commitment and behavior change processes include *values* and *committed action*, plus, again, *contact with the present moment* and *self as context*. A brief review suggests that the insights derived from mindfulness practice predominate in assisting clients towards psychological flexibility. *Acceptance*: interventions to demonstrate the futility of avoidance or control strategies, and to promote choice and action when change is possible. *Defusion*: to separate the thought from the thinker. *Contact with the present moment*: to reveal that "now" is when one is connected to living, both its pain and its vitality and infinite possibilities. *Self as context*: to demonstrate that one's awareness is larger than any given self-concept, e.g., that one is bigger than the bad or good or suffering version of the self. *Values*: to help clarify and choose values and goals, and to understand what one might do as well as what may need to be overcome to move towards them. *Committed action*: to establish a pattern of behavior driven by values and taking place in the present moment.

ACT intentionally does not include explicit meditation practices. However, principles or facets have been extracted from the meditative experience, and are presented as experiential exercises, metaphors, paradoxes, stories, and the like — many of which are intuitively shared or approximated by teachers within the other interventions. The result is a kindred sense, an identification of ACT as an MBI. Further, ACT's growing base of empirical evidence and continually widening range of applications, including group approaches, contribute to the overall interest in and expansion of MBIs.

Psychodynamic and Other Psychotherapies

As we will see in Chapter 2, the history of engagement with contemplative practices from both the West and the East is much longer in psychotherapies outside the cognitive-behavioral tradition, with the particular influence of Buddhist philosophy, psychology, and practice associated with mindfulness assuming considerable importance in their development or elaboration after World War II of recent developments will add to the evidence of need for competent professionals to teach mindfulness.

The psychodynamic therapies, from the beginning, were in touch with the contemplative traditions — implicitly and explicitly. Although Freud claimed to be constitutionally incapable of the meditative/mystical "oceanic feeling" (1930/1961, p. 65), the disposition of "evenly-suspended attention" he prescribes for the analyst (1912/1953, p. 111) is a marvelous intuition of the almost inestimable value of mindfulness in the therapeutic encounter, which is just now a subject of empirical research (e.g., Grepmair et al., 2007). Jung, on the other hand, was constitutionally predisposed to engagement with contemplative practice. He used "yoga exercises" for decades to help him quiet his emotional reactivity enough to work with the material arising in his unconscious (1965, p. 177), was acquainted with a number of Eastern traditions, and was in dialog with the contemporary Zen Buddhist thinkers and practitioners D. T. Suzuki and Shin'ichi Hisamatsu (e.g., Meckel and Moore, 1992). The pragmatism inherent in these early manifestations also characterizes the latest wave of influence of Buddhism on psychodynamic clinical approaches. As the discourse about meditation and mindfulness heated up in the 1990s, Mark Epstein's *Thoughts without a Thinker* (1995) was published, with the *imprimatur* of a foreword by the Dalai Lama, bringing a higher cultural profile to the idea that analytic psychotherapy and meditation practice are complementary — that each can provide tools and insights to make the other more fruitful. And mindfulness is singled out:

> It is through mindfulness practices that Buddhism most clearly complements psychotherapy. The shift from an appetite-based, spatially conceived self preoccupied with a sense of what is lacking to a breath-based, temporally conceived self capable of spontaneity and aliveness is, of course, one that psychotherapy has come to envision. It is one of the most significant paradigm shifts to have taken root in psychoanalytic theory in recent years and is one of the reasons why the Buddha's message is now so appealing to the therapeutic community" (p. 147).

Further, the practicality and willingness to confront the strengths and weaknesses of both paths, evidenced by Jeffrey Rubin in *Psychotherapy and Buddhism: Toward an Integration* (1996), and by the contributors to Jeremy Safran's (2003) *Psychoanalysis and Buddhism: An Unfolding Dialog,* for example, suggest a level of commitment beyond fad or fashion.

Attachment theory and research have done much to shape relational and intersubjective approaches to psychotherapy, and to precipitate an interest in mindfulness practice. Just as a child's attachment to the caregiver — a co-created and sustained relationship — may become a physically and emotionally secure base from which the child can explore her inner and outer worlds to learn and grow, so the therapist and client can co-create a relationship that allows new learning and growth in the direction of freedom and health. In seeking something more than interpretation to account for change in psychotherapy, the Boston Change Process Study Group (Lyons-Ruth and BCPSG, 1998) propose an "implicit relational knowing" developed as the two members of a caregiver — child or therapist — client dyad are present to each other in encounter after encounter. A focus of research and clinical interest, then, is these moments of meeting, always in the present moment, explored at book length by BCPSG member Daniel Stern (2004). This is, of course, the moment into which mindfulness practice is an instrument of exploration, leading the attachment-based psychotherapist David Wallin (2007) to suggest that mindfulness training is essential for the therapist and useful for some clients. As a sidelight, Wallin's approach supports the sense that there is a growing need for competent professionals to teach mindfulness, as he comments that the clients to whom he recommends mindfulness training value the structure and support of a group or class.

In addition, mindfulness is historically ingrained in a panoply of other approaches to therapy, particularly those that were birthed or came of age in the earlier surge of interest in meditative practices in the 1950s and 1960s. The privileging of present-moment experience and embodied knowing in today's mindfulness-based approaches resonates with the practice traditions of existential, Gestalt, transpersonal, humanistic, and systemic therapies, as well as the expressive and body-based therapies. Possibly, all of these approaches will benefit from the multifaceted ways in which empirical evidence for the efficacy of mindfulness is accumulating. Certainly, these approaches could have much to contribute to the development of a mature pedagogy of mindfulness and an expansion of the ranks of professionals teaching mindfulness.

Neuroscience

The rising visibility of neuroscience, as evidenced by, for example, the U.S. government's naming the 1990s "The Decade of the Brain," has sought to build bridges of shared research and practice across medical and mental healthcare disciplines. Further, it has engendered connections to the broader domains of culture — the arts, religion, the social sciences, and education, all benefit from the insights of this new perspective on and new vocabulary for the ways we experience ourselves and our world. Likewise, neuroscience would benefit from the acceptance of insights from the arts, religion, and social sciences. For example, the new perspectives on how relationships influence infant, child, and adult brain development (e.g., Siegel, 1999; Cozzolino, 2006) continue to add new dimensions to psychotherapy, particularly within relational and systemic approaches. And the discovery of mirror neurons (Gallese et al., 1996; Rizzolatti, 2008; Iacoboni, 2008) which provide our capacity to simulate other people's subjective experiences, is illuminating our understanding of embodied knowing, language, empathy, group dynamics — in fact, a great many of the concerns of this book, as you will see.

It is logical that a major stream of neuroscience research would arise from the confluence of the newest technologies of imaging and measurement and the ancient technologies of introspection and transformation. And that certainly has been the case. Much of the awareness in the culture at large of the linkage of contemplative practices and neuroscience come from that wonderful flagship of scientific — contemplative dialog, the Mind and Life Institute, through which the Dalai Lama and leading international scientists began meeting privately to explore the intersections of Buddhist philosophy and practice with contemporary scientific theory and experimentation. Begun in the late 1980s and meeting biennially, by 1990 the group had begun collaborations on contemplative neuroscience using highly accomplished meditators, monks, as subjects; now monks are scientific collaborators, and, in fact, the curriculum at the Dalai Lama's monastery now includes training in western science. Perhaps the neuroscientist Richard Davidson's research on emotion has the highest profile of the outcomes of such collaborations, as the public meetings of the Mind and Life Institute with His Holiness in attendance have produced the kind of publicity that helps to bring ideas into cultural currency, capturing media interest, including front page space in major newspapers like the *New York Times*, and cover stories in respected general interest magazines, such as *Newsweek*, and *Time* (Goleman, 2003; Kalb, 2003; Stein, 2003). Davidson's work with the monks generated further empirical support for the concept of neuroplasticity, the idea that, contrary to long-held scientific dogma, the adult brain can create new functioning neurons and actually change. Further, it showed that the dramatic differences brought about by years of intensive meditation practice — particularly on compassion — resulted in much greater activation of areas in the prefrontal cortex associated with "positive" or "approach" emotions. The suggestion, therefore, is that it is actually possible to change one's brain, even one's disposition, by practicing meditation.

There is a unique, controlled study — a collaboration by Davidson et al. (2003) — that reflects and reinforces much of what you have read so far. The study, using employees recruited from a biotechnology firm as subjects, was designed to investigate longer term changes in physiology that may be brought about by training in mindfulness, using the 8-week MBSR program. Specifically, they predicted that the subjects who received mindfulness training would show reduced trait anxiety (essentially, less nervousness and worry) and increased disposition towards positive emotion (in effect, more happiness). They measured this immediately after the 8-week course and four weeks later with an anxiety questionnaire and recordings of brain electrical activation in the left anterior regions of the prefrontal cortex that reflect positive emotions and a more positive "set point" for emotional response. Further, they expected that the immune systems of the more mindful subjects would respond more strongly to a challenge. They investigated this by giving subjects an influenza vaccination at the end of the eight weeks and measuring the level of antibodies generated in response at about one month and two months after the course.

Results were very much as they predicted (Fig. 1.1a–c). Compared to the control group (who actually took the course later), the subjects who had been trained in mindfulness through MBSR showed significantly less trait anxiety at the end of the course (time 2) and four months later (time 3), and also showed signifi-

Chart 1a Reduction in mean trait anxiety

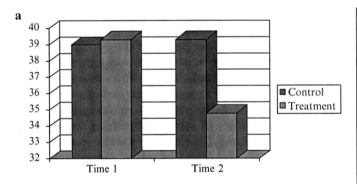

Chart 1b Means of asymmetric brain activation

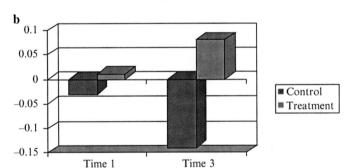

Results of a study by Davidson, Kabat-Zinn, and colleagues (2003) show that healthy subjects who completed an 8-week MBSR course reported that they were less nervous and worried day to day (Chart 1a). The electrical activity in their brain showed that they had shifted their "emotional set point" more towards the positive (Chart 1b). And their immune systems responded more strongly to threat of infection than the control subjects (Chart 1c).

Chart 1c Means of antibody rise

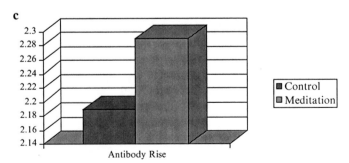

cantly greater left-sided brain activation at the two post-course measurement times. Response to the flu vaccine again reflected significant differences between the groups.

The question arising, then, is a happy one: Who wouldn't want to worry less, be closer to happiness, and have a greater capacity for staying healthy? The potential demand is enormous, which is a concise way of answering the original question of *why* one would teach mindfulness as a professional. And further, it sets up the next question of *who* would, could, or should teach.

Mindfulness training reduces anxiety, makes emotional disposition more positive, and improves immune function.

Who? Confronting Considerable Confusion

Just looking across the four MBIs that are drawing the most professional and cultural attention in this moment — MBSR, MBCT, DBT, ACT — we see a wide disparity in the characterization and expectations of the professional who teaches mindfulness. Based on the abstract, theoretical positions staked out in the literature for each intervention, there appears to be a continuum of *who* — running from a teacher with a total existential commitment to the embodiment of mindfulness in the world, to a professional with a basic understanding of the principles of mindfulness and a one-step-ahead-of-the-client experiential knowledge of certain techniques. Yet, despite the "official" positions, the nearly unavoidable personal encounters with the transformative potential of mindfulness practice inherent in all the interventions seem to be bringing the expectations and actions of developers and practitioners of every stripe closer and closer together. Among professionals, there is a shared unease — with different questions and resistances, to be sure — about defining a teacher.

In MBSR, the minimum expectations for the *who* of the teacher are mapped out in the guidelines for entry-level teachers in the MBSR program at the Center for Mindfulness at the University of Massachusetts Medical School (Santorelli, 2001a). The minimum educational requirement is a Master's degree in the social sciences, health sciences, education, or related fields, suggesting that the capacity for critical thought cultivated in graduate education is valuable, as is a knowledge base that offers perspectives on how people work individually and in groups. Plus, specific education in MBSR would include the 7-day residential Professional Training in Mindfulness-Based Stress Reduction in Mind-Body Medicine with Jon Kabat-Zinn and Saki Santorelli. The expectation for mindfulness training and commitment is striking: a 3-year history of daily meditation practice; participation in two 5-day or longer mindfulness retreats in the Theravada or Zen traditions; three years of body-centered practice, such as Hatha yoga. The existential commitment to mindfulness as a way-of-being is strongly implied in these criteria. Santorelli (2001b) makes it explicit that the demand for ongoing practice is not so much about learning to teach *how to* as it is about the teacher's *presence* — "...an authentic embodiment of this commitment to be awake to one's life no matter what is occurring" (p. 11–8:1). The willingness to live mindfully allows teachers to connect deeply, empathically, compassionately with their students. So, as Santorelli notes (2001b, p. 11–8:4), "When patients feel this unspoken connection with their instructor, it offers them the possibility of feeling the same kind of warm connection with themselves." Thus, the person, the *being,* of the teacher is what does the teaching in MBSR. Santorelli's (2001b, p. 11–85) summation is an epiphany: "For me and all of us at the clinic, this is nothing less than a lifetime's work."

In MBCT (Segal et al., 2002), the educational expectations of a professional degree/license in counseling or psychotherapy, plus training in cognitive therapy and group dynamics, is shaped by the specifically therapeutic outlook of the intervention. The signal requirement for therapists of "having your own practice" (p. 83) comes directly from the developers' failed attempts to teach without it, as well as with their positive experiences with MBSR teachers. The requirement of "having your own practice" has, perhaps, a more pragmatic justification in MBCT than in MBSR, as the foreground reason is to experience what it is you are teaching — to be a swimmer teaching swimming, to use the MBCT analogy. Yet, beyond that, there is an acknowledgement of the ideal of teachers "embodying" the way of being they present to their patients. The implied existential commitment is still strong.

In DBT (Linehan, 1993a,b), educational expectations are shaped by the identity of DBT as a manualized therapy delivered within a specific tradition. As to mindfulness practice for the therapist, the "rubrics" are different from MBSR and MBCT. There is no requirement that the therapists have their own practices, although they are expected to practice and have experiential knowledge of the DBT mindfulness skills activities. As well, occasional formal practice is built into the overall program. Weekly consultation team meetings begin with a mindfulness practice led by one of the therapists. There also appears to be a philosophical resistance about asking the therapist for the kind of commitment that is assumed in MBSR. There is an understanding that mindfulness practice can help the therapist maintain the balanced stance between change and acceptance, nurturing and benevolent demanding, and unwavering centeredness and compassionate flexibility that makes DBT effective. Yet, because Linehan (Dimidjian and Linehan, 2003) privileges the spiritual (religious) roots of mindfulness, she feels that asking a therapist to undertake a personal commitment to daily practice and regular retreats is "outside the bounds of what a therapeutic model can require." She has, however, also suggested (2001, cited in Welch et al. 2006) that both a connection with a mindfulness teacher, either in person or through reading, and a connection with a practice community could be "the most important element of a therapist's training" (p. 123).

In ACT, again, the educational expectation is congruent with the identity as a therapeutic intervention. As to therapist mindfulness practice, there is no specific requirement. It is as if, as the Melbourne Academic Mindfulness Interest Group (2006, p. 291) has noted about ACT, "Mindfulness from this perspective has a coherent theoretical model and the ideas are easily conveyed to the 'student' by a practitioner who practices little or not at all." Yet, Strosahl et al. (2004) note that core competencies of the ACT therapist is to be able to contact the ACT "space" of mindfulness and to be able to model the skills and benefits of getting in contact with the present moment. To help in developing these competencies, Strosahl et al. (2004) suggest the ongoing study and practice of ACT techniques, including ACT intensive retreats, and attendance at mindfulness retreats, which are characterized as "good for contacting the ACT 'space', less useful with ACT techniques" (p. 57). Here, again, is an implicit acknowledgement of the power and value of the teacher's way of being.

In the psychodynamic and other psychotherapies, the identity of a mindfulness teacher repeats the spectrum of possibilities, with implications for the level of existential commitment and, relatedly, commitment to ongoing practice. At one end of the spectrum we could locate Jeffrey Martin's (1999) conceptualization of mindfulness as a common factor in all psychotherapy. For Martin, mindfulness is identified with psychological freedom, in which the potentially problematic permanent sense of self is softened, and it is possible to explore experience in fresh, nonhabitual ways. It arises in collaboration with the client, facilitating insight, self-acceptance, and change. In this view, which is entirely secular, nonhistorical, and integrative, every therapist is implicated as an informal teacher who may choose to make mindfulness more or less explicit in her work. As Martin puts it, "In a sense, mindfulness is right under our feet when we and our patients are doing our best work" (p. 310). At the other end of the spectrum, we would place mindfulness teachers trained within spiritual traditions who are also psychotherapists, such as Jack Kornfield, Sylvia Boorstein, or Tara Brach within the Western Vipassana Buddhist tradition, in whom the two identities seem fused. We can also place at this end other contemporary Westerners who are not necessarily therapists but who have trained and been authorized to teach within particular traditions. Many of these Westerners trained with Asian teachers, often in Asia, although that generation is now giving way to a younger generation of "home grown" Western-trained teachers.

The Decision to Teach. Any professional who might consider teaching mindfulness, then, will approach such a decision from a set of expectations and an identity somewhere along the continuum in Fig. 1.1. For anyone considering this work, there's natural location between the total existential commitment of an MBSR teacher or the privileged position of a teacher within a specific lineage on one end, and the polished professional or the inherently mindful therapist on the other. The precise location on that continuum potentially will reflect both what draws the professional to mindfulness and how difficult the decision will be to actively teach.

Professionals who are nearer the existential commitment end of the continuum will likely be drawn by the resonance of mindfulness practice with their life experiences. This might include those who have histories of physical and or psychological suffering moderated through engagement with spiritually based practices as well as through medical or psychotherapeutic interventions. Such a person may conceive the mindfulness teacher's role as *extra*-ordinary; may see the teacher as responsible for a powerful, enduring transformation in the other — a *metanoia*, a conversion, a healing. The person may know through her own encounters with

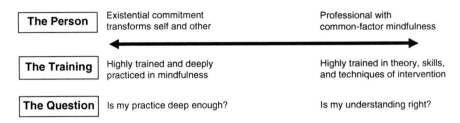

Fig. 1.1 *Continuum of the* who *of teaching mindfulness as a professional.* The view or construct of the mindfulness teacher in a wide range of interventions or approaches could be located on this continuum between the existential commitment of one's personal life to ongoing investigation and transformation in order to help others do the same, and the polished professionalism that demands clinical perfection. In either case, and everywhere in between, the questions of *Who am I?* and *What do I know?* may engender enthusiasm or resistance to the possibility of teaching.

mindfulness that students internalize their teacher, and that an affective connection can be created that neither time nor distance will diminish. For that person, then, the decision to assume the role of teacher is inherently fraught with an inner turmoil, a wrestling with feelings of overwhelming responsibility and perpetual inadequacy. The decision is layered with assumptions about what a teacher with a capital "T" is: with essential questions of training, lineage, authorization to teach, and fidelity to received views and practices becoming ever more insistent.

Professionals at the common factor end of the continuum initially may be drawn by the novelty, excitement, and evidenced effectiveness of the MBIs. The decision to become a teacher may first engage the professional interests and persona of the

---

How do I dare to assume a teaching role? and *Do I — could I ever — have what it takes?* to *Is my practice strong enough?* and *Who says?* to *How much is really at stake when I work with others — just the reduction of symptoms or the fate of an eternal soul?*

---

person, so that the weighting of time and financial investment, the strategies of differentiation in the market, and the needs of the populations served may take precedence over the more existential considerations of personal transformation and vocational calling. The questions arising first:

What do I know? and Do I Know It well enough to teach It?

This is not to say that the existential commitment dimension does not play a part in every decision. Certainly, once the person has investigated any of the interventions on a deep enough level, questions of personal readiness to teach arise to play a significant part in the pursuit of training and experience — and often an encounter with a resistance to begin teaching. It may be informative to look at the ways that the backgrounds and histories of the MBIs have shaped specific definitions of and attitudes towards the person of the mindfulness teacher. MBSR and DBT could be located at very different points on the continuum in Fig. 1.1, yet, both are uneasy about the *who* of teaching. As we will see, that unease stems from the particular traditions of mindfulness training privileged by the developers.

The extent of commitment expected of the MBSR teacher has been encapsulated by Jon Kabat-Zinn (2002) in a quote from T. S. Eliot's *Four Quartets:*

"A condition of complete simplicity/(Costing not less than everything)."

The MBSR conceptualization of the person of the teacher can be seen as a version of the *ad hoc* teacher selection process of Western Vipassana practitioners. Rawlinson (1999) gets the pith of it as he discusses how Jack Kornfield, ordained and trained within a traditional Asian Vipassana lineage, and Joseph Goldstein, trained as a layperson mostly by lay teachers, are judged as equal. "People do not think that one is superior or inferior because he has or has not been a member of a traditional *bhikkhu sangha.* It is depth of Vipassana practice that counts, not how one got there or where one comes from" (p. 590). Even more crisply, Rawlinson (1999, p. 590) notes a principle: "the only credentials that are of any value are practice and experience." Kabat-Zinn's training in both Zen and Vipassana have had a profound influence on both the form and formless elements of MBSR. MBSR's ties to the Western *Vipassana sangha* are close. Vipassana retreats (and, parenthetically, Zen retreats) are recommended for MBSR teacher training (Santorelli, 2001b). In fact, in 2008, a silent retreat specifically for MBSR and MBCT professionals was a joint benefit for the UMASS Center for Mindfulness (CFM) and Insight Meditation Society (IMS) — a flagship retreat center of the Vipassana sangha, founded by Joseph Goldstein, Sharon Salzberg, and Jack Kornfield — with Jon Kabat-Zinn and John Teasdale representing MBSR and MBCT and Cristina Feldman, an IMS guiding teacher, representing IMS. It is not surprising, therefore, that the emphasis on readiness to teach in MBSR comes from faith in depth of practice and experience. This has been tempered somewhat by a worldly pragmatism. There is a very conscious and insistent recognition in MBSR that more is not always better: "We have had instructors with five or six years of meditation experience who do very well in the classroom. Conversely, we have met people seeking jobs who have twenty or more years of meditation practice in their background who we did not feel at the time were capable of teaching in the class-room" (Santorelli, 2001b, p. 11–8:4). Yet the faith in practice is strong, so it is unsurprising that individual reluctance to teach MBSR resounds with the question:

Have I practiced enough to be ready to teach?

DBT's development was influenced by different mindfulness practice traditions. Marsha Linehan (2008) discusses it in terms of both her ongoing Zen training and the training she received as a spiritual director in the Christian tradition early in her career. These two influences can be seen to shape the very different questions and resistances that arise about the *who* of the mindfulness teacher in DBT. Western Zen is far more lineage-oriented than the *Vipassana sangha*. In Zen — to risk making a very technical process overly simple — a student may, depending upon the level of practice attainment judged by the teacher, be given a particular level of authority to train others. The highest level of authority given is to be named a *Dharma* heir by a master, and thereby be able to authorize teachers and name heirs oneself. This method of recognized succession is considered by some to be a direct link back through the generations to the historical *Shakyamuni Buddha*, implying an unbroken transmission of the teachings. Within this view, then, any change, contamination, or watering-down of what is taught and the way it is taught would be problematic, threatening the authority and integrity of the community — teachers and students alike.

With such a background view, Linehan's resistance and questions about professionals as mindfulness teachers, then, first focus on adherence and competence in delivery of the intervention. DBT's skill-based approach to teaching and learning mindfulness, developed by Linehan in association with her Zen teachers, is a way of addressing these concerns, as is the requirement for regular meetings of DBT therapists in a "community" that functions not just for peer support, but also oversight and reinforcement of protocols. Also, it is interesting to note that Dimidjian and Linehan (2003) suggest that engaging with spiritual teachers of mindfulness acknowledged within traditions to understand how they teach and recognize teaching competence in their students may provide guidelines for the mindfulness-based clinical interventions. The second focus of resistance and questions can be found in Linehan's Roman Catholic religious background and her early training in spiritual direction. She attended the program at the Shalem Institute, which, while ecumenical, arose within the small "c" catholic Christian tradition in which questions of authority, lineage, and "truth" of teachings are salient. In fact, the doctrine of "apostolic succession," in which Bishops are supposed to be created by other Bishops in an unbroken chain of laying on of hands that extends back to the 12 apostles, parallels the Zen lineage model. Again, concerns of adherence and competence arise, but more important still in this tradition is the character of the spiritual director — the person of the teacher. Shalem's founder Tilden Edwards (1980) is deeply concerned with this question. He interviewed 29 spiritual leaders to create a consensus delineation of the qualifications for a spiritual director. The consensus revealed two sets of qualities (p. 126):

1. "Personal spiritual commitment, experience, knowledge, and humility, and an active discipline of prayer/meditation."
2. "The capacity to be caring, sensitive, open, and flexible with another person, not projecting one's own needs or fostering long-term dependency."

In such a description, we see inherent expectations for a limitless, ceaseless engagement in the investigation and transformation of one's own life and the lives of others. Therefore, we can see how, in the DBT view, this may seem too intimate, too personal, too spiritual of an undertaking to require of most clinicians.

Wherever and however we find ourselves as teachers or potential teachers, we face, perhaps at first, perhaps forever, the push and pull of the questions of *Who am I?* and

What do I know? As we will see in Part 2, these are the questions of our authenticity and authority. How you work with these questions, how you ultimately decide to begin teaching, is — up to you! It may help, though, to learn how others came to take up this work.

Who Becomes a Teacher? Professionals who are teaching mindfulness now come from a surprising array of educational and professional backgrounds. They have found their way from hard science or religious life, from nursing or the business world, from teaching or therapy. And they have arrived at the decision to teach after journeys that are very different as well. For one, it may have been a personal crisis that ignited the process, for another, a professional insight. The sense of calling may have been anything from a whisper to a shout. In the capsule autobiographies below, you may find some connections. Perhaps you'll find some inspiration for beginning your own journey, or perhaps some affirmation for the direction you've already chosen.

DIANE REIBEL, CO-AUTHOR: FROM RESEARCHING THE HEART TO HEALING IT

In the mid-1980s I was an Assistant Professor in the Department of Physiology at Jefferson Medical College, investigating cardiac metabolism and function. My research was funded by the National Institutes of Health (NIH). I was presenting regularly at scientific meetings, publishing scientific papers, and teaching cardio vascular physiology to medical and graduate students. This time of my life was highly successful and stressful professionally. I became ill with an immune disorder, and was in chronic physical pain. I suffered emotionally as well, with the uncertainties of whether my illness would progress, and whether I would be able to care for my child, have more children, and continue my career.

After batteries of medical tests, repeated visits to specialists, and an exhausting array of conventional medical treatments, I was told to "learn to live with the pain." Despite all my years of higher education, that was learning I had never approached. But I made a beginning. Although as a scientist I was skeptical, I explored alternative medicine, trying biofeedback, hypnosis, and meditation for pain management. After practicing meditation for several months I found that I was struggling less emotionally and experiencing a general sense of well-being even in the midst of my chronic illness. I continued to meditate regularly for two years.

Reflecting on my first hand experience of the benefits of meditation and other mind/body techniques, I became interested in learning more about the use of these modalities in healthcare. So, in true scientist fashion, I sought out more information through professional conferences. At a behavioral medicine conference, the workshop on biofeedback that I originally signed up for was canceled, so on an impulse I shifted to something that was new to me — a workshop with Jon Kabat-Zinn on Mindfulness-Based Stress Reduction. The experience moved me deeply. It fueled my personal meditation practice. It also gave me some hard evidence that mindfulness was beginning to be integrated into mainstream medicine.

With continued practice through the years, mindfulness became a way of life. Life became richer and fuller. My health improved. And my passion for wanting to share mindfulness meditation with others grew. I let go of my academic position to embark on a new career. I attended professional trainings with Jon Kabat-Zinn and began teaching MBSR at cardiac rehabilitation centers in local hospitals — keeping some continuity with my life experience. After I had been teaching MBSR primarily to cardiac patients for about four years, a former colleague of mine at Jefferson asked me if I would run a stress reduction program for medical students. So I closed the circle, going back to Jefferson to teach medical students again. But this time teaching meditation. Following the success of the pilot course, MBSR was soon integrated into the medical school curriculum. I was offered a faculty position and found myself back on staff at Jefferson, now as Director of the Stress Reduction Program at the Center for Integrative Medicine, developing and teaching MBSR programs for patients. My research background came in handy as we began to study the effects of MBSR, both in our medical students and the patient population.

The Stress Reduction Program has grown over the years to include programs for patients, healthcare professionals, corporations and nonprofit organizations, students, and the homeless. Our research involvement has grown as well, and currently we are funded by NIH to study the effects of MBSR on immune function.

I have been living my passion for the practice and teaching of mindfulness, both of which have nourished me in ways I could never have imagined. I would like to give a personal thanks here to Saki Santorelli of the UMASS Center for Mindfulness for his fierce, loving presence. Many years ago, Saki sat with me in the hallway at a professional training retreat as I tried to control uncontrollable tears. I will never forget his invitation to me to uncover my face and hold nothing back. I have sat with many people since then and shared the same invitation, offering them a healing presence as they dive into the river of grief. Each time, I feel Saki's presence and his reassuring words that my personal longing for "eyes of compassion" will come as I continue on this path of awakening.

In describing my career change, one of my colleagues said that I have gone from being a heart researcher to a heart healer. Whether in practice or teaching, mindfulness is very much about healing the heart.

TOM: CREATING A MORE COMFORTABLE MEDICAL PRACTICE

My interest in MBSR arose out of concern for my own cardiovascular health. I have a very strong history of cardiovascular disease on both sides of my family. Both my parents died before age 60. As a physician, I paid close attention to information about prevention of cardiovascular disease and practiced those preventive measures. I read Dr. Dean Ornish on the benefits of meditation and yoga for cardiovascular disease management, and sought out these modalities. I found yoga to be a very joyful practice, much more than a workout.

About 10 years ago, following my older brother's coronary artery bypass surgery at age 54, I sought out instruction in MBSR. My experience with a 7-day MBSR program with Jon Kabat-Zinn and Saki Santorelli was profound. It provided an opportunity to be immersed in the present moment, attending to the breath in the body for long periods in a large room full of other seekers. (Plus, the program qualified as accredited continuing medical education, a gold standard of intellectual respectability for physicians!).

Being mindful grew in importance as I engaged in my medical practice, which focuses on neurodevelopmental disabilities. It reduces my stress level and enables me to have a stress reducing effect on my patients and their parents during our interactions and discussions in the office. I came to learn this in surprising ways. I found myself abandoning my usual reserved, slightly ironic, "professional" demeanor, and becoming more direct. I got more comfortable pausing to find the right word. I began to feel freer to abandon a set agenda for an appointment and to turn my attention jointly with parents and children to what was concerning them at the moment. In situations with patients and their families where there seemed to be unacknowledged tensions or feeling of anger in the room, I became more likely to express my perception of this. This often led to open, fruitful discussions about problems that might otherwise not have come up.

I have come to see stress reactivity as a very significant neurodevelopmental issue. This awareness has helped me develop a more refined, practical framework for developing treatment plans for children and families. I have given formal presentations for families regarding mindfulness practices. I frequently bring up and teach mindfulness and yogic breathing techniques for stress management. Yet, the bigger effect on my medical practice has been the arising of awareness in the present moment.

As I dictate this note, I recall the last patient I saw, a 7-year-old boy. He stated a preference for having his mother in the room. I was uncomfortable with this, but proceeded. As we spoke, I noted his hesitant speech and rigid body posture. I proposed that we move to another room for one-to-one interview. As he sat in the room, away from his mother and two younger sisters, I watched his shoulders drop, saw his face become more relaxed, and listened as he began speaking in much greater detail with much more fluency. I felt my own sense of ease as well. The value of present-moment awareness was confirmed once again. So, mindfulness informs in my life, both in and out of my medical practice.

JULIE: BRINGING MINDFULNESS TO AT-RISK STUDENTS

I am a Licensed Social Worker and Certified School Psychologist. I have worked in the field of mental health for more than 20 years, and have provided clinical services to adults, children, adolescents, and families in a variety of settings. I took my first MBSR course five years ago and found it very helpful with managing my own chronic pain and general life stressors. My personal involvement in mindfulness practices has grown considerably since then, as has my desire to bring mindfulness practices into my work with others.

I am currently working in an elementary and middle school, leading skill-building groups with children who are identified as "at-risk," as well as working with teachers and staff to improve overall school climate. The schools are located in urban neighborhoods beset by poverty and gang violence. Many children do not play outside because they do not feel safe. At least once a month, the administrators at the elementary school cancel outdoor recess because of neighborhood violence. Not surprisingly, many children and teachers do not feel safe in school.

It became apparent to me that the children were trying to function in school while dealing with chronic and often pervasive life stressors without the coping strategies to manage them. It was also apparent that many teachers were struggling over how best to support and teach the students. Keeping in mind how useful mindfulness practices have been in my life, I began to integrate mindfulness activities and practices into the groups I lead. I also began to introduce mindfulness practices during the teacher trainings. The feedback I have received from both groups has been overwhelmingly positive.

YAACOV: INTEGRATING JEWISH SPIRITUALITY WITH PSYCHOLOGY AND MINDFULNESS

My interest in meditation began during my college days. I didn't know anyone who meditated, so I tried to learn through books. The written exercises didn't seem to get me anywhere, so I gave up. I began doing a series of spiritual meditations which I found engaging and meaningful. Those meditations continue to be part of my spiritual practice. While attending graduate school, studying psycho-educational processes, I became involved in the human potential movement. I was exposed to and began practicing mindfulness in a very informal way — not sitting meditation, just bringing myself back to the present moment as often as I could throughout the day. Walking and jogging became the primary activities I used to practice mindfulness.

After receiving my doctorate and rabbinical degrees, I began to become more involved in counseling and therapy. On a personal level, I worked at integrating what I knew about psychology, mindfulness, and spirituality. As a therapist, I was continually challenged to bring myself into the moment and to do whatever I could to facilitate the same for my clients. Finally, about 10 years ago I began a formal mindfulness practice and received training in MBCT and ACT. These approaches were instrumental in helping me integrate mindfulness with my therapy practice. Much of the therapy I now do is mindfulness-based, and I lead two or three MBCT groups a year.

My mindfulness practice has also influenced my approach to spirituality. The ACT understanding of the psychological processes involved in meditation has been a wonderful inspiration and has deepened my understanding of the processes involved in a program I have developed, which integrates psychology, mindfulness, and spirituality.

DON McCOWN, CO-AUTHOR: FROM BUSINESS TO WHOLENESS

My engagement with the contemplative traditions began in my rather troubled ado-
lescence in the ferment of the late 1960s and early 1970s. As a middle child
between two developmentally disabled siblings in a family that struggled to cope
with its challenges, sadness and suffering dominated my experience. Depression
was a close companion.

To help understand and (somewhat) assuage what was happening with me, I
investigated the traditions that suggested themselves by birth, by friends, and by the
compulsive reading that placates an unquiet mind. The esthetic glory of the liturgy of
the Episcopal tradition into which I was born was a focus of my adult life for decades,
and my private prayer, rooted in the very homely English spirituality of the fourteenth
century (Julian of Norwich, Margery Kempe, *The Cloud of Unknowing*) looped and
flowed, pushed by Alan Watts's and Thomas Merton's books, in and out of the Asian
traditions. Psychotherapy of various flavors was a constant undercurrent, as well,
including work with a therapist who brought meditation into our sessions and encouraged me to be focused and regular with practice. That helped immeasurably.

This was one stream of my life. In the other, I worked in advertising for a
Fortune 100 corporation, and then as a creative executive in an advertising agency.
The 1980s and 1990s were filled with career stress and the tensions of childrearing
and a maturing marriage. As I struggled for balance at work and at home, I came
to rely on my spiritual practices more and more. But I couldn't find a way to bring
the two streams together in a meaningful way.

More by convenience than design, it seemed, I was drawn from the little meditation group at my parish church into the Shambhala center just a few blocks from
my office. I attended workshops, trainings, and retreats. But mostly I sat. In the
empty shrine room. Every possible day at lunchtime. Then one day, on the brochure
table, I found a catalog for a Master's program in Applied Meditation Studies at
the Won Institute, a brand new venture at a Won Buddhist seminary. It felt right.
I thought I would shift my career into corporate communications consulting based
on meditation! At last, that would bring my two streams together. I began the highly
experiential program, which included a meditation practice class or a moving meditation class before every academic class, as well as two 10-day retreats.

For the two-semester practicum in my second year. I worked in the MBSR program at the Jefferson-Myrna Brind Center of Integrative Medicine, with Diane
Reibel. I developed a *Mindfulness at Work* program, and was quickly able to sell a
few workshops, which Diane and I co-led, and I later taught solo. I was also a
participant-observer in the 8-week patient courses. I was indelibly impressed with
how — by week three! — many patients began to carry themselves differently.

Something shifted in me. I felt drawn to the work with patients, yet reticent
about undertaking it. I had helped my own suffering in deep ways, but could I
possibly help others? I attended the 7-day professional MBSR training with Kabat-
Zinn and Santorelli, and returned only more sure that I was not prepared to teach
patients. I graduated from the Won Institute and began a year-long internship in the
Jefferson program, running workshops and classes in the workplace, and co-teaching

in patient classes, and at last teaching on my own. Advanced MBSR training and supervision built my confidence. But simply staying connected to my own practice, and making my teaching my own, built it more.

The workplace and academic courses that I teach are satisfying. Yet it's been the work with patients that has transformed me. So, to go further and deeper, I took a clinical social work degree, to help families with children with developmental disabilities. With mindfulness. There's a wholeness to my life now, and, with practice, I even experience it sometimes.

Paradox

The More We Know About Mindfulness-Based Interventions, the Less We Know About Mindfulness Teachers

Public dialog around the *who* and the *how* of teaching mindfulness has been cramped by the same forces that are bringing mindfulness further and further into the mainstream and creating the demand for more and more teachers. Worldwide, the clinical research enterprise has been building a strong evidence base for MBIs. It has been a marvelous boon to all of us, researchers, teachers, and patients alike. Yet here's the thing of it — it's all been happening inside the modern scientific paradigm, the land of *either — or*, where every confounding influence must be neutralized or controlled. Mindfulness teachers, though, have been working outside that paradigm, in the land of *both-and*, where new possibilities arise moment by moment and the placebo effect is a welcome guest, or even host.

The "gold standard" research model of randomized clinical trials holds great sway in Western biomedical culture. There is an endless loop, a self-reinforcing cycle, an embeddedness in the system that is shaped and maintained by the funding sources for research and the expectations of healthcare payers. Criticism from within the system is rare (e.g., Beutler et al., 2004; Blow et al. 2007; Lebow, 2006; Wampold, 2001), but comes right to the points that touch mindfulness teachers as they attempt to grow and develop. First, the dominant paradigm assumes that the *ingredients* of an intervention are significantly more important than the *person* delivering the ingredients. From that assumption, it follows that manualized models and fidelity measures will control for "therapist effects" or "operator effects" and spotlight the efficacy of the ingredients.

All of this has allowed the secondary needs of researchers to overshadow the primary needs of teachers and students. The research on MBIs is the sunny side of the mountain — warm, inviting, and a topic of much animated discussion. The pedagogy of mindfulness, then, is the shadow side — forbidding, less explored, and spoken of only in small groups and rarely above a whisper. It has been suggested (McCown & Wiley, 2008, 2009) that robust public dialog must be engaged between the two "sides," which are not opposed but interdependent. In fact, many researchers are also teachers (or vice versa). Such a dialog would involve accommodating both researchers' requirements for *fidelity* — the strict reproduction of a specific curriculum and structure of an intervention — and teachers' desires for *integrity* — the authentic response to the moment-to-moment context in delivery of an intervention. We trust that the community will take this book as a contribution to the dialog.

How? Entering a Mystery

To someone looking into the community of practitioners using MBIs, the *how* of teaching would be a black box. The public discussion of the pedagogy of mindfulness is either hidden inside highly experiential training programs, or transformed into specific scripts and concrete moves in manuals and workbooks. Further, the unique environment of the group setting, although of central importance to most of the interventions, is more or less disguised within a requirement for the teacher to have some generic knowledge and experience of group development and dynamics. The issues raised here result from a combination of factors embedded in the construction of the most recent MBIs. Three of those factors are particularly salient and could drive the professional dialog we hope this book will help engender: (1) the varied conceptualizations of the person of the teacher within the interventions; (2) the institutional and financial influences that privilege empirically validated, and preferably manualized approaches to psychotherapy; (3) the overshadowing of the group experience due to a focus on measurement of individual outcomes.

Experiential Training

Teacher development in MBSR and MBCT, for example, is weighted towards development of the teacher's personal practice and transformation of her way of being, because the teacher's presence is deemed central to how the class learns. The authors are products of the MBSR training program, and can attest to the powerful influence the courses have had on who they are. The pedagogical approach taught in the program reflects an eclectic pragmatism, drawing on a wide range of medical, psychotherapeutic, educational, and anthropological-sociological insights and techniques. Integration is not theoretical, but, rather, pragmatic and personal. It is expected that each teacher will integrate the ideas that resonate most into her practice and presence when teaching. Certainly, a teacher developed in this way can have a profound effect on students through the dimension of her being.

Santorelli (2001b) also identifies another dimension of teaching that he deems equally important — the ability to bring the experience of mindfulness into language that can affect others; that is, the ability to "eff" the ineffable. While, again, personal mindfulness practice is essential, two specific pedagogical skills are also implied. First, a teacher must have a capacity to think conceptually about the experience of mindfulness. She must be able to take a question or observation from anyone in the class at anytime, and place it within some workable theoretical scheme of how students learn, grow, and develop their mindfulness practices, in order to consider a response. Only then can she bring the second skill to bear, the ability to create within each class a highly evocative shared vocabulary of terms, metaphors, and allusions — to the class's history together, as well as to stories, poems, and personal anecdotes — that will help make her points in very concrete, affecting ways. In the teacher trainings, with their experiential focus, these skills are developed implicitly; the conceptual knowledge becomes available to each individual teacher in an idiosyncratic way, and is likely to be embedded within the context of the intervention's curriculum.

This individual, implicit approach is effective and logical, particularly given the dominance of manualized models. However, it can also be seen as having a restrictive effect on development of both the individual teacher and the larger community of professionals teaching mindfulness. Without a well-articulated and integrated theoretical account of the important lines of development of mindfulness skills in the class, it is difficult for individual teachers to critique and refine their own pedagogical efforts, and, as well, critique and refinement of the curricula and general approaches to teaching across the community of professionals teaching MBIs are also hindered, as dialog is difficult without a shared outlook and vocabulary.

Manualization

The pairing of a highly practiced and trained teacher with an empirically validated and refined manualized intervention may consistently produce the predicted positive outcomes. These conditions are ideal. Under such conditions, teacher and intervention may mesh closely enough to generate powerful innovations. This is suggested in ACT (Hayes and Strosahl, 2004), in which the ideal therapist ultimately does not rely on set pieces and technique, but improvises a unique intervention tailored to the shared history and the present-moment situation in the flow of the session. This, it is noted, requires a deep understanding of ACT theory as well as extensive experience. As we trust has been revealed, all the MBIs are aligned, ultimately, on the existential commitment of the teacher, regardless of their individual positions on demands for specific formal practice.

In essence, the manuals come alive when they are connected to the practice, or, in ACT terms, the "space," of mindfulness. Yet, the growth in demand for professionals to teach MBIs mitigates against the ideal pairing as the norm. The prospect of teachers working with less training and theoretical understanding increases as demand rises. The words of the manuals could easily lose their liveliness — a haunting thought. Again, if the community can work to make explicit and to refine the learning that is implicit in each teacher's development, perhaps teachers can grow to competence more quickly.

The Barely Visible Group

The group format dominates the MBIs, yet, we know very little about the importance of that format. This is due in great part to the conventions of the empirical research model in use, which prefers to observe outcomes for individuals. To make the point, all of the data reported in the studies in the two meta-analyses discussed earlier are based on measures of individual participants. It is also interesting to note that the empirical record on correlations between individual mindfulness practice by subjects and improvements in outcome is ambiguous (compare, e.g., Carmody and Baer, 2008 and Davidson et al., 2003).

Across the MBIs, it is suggested that adequate understanding of the development and dynamics of a mindfulness class, can come from a group therapy or adult education perspective (Santorelli, 2001a; Segal et al., 2002; Hayes and Strosahl, 2004). Dissenting voices such as Allen et al. (2006) suggest that "there may be some unlearning to do" (p. 292), particularly because the teacher's embodiment of mindfulness is an unusual influence on the group. Dimidjian and Linehan (2003), noting the historic prevalence of group-oriented teaching and practice across spiritual traditions, go so far as to suggest that, "It may be important for future research to address whether the group format is an essential quality of teaching mindfulness in the clinical context" (p. 169). If research shows this to be true, they further suggest that teaching in those circumstances would demand unique skills and techniques, which might best be developed in concert with master teachers from spiritual traditions that use mindfulness.

This area of mindfulness pedagogy has been but barely visible: under-researched, under-theorized, and under-taught. In our experience in teaching, and in helping other professionals to develop their teaching, mindfulness-based groups are distinctive in the ways they develop over time, and in the ways they respond moment by moment to the needs or actions of their members. Much of the discussion in debriefing after a class with an intern or a practicum group is prompted by the changes the group went through, prompted by group practices, encounters of individuals in the group, or dyadic exchanges with the teacher with the group as witnesses and context. The teacher's role in the group is crucial — as the word suggests, there's a crossroad formed with every decision — and it deserves a vital place in the discussion of mindfulness pedagogy.

From Questions to Dialog

Why and *Who* and *How* are certainly insistent questions. Perhaps this survey of them has helped to ground you in the instability of this cultural moment. If you have read this far, you may feel that *why* is obvious, and the evidence just keeps pouring in. *Who*, however, may be more of an open question. Maybe even more of a personal question. To invoke T. S. Eliot once again, this time from *The Lovesong of J Alfred Prufrock*:

"Do I dare/Disturb the universe?"

Finally, *how* is still unanswered. It's why you're still reading. It's also your invitation to join a community, and a dialog, and to keep going.

With this book, we intend to deepen discussion around the *who* and *how* of teaching mindfulness as a professional. We intend to engage everyone, all across the community. We are staying with the core questions involved in teaching, the basics of *who* and *how* that transcend the specific interventions, even as they multiply, grow, and change. We're not proposing that what we describe here is the right way or the best way to consider these two questions. We're simply professionals who are deeply engaged in teaching because we find ourselves so deeply nourished by it, and who want to grow and learn in the most direct and powerful ways, by teaching others, and by sharing in open dialog. We invite you to join us.

In Part Two, we'll offer our understanding, from what we know inside and what we've learned from outside, of *who* it is that teaches. We'll try to help you get in touch with your *authenticity, your authority, and the friendship* that you can bring to help others. In Part Three, we'll outline best practices that we've developed ourselves and collected in our dialogs with other teachers. We'll lay out the theories that underpin our approach to pedagogy, not because we believe they're profound, or even correct, but because we find them helpful in the moment in the classroom to ground us and guide us. We'll consider just what the mechanisms are that make a mindfulness class "work" as a group, and how to use them to ensure optimum learning. We'll look at the essential teaching intentions for mindfulness practices, to help maintain continuity and fidelity when you must shift, adapt, or change your curriculum to meet challenges of unique times, places, contingencies, or populations. And we'll cover the real nuts and bolts of this unique vocation, giving you information on equipment and processes for making your own recordings of mindfulness practices. We'll even provide sample scripts for the core practices, and share with you a selection of our favorite activities, and ideas for working with challenging groups and individuals. And we hope that at some point you'll share your insights and experiences with us as well.

First, though, we need to build a bit more scaffolding. Our teaching is located at a certain time and place in our culture, so we'll provide a brief overview of the history of the cultural shifts that have allowed mindfulness to move further and further into the mainstream of healthcare — and the rest of society as well. And, of course, we need to understand just what we mean — in this book — by the term *mindfulness*. Then we can start. So, let's get going.

Chapter 2
A History Exercise to Locate "Mindfulness" Now

The practice of mindfulness is an experience that from a certain perspective is inexpressible. You gain a *tacit* knowledge of it that is yours alone; you "know more than [you] can tell," as Michael Polanyi (1966) phrases it. Yet, from a different perspective, the practice is also a product of all the communications that you have around your experience. Your *explicit* knowledge, what you *can* tell, is co-created in relationship with all of those with whom you share your experience now or in the future, from your mindfulness teachers and fellow students, to your colleagues and supervisors in working with mindfulness-based interventions, to the clients or patients that you teach. This co-creation takes place most obviously in verbal language. You learn from a talk or a book by a teacher, a conversation with a colleague, or a dialog with a client. But the nonverbal dimensions are also important. There is much to be learned from a teacher's posture, gestures, tone of voice, and rate of speech, or from the way a colleague meets your eyes, or from the quality of the pause before a supervisor responds in a tense moment. So, within such relationships, within your own small community, there is an evolving discourse, through which you learn to better understand and, thereby, better express your tacit knowledge of mindfulness practice. Further, it is within such a community and its discourse that you are learning, or will learn, to teach mindfulness as a professional.

The small community, even in an isolated place, is meaningfully connected in its discourse to larger communities of discourse and practice. For example, an MBSR program at a local hospital is connected to the MBSR community and its founders and senior teachers through ongoing personal relationships supported by writings, recordings, retreats, trainings, and conferences. There is a further connection to the discourse of all the mindfulness-based interventions, which are increasingly associated (e.g., Baer, 2006; Didonna, 2009; Hayes et al., 2004). From there, it is anticipated that teachers and practitioners make connections as well to the valuable insights and long history of mindfulness and acceptance within the psychodynamic, humanistic, and experiential psychotherapies. Last, but perhaps most important, connections may be made even further out into the many other cultures of spiritual practice. In the current discourse of mindfulness-based interventions, these cultures are predominantly Asian in origin, specifically certain forms of Buddhism

D. McCown et al., *Teaching Mindfulness: A Practical Guide for Clinicians and Educators*, DOI 10.1007/978-0-387-09484-7_2, © Springer Science+Business Media, LLC 2010

that have become popular in the West. It should be remembered that Judaism, Christianity, Islam, Jainism, and Sufism could be easily connected as well, as is evident in Linehan's work and in the work of many individual teachers within the interventions.

To teach effectively, it serves well to have awareness of the history, language, images, metaphors, and assumptions of the current discourse of mindfulness. That is the reason for this chapter. We present here a sketch of how the context in which you are learning to practice and teach has been shaped historically by a rapprochement of Western and Eastern philosophical, religious, medical, and psychological thought over the past two centuries. Given space limitations and our very pragmatic intentions, what follows is not meant as an exhaustive critical analysis. Rather, it serves two parallel purposes. First, it provides essential background for the attempt at defining mindfulness that occupies in Chapter 3. Second, it acts as an appreciation of how our Western culture, particularly in the United States, got to this exciting moment in history, and offers some jumping-off points for deeper exploration of this discourse within which you are teaching, or will teach, as a professional.

Early Encounters

It is possible to date a European intellectual connection to Eastern spiritual thought and practice as early as the ancient Greek histories of Herodotus, Alexander the Great's Indian campaign in 327–325 BCE (Hodder, 1993), or, to Petrarch's mention of Hindu ascetics in his *Life of Solitude*, written during 1345–1347 (Versluis, 1993). A more substantive start, however, would be 1784, which marks the founding by British scholars and magistrates of the Asiatic Society of Bengal, from which quickly flowed first translations of Hindu scriptures directly from Sanskrit texts into English. Sir William Jones was the preeminent member of the group. His tireless work included translations of Kalidasa's *Sakuntala* (1789), Jayadeva's *Gitagovinda* (1792), and the influential *Insitutes of Hindu Law* (1794). His early tutor in Sanskrit, Charles Wilkins, holds the distinction of making the first translation of the *Bhagavad Gita* (1785). In 1788, the group founded a journal, *Asiatik Researches*, widely circulated among the intelligentsia, including the second U.S. President John Adams, an enthusiastic subscriber (Hodder, 1993; Versluis, 1993). The effect of this flow of scholarly and objective information about Indian culture and religion began a profound shift in Europe's view of the East: "from the earlier presupposition of the East as barbarous and despotic, to a vision of an exotic and highly civilized world in its own right" (Versluis, 1993, p. 18).

The new language, ideas, images, and narratives embedded in such texts immediately touched something in poets, philosophers, and artists, particularly in England and Germany — powerful influences on the development of American culture. In England, the Romantics embraced all things "Oriental" as a celebration of the irrational and exotic. Their use of the scriptures, stories, lyrics, and images becoming ever more available to them from Hinduism, Buddhism, Confucianism, and Islam was not discrete, but rather an amalgam. Their drive was not for a practical use of these new elements of discourse in expressing some tacit knowledge heretofore inexpressible; to the contrary, as Versluis (1993) notes, "their Orientalism was not serious but rather a matter of exotic settings for poems" (p. 29). The later confounding of international relations by "Orientalism" (Edward Said) was an unforeseen serious consequence. Herder, Goethe, and the Romantics who followed them in Germany found "Oriental" thought a refreshing alternative to the stifling rationality (and then nationality) of their time. Yet, again, their usage of the new material available was not entirely pragmatic. Their philosophical and poetic insights could have been expressed in the preexisting discourse of Christian mysticism, Neo-Platonism, and Hermeticism and the charismatic movement. What the use of Oriental religious discourse by a poet of spiritual power such as Novalis (Freidrich von Hardenberg) did do was to suggest that the full range of Eastern and Western religious expression pointed to a Transcendent reality, and that all — *in essence* — offered truth (Versluis, 1993). It is this last point that brings us to America, to the Transcendentalists, and, at last, the pragmatic use of the Eastern discourses to better understand and express a personal tacit knowledge.

In writers such as Ralph Waldo Emerson and Henry David Thoreau, and the utopian vision of the Transcendentalist Old Concord Farm and other communities, the influence of Eastern thought is evident (Brooks, 1936; Versluis, 1993; Hodder, 1993). Through the *Dial,* their journal that did much to shape American Transcendentalism, they brought out translations of Hindu, Buddhist, and Confucian texts, and of the Sufi poets, such as Hafiz, Rumi, and Saadi. In these "transcendentalations" a new, rich brew began to find ways to give voice to tacit experience.

It is possible to see both Emerson and Thoreau as both natural (and learned?) contemplatives whose entwined literary and spiritual lives reflect experiences that demanded a larger discourse than the West provided for more explicit understanding and more elaborated communication. Emerson's early (1836) essay, "Nature," written before his deep engagement with Eastern thought, contains a description of such an experience:

> Crossing a bare common, in snow puddles, at twilight, under a clouded sky, without having in my thoughts any occurrence of special good fortune, I have enjoyed a perfect exhilaration. Almost I fear I think how glad I am. In the woods, too, a man casts off his years, as the snake his slough, and at what period so ever of life is always a child. In the woods, is perpetual youth. Within these plantations of God, a decorum and a sanctity reign, a perennial festival is dressed, and the guest sees not how he should tire of them in a thousand years. In the woods, we return to reason and faith. There I feel that nothing can befall me in life, — no disgrace, no calamity, (leaving me my eyes,) which nature cannot repair. Standing on the bare ground, — my head bathed by the blithe air, and uplifted into infinite space, — all mean egotism vanishes. I become a transparent eyeball. I am nothing. I see all. The currents of the Universal Being circulate through me; I am part or particle of God.

As Emerson began reading the amalgam of Oriental writings in earnest, which consumed him for the rest of his life, his enterprise became the essentialization (distillation) and integration of the insights that supported his experience and vision on both a personal and a cultural scale. Versluis notes that, "For Emerson… the significance of Asian religions — of all human history — consists of assimilation into the present, into this individual here and now" (1993, p. 63). He was reading and feeling and thinking his way towards a universal, literally unitarian religion. (Imagine if the early New England settlers had not thought to provide "Commons" as the centerpieces of their settlements as spiritual practices evolved from Puritanism to Congregationalism to Unitarianism.).

It seems Thoreau had a different enterprise under way, using the same materials. Where Emerson was grappling with universals and theory to make sense of his world, Thoreau was intent that particulars and practice would make sense of his own world. Though he had only the translated texts to guide him, he did more than just *imagine* himself as an Eastern contemplative practitioner. He wrote to his friend, H. G. O. Blake, in 1849, "… rude and careless as I am, I would fain practice the yoga faithfully… To some extent, and at rare intervals, even I am a yogin" (quoted in Hodder, 1993, p. 412). Thoreau offers descriptions of his experience, such as this from the "Sounds" chapter of *Walden*:

> I did not read books that first summer; I hoed beans. Nay, I often did better than this. There were times when I could not afford to sacrifice the bloom of the present moment to any work, whether of the head or hands. I love a broad margin to my life. Sometimes, in a summer morning, having taken my accustomed bath, I sat in my sunny doorway from sunrise till noon, rapt in a revery, amidst the pines and hickories and sumachs, in undisturbed solitude and stillness, while the birds sang around or flitted noiseless through the house, until by the sun falling in at my west window, or the noise of some traveler's wagon on the distant highway, I was reminded of the lapse of time. I grew in those seasons like corn in the night, and they were for me far better than any work of my hands would have been. They were not time subtracted from my life, but so much over and above my usual allowance. I realized what the Orientals mean by contemplation and the forsaking of works.

Like Emerson, Thoreau read the "Orientals" back into his own experiences, to help express that which was inexpressible without them. A journal entry from 1851 states that "Like some other preachers — I have added my texts — (derived) from the Chinese and Hindoo scriptures — long after my discourse was written" (quoted in Hodder, 1993, p. 434). That original inarticulate discourse of ecstasy in nature was capable of transformation with the insights he found in the translations of Jones and Wilkins. It was the here-and-now value of the new language, images, and stories that counted. An emphasis on the moment-to-moment particulars of nature and his own experience was the central concern of his later life. He became, in his own words, a "self-appointed inspector of snowstorms and rainstorms," which is, perhaps, as cogent a description of a mindfulness practitioner as any from the Eastern traditions.

While India and, particularly, Hindu thought have taken the prime place in the discussion so far, America's engagement with the East by the middle of the nineteenth century also included East Asian culture, with Chinese, Korean, and Japanese arts, literature, and religion — including the Buddhism of these areas — shaping the intellectual direction of an emerging American modernism. For example, the work of Ernest Fenollosa, American scholar of East Asian art and literature and convert to Tendai Buddhism, brought this spirit into wider intellectual discourse (Bevis, 1988; Brooks, 1962). Fenollosa represents a more specific, scholarly, but no less engaged, use of the East by an American. A few lines from Fenollossa's poem, "East and West," his Phi Beta Kappa address at Harvard in 1892, reflect a growing need of Western thought for contemplative space. Addressing a Japanese mentor, Fenollossa says, "I've flown from my West/Like a desolate bird from a broken nest/ To learn thy secret of joy and rest" (quoted in Brooks, 1962, p. 50).

At Fenollossa's death, his widow gave his unpublished studies of the Chinese written language and notebooks of translations from the classical Chinese poet Li Po to the American poet Ezra Pound, for whom a whole new world opened. Pound's Chinese translations drawn from Fenollossa's work radically transformed the art of the time. Indeed, Pound had, arguably, the most powerful influence of any single poet in shaping the poetry, not only of his modernist contemporaries, but of the generation that would come to maturity in the middle of the twentieth century.

While Pound's use of Eastern influences was mainly stylistic, a very different sort of poet, Wallace Stevens, used his own encounter with the East — studying Buddhist texts and translating Chinese poetry with his friend the scholar-poet Witter Bynner — to better understand and express his tacit experience (Bevis, 1988). Perhaps "The Snow Man," an early poem (written in 1908 and first published in 1921), suggests this (Stevens, 1971, p. 54).

> One must have a mind of winter
> To regard the frost and the boughs
> Of the pine-trees crusted with snow;
>
> And have been cold a long time
> To behold the junipers shagged with ice,
> The spruces rough in the distant glitter
>
> Of the January sun; and not to think
> Of any misery in the sound of the wind,
> In the sound of a few leaves,
>
> Which is the sound of the land
> Full of the same wind
> That is blowing in the same bare place
>
> For the listener, who listens in the snow,
> And, nothing himself, beholds
> Nothing that is not there and the nothing that is.

Here is the description of an undeniably meditative stance, using an image from the poet's Connecticut landscape, and rhetoric from his East Asian studies, perhaps. Yet, it is possible that this is *also* an articulation of personal experience. Stevens did not study meditation formally, but, like Thoreau, he was a prodigious walker. In any season or weather, a perambulation of 15 miles or so — in a business suit — was a common prelude to writing (Bevis, 1988). This is neatly captured in a few lines from "Notes for a Supreme Fiction": "... Perhaps/The truth depends on a walk around a lake,// A composing as the body tires, a stop/To see hepatica, a stop to watch/ A definition growing certain and// A wait within that certainty, a rest/In the swags of pine trees bordering the lake ..." (Stevens, 1971, p. 212).

A transparent eye-ball. An inspector of snowstorms. A mind of winter. These are powerful metaphors to describe experiences that sought and found elaboration through encounters with Eastern thought. For these individuals, there was a willingness to use whatever comes to hand — from whatever culture or tradition suggests itself or is available — to understand what is happening in the here and now. This reflects a perennial American pragmatism, which endures today in much of the discourse of the mindfulness-based interventions: Hatha yoga mixes with Buddhist meditation, while Sufi poetry and Native American stories illuminate teaching points, and the language of the Christian and Jewish contemplative traditions hover in the background.

In the same early time frame we've been discussing, a more specific connection to Buddhism began developing, as well. Of the major traditions in the Oriental amalgam, Buddhism appears to have been the least understood and the most scorned during the earlier part of the nineteenth century. Reasons include Christian defensiveness and hostile reporting from the mission field; a portrayal of Buddhist doctrines as atheistic, nihilistic, passive, and pessimistic; and, even, the contagious anti-Buddhist biases of the Hindu scholars who taught Sanskrit to the English translators of the Asiatic Society of Bengal (Tweed, 1992; Versluis, 1993). The "opening" of Japan with Commodore Perry's visit in and the subsequent travels, study, and writing of American artists, scholars, and sophisticates, including Ernest Fenollossa, Henry Adams (great-grandson of aforementioned John Adams), John LaFarge, and Lafcadio Hearn, who all had direct contact with Buddhism did much to increase interest and sympathy for Buddhism. Then, the 1879 publication of *The Light of Asia,* Edwin Arnold's poetic retelling of the life of the Buddha, drawing parallels with the life of Jesus, turned interest into enthusiasm. Sales estimates of between 500,000 and a million copies put it at a level of popularity matching, say, *Huckleberry Finn* (Tweed, 1992) or the number-one bestseller of that time, *Ben Hur*, by retired Civil War General Lew Wallace.

Buddhism became a new possibility for those at the bare edge of the culture who intuited the tidal shift of Christian believing that Matthew Arnold had poignantly articulated in "Dover Beach" in 1867:

The Sea of Faith
Was once, too, at the full, and round earth's shore
Lay like the folds of a bright girdle furled.
But now I only hear
Its melancholy, long, withdrawing roar,
Retreating, to the breath
Of the night-wind, down the vast edges drear
And naked shingles of the world ...

And for some, Buddhist belief became a formal identity. Madame Blavatsky and Henry Steele Olcott, founders of the Theosophical Society (and the alternative practice of Theosophical Medicine), were long engaged with Buddhism, and in Ceylon in 1880, made ritual vows in a Theravada temple to live by the five precepts and take refuge in the Buddha, the teachings, and the community. The most powerful event, however, was the face-to-face encounters with Buddhist masters afforded by the Parliament of World Religions, particularly the Theravadin Anagarika Dharmapala and the Rinzai Zen Master Soyen Shaku. Both of these teachers continued to raise interest in Buddhism through subsequent visits. In fact, Soyen Shaku bears significant responsibility for popularization of Buddhism through the present day. The vision of Buddhism that he presented jibed perfectly with the early modern scientific and moral outlooks. The themes he presented — "an embrace of science combined with the promise of something beyond it, and a universal reality in which different religions and individuals participate, but which Buddhism embodies most perfectly" (McMahan, 2002, p. 220) still resonate. (These themes resonate with contemporary reconciliation of ancient, traditional ayurvedic precepts with quantum mechanics and fundamental particle physics in the formulations of Maharishi Ayurveda.) He also had a "second generation" impact through the 1950s and 1960s, as he encouraged his student and translator for the Parliament visit, the articulate Zen scholar D. T. Suzuki, to maintain a dialog with the West through visits and writing (Tweed, 1992; McMahan, 2002).

It is important to note that the character of Buddhist "believing" during this period was just that — an engagement with philosophy and doctrine, a search for a replacement for the Judeo — Christian belief system that some felt was no longer sustaining. Consider that two other Buddhist "best sellers" beside Arnold's *The Light of Asia* were Olcott's *Buddhist Catechism* and Paul Carus's *The Gospel of Buddha,* whose titles even reflect a Christian, belief-oriented approach to Buddhism. In the best Evangelical Protestant tradition comes the story of the first "Buddhist conversion" in America. In Chicago in 1893, Dharmapala was speaking on Buddhism and Theosophy to an overflow crowd in a large auditorium. At the end of the talk, Charles Strauss, a Swiss-American businessman of Jewish background, stood up from his seat in the audience and walked deliberately to the front. One can imagine the hush and expectancy. As planned in advance, he then — to use an Evangelical Protestant phrase — accepted Buddhism, repeating the refuge vows for all to hear (Tweed, 1992; Obadia, 2002).

The connection of most of the two or three thousand Euro-American Buddhists and the tens of thousands of sympathizers at this time (Tweed, 1993) was, with a few exceptions, intellectual. The popular appeal of Buddhism was as a form of *belief*, not as a form of spiritual *practice*. According to Tweed (1993), the fascination with Buddhist believing reached a high water mark around 1907, and declined precipitously thereafter. A small nucleus of Euro Americans interested in the academic or personal study of Buddhism maintained organizations and specialized publishing, but few Asian teachers stayed in the United States, and impetus for growth was lost. Dharmapala, in 1921, wrote in a letter to an American supporter, "At one time there was some kind of activity in certain parts of the U.S. where some people took interest in Buddhism, but I see none of that now" (In Tweed, 1993, p. 157). Charges by the status quo religious and cultural powers that Buddhism was passive and pessimistic — terrible sins in a culture fueling itself on action and optimism — drowned dissenting Buddhist voices.

Three Buddhisms in America It is important to note that the narrative that has shaped the discourse of mindfulness among professionals today sidelines the story of ethnic Asian Buddhism in America. Religion scholar Richard Hughes Seager (2002) describes three Buddhisms in America:

1. Old-line Asian-American Buddhism, with institutions dating back into the nineteenth century;
2. Euro-American or convert Buddhism, centered in the Westernized forms of Buddhism — often generically parsed as Zen, Tibetan, and Theravada (or Vipassana or Insight), which are centered on meditation practice; and Soka Gakkai International, an American branch of a Japanese group, which with a rich mix of Asian-Americans, Euro-Americans and substantial numbers of African-Americans and Latino-Americans is the most culturally diverse group, and is centered on chanting practice rather than meditation; and
3. New immigrant or ethnic Buddhism, which is most easily parsed by the country of origin.

In the Aftermath of World War II

The applications of Eastern thought to Western experience developed a powerful momentum immediately following the Second World War. Western soldiers, many drawn from professional life into active duty, were exposed in great numbers to Asian cultures, from India, Burma, and China. In Japan, physicians, scientists, and artists and intellectuals who held posts in the occupation forces were exposed to a culture that included the esthetic, philosophical, and spiritual manifestations of Japanese Buddhism, particularly its Zen varieties. Some stayed to study, and East — West dialogs that had been suspended were resumed, such as with D. T. Suzuki and Shinichi Hisamatsu. Most important for the discourse of mindfulness in medicine and psychotherapy, American military psychiatrists were exposed to Japanese psychotherapy, particularly that developed by Shoma Morita, which is based on a paradox that had enormous repercussions in Western practice. Instead of attacking symptoms as in Western approaches, Morita asked his patients to allow themselves to turn towards their symptoms and fully experience them, to know them as they are (Dryden and Still, 2006; Morita, 1928/1998).

Morita therapy was of interest and intellectually available to those Westerners in Japan for two powerful reasons. First, it is a highly effective treatment for what Western practitioners would identify as anxiety-based disorders; reports of cured or improved rates greater than 90% are common (Morita, 1928/1998); Reynolds, 1993). Morita developed a diagnostic category of *shinkeishitsu* for the disorders he targeted, which he describes as anxiety disorders with hypochondriasis (Morita, 1928/1998). Second, Morita did not develop his work in cultural isolation. Working contemporaneously with Charcot, William James, Freud, and Jung, Morita read, referenced, and critiqued Western developments. He was particularly interested in the therapies that paralleled his own in certain ways, such as Freud's psychoanalysis, S.Weir Mitchell's rest therapy (also rest cure, "west cure', and Nature Cure), Otto Binswanger's life normalization therapy, and Paul DuBois's persuasion therapy (Morita, 1998). It integrated East and West — from an *Eastern* perspective.

While the entire regimen of Morita therapy, a four-stage, intensive, residential treatment (see sidebar) has rarely been used in the Unites States, — David Reynolds (1980, 1993) has adapted it and other Japanese therapies for the West — two of its basic insights had immediate and continuing effects. First is the paradox of turning towards rather than away from symptoms for relief. Second is the insistence on the nondual nature of the body and mind. Although the influence of Zen is easily seen in his therapy, Morita did not wish to promote a direct religious association, fearing that it might be seen as somehow less serious, exacting, and effective (LeVine, 1998). Paradoxically, perhaps the Zen connection actually drew the interest of the Westerners.

MORITA THERAPY: *MUSHOJU-SHIN* AND THE STAGES OF TREATMENT.

In the nutshell version of Morita therapy, the Zen term *mushoju-shin* points to the end, or the beginning. It describes a healthy attention. In Morita's (1928/1998) metaphor, it is the attention you have when you're reading while standing on the train. You must balance, hold the book, read, remember the next station, and be aware of others. That is, you cannot focus on any one thing too tightly. You must be willing to be unstable, open to whatever happens, and able to respond and change freely. In short, you are not "self" focused, rather, mind = body = environment are one. "This is the place from where my special therapy begins" (p. 31), says Morita. It is also the place that Morita therapists are required to inhabit as they work.

First Stage: Isolation and rest (5–7 days).

Disposition: After careful assessment to ensure safety, patients are isolated and asked to remain in a lying-down posture, except to use the bathroom.

Instructions: Experience the anxieties and illusions that arise; let them run their course, without trying to change or stop them.

Purpose: There is a Zen saying that if you try to eliminate a wave with another wave, all you get is more waves, more confusion. This becomes clear.

Second Stage: Light occupational work (5–7 days).

Disposition: Isolation is maintained; no conversation or distractions. Sleep is restricted to 7 or 8 hours a night. Patients must be working during the day, and may not return to the room to rest.

Instructions: Move gently into mental and physical activity again, tidying the yard by picking up sticks and leaves, and moving into more effortful activities over time. Allow physical and mental discomfort to be just as it is.

Purpose: Breaking down the "feeling-centered attitude," by deemphasizing judgments of comfort and discomfort; promoting spontaneous activity of mind and body.

The Zen Boom

Zen had a double-barreled influence in the United States, particularly in the postwar "Zen boom" years of the 1950s and 1960s, touching both the intellectual community and the popular culture. With the first barrel, it had significant impact on the serious discourse of scholars, professionals, artists, and Western religious thinkers. One person was so profoundly influential in conveying the spirit of Zen that he epitomizes this impact: D.T. Suzuki. As a young man, you'll remember, Suzuki had played a role in the Buddhist enthusiasm of the 1890s and 1900s, as translator for Soyen Shaku. Suzuki had then lived for a time in the United States, working for Open Court, a publishing company specializing

> *Third Stage: Intensive occupational work* (5–7 days).
> Disposition: As in stage two.
> Instructions: Patients are assigned more strenuous labor, such as chopping wood and digging holes, and are encouraged to do art or craft projects that please them and to be spontaneous.
> Purpose: Learn to be patient and to endure work, build self-confidence, and own their subjective experiences.
>
> *Fourth Stage: Preparation for daily living* (5–7 days).
> Disposition: Patients may interact purposefully with others but not speak of their own experience, and may leave the hospital grounds for errands.
> Instructions: The work and activities are not chosen by the patient.
> Purpose: Learn to adjust to changes in circumstances; to not be attached to personal preferences. Prepare for return to the natural rhythms of living.

in Eastern thought, and had married an American woman. After the war, Suzuki returned to the West, where he continued to write books of both scholarly and popular interest on Zen and Pure Land Buddhism, traveled and lectured extensively in the United States and Europe, maintained a voluminous correspondence, and affected an incredibly varied range of thinkers. Three short examples give a glimpse into the effects of Suzuki's Zen on intellectual discourse: Thomas Merton, John Cage, and Eric Fromm.

The Trappist monk Thomas Merton was greatly influenced by Suzuki's work — which he had first known in the 1930s before entering the Monastery. An engagement with Eastern religious and aesthetic thought — particularly Zen, and particularly through Suzuki's work — shaped Merton's conception of and practice of contemplative prayer, which has had a powerful influence on Christian spiritual practice to the present day (e.g., Merton, 1968; Pennington, 1980). Merton began a correspondence with Suzuki in 1959, asking him to write a preface for a book of translations of the sayings of the "Desert Fathers." Merton's superiors felt such collaboration in print was "inappropriate," yet in practice, they encouraged Merton to continue the dialog with Suzuki, one telling him, "Do it but don't preach it" (Mott, 1984, p. 326). This stance represented a reversal of the earlier Buddhist fusion of *belief* without *practice*. The dialog did indeed continue, each endeavoring to explore and understand Christianity and Zen from their own perspectives. The relationship meant so much to Merton that, although his vocation had kept him cloistered in the Monastery of Gethsemane in Kentucky from 1941, he sought and gained permission from his Abbott to meet Suzuki in New York City in 1964, Merton's first travel in 23 years (Mott, 1984; Merton, 1968; Pennington, 1980). Suzuki summed up the burden of their two long talks this way: "The most important thing is Love" (Mott, 1984, p. 399).

The composer John Cage, who was deeply influenced by Hindu, Buddhist, and Taoist philosophy and practice, regularly attended Suzuki's lectures at Columbia University in the 1950s. His statement that in choosing to study with Suzuki he was choosing the elite — "I've always gone — insofar as I could — to the president of the company," (Duckworth, 1999, p. 21) — suggests the value of Suzuki's thought to him and to much of the avant garde. The Zen influence on Cage's work is captured in his conception of his compositions as "purposeless play" that is "... not an attempt to bring order out of chaos, nor to suggest improvements in creation, but simply to wake up to the very life we are living, which is so excellent once one gets one's mind and desires out of the way and lets it act of its own accord" (Cage, 1966, p. 12). Suzuki's expansive sense of play is reported by Cage (1966) in an anecdote: "... an American lady said, 'How is it, Dr. Suzuki? We spend the evening asking you questions and nothing is decided.' Dr. Suzuki smiled and said, 'That's why I love philosophy: no one wins'" (p. 40).

The psychoanalyst Eric Fromm was one of many in the psychoanalytic community of the time to be drawn by Zen and Suzuki's exposition of it. At a conference held in Mexico in 1957 entitled "Zen Buddhism and Psychoanalysis," which was attended by about fifty psychoanalytically inclined psychiatrists and psychologists, Suzuki was a featured speaker, and engaged in dialog particularly with Fromm and the religion scholar Richard DeMartino. A book of the lectures was published after the conference (Fromm et al., 1960). Fromm suggests that psychoanalysis and Zen both offer an answer to the suffering of contemporary people: "... the alienation from oneself, from one's fellow man, and from nature; the awareness that life runs out of one's hand like sand, and that one will die without having lived; that one lives in the midst of plenty and yet is joyless" (p. 86). The answer, then, would not be a cure that removes symptoms, but rather *"the presence of well being"* (p. 86; Fromm's italics). Fromm defines well being as "... to be fully born, to become what one potentially is; it means to have the full capacity for joy and for sadness or, to put it still differently, to awake from the half-slumber the average man lives in, and to be fully awake. If it is all that, it means also to be creative; that is, to react and respond to myself, to others, to everything that exists ..." (p. 90). For Fromm, the work was not just to bring the unconscious into consciousness, as Freud suggested, but rather to heal the rift between the two. What was most intriguing for Fromm in the possibilities Zen offered for such a project was *koan* practice — the use of paradoxical or nonrational questions, statements, and stories to back the student's ego-bound intellect against a wall, until the only way out is through. This process of amplifying the root contradiction of ego-consciousness, leading to its overturning — *satori*, or enlightenment — was the subject of DeMartino's contribution to the conference and book. Fromm drew a parallel between this process and the work of the analyst, suggesting that the analyst should not so much interpret and explain, but rather should "take away one rationalization after another, one crutch after another, until the patient cannot escape any longer, and instead breaks through the fictions which fill his mind and experiences reality — that is, becomes conscious of something he was not conscious of before" (p. 126).

Love, play, and well-being: it was not just Suzuki's erudition that attracted so many, it was his embodiment of what he taught. Alan Watts, the scholar-entertainer to whom we shall turn next, who got to know Suzuki at the Buddhist Lodge in London in the 1920s, described him as "… about the most gentle and enlightened person I have ever known; for he combined the most complex learning with utter simplicity. He was versed in Japanese, English, Chinese, Sanskrit, Tibetan, French, Pali, and German, but while attending a meeting at the Buddhist Lodge he would play with a kitten, looking right into its Buddha nature" (Watts, 1972). Suzuki should have the last word on his way of being, and what he wished to communicate to others (Fromm et al., 1960):

> We cannot all be expected to be scientists, but we are so constituted by nature that we can all be artists — not, indeed, artists of special kinds, such as painters, sculptors, musicians, poets, etc., but artists of life. This profession, "artist of life" may sound new and quite odd, but in point of fact, we are all born artists of life and, not knowing it, most of us fail to be so and the result is that we make a mess of our lives, asking, "What is the meaning of life?" "Are we not facing blank nothingness?" "After living seventy-eight, or even ninety years, where do we go? Nobody knows," etc., etc. I am told that most modern men and women are neurotic on this account. But the Zen-man can tell them that they have all forgotten that they are born artists, creative artists of life, and that as soon as they realize this fact and truth they will all be cured of neurosis or psychosis or whatever name they have for their trouble (p. 15).

Certainly, such a vision of unfettered creativity and immediate relief from the pains of living would be resonant in postwar American culture.

It should be noted, however, that in the 1950s and 1960s, despite his tremendous stature, Suzuki was also criticized — accused by the *academic* Buddhist community as a reductionist "popularizer" of Zen — and dismissed by the *practice* community as one who did not sit in meditation with enough discipline and regularity. On one hand, these may be valid charges, yet on the other, they may be significant reasons for Suzuki's influence. This was a time when Western intellectuals were in search of new rhetoric and new philosophy to help express and ground their shifting experiences and intuitions; for many, it was a time of wide-ranging dialog, of exploring possibilities, of framing a debate, rather than a time of grounding, of digging in, of focus on details. Indeed, the charges might simply be moot, when Suzuki's enterprise is cast in the mode of his teacher Soyen Shaku, or even the mode of Ralph Waldo Emerson, of attempting to universalize spiritual experience. In his dialog with Christian mysticism, for example, Suzuki (1957) found it possible that "Christian experiences are not after all different from those of the Buddhist" (p. 8).

The Boom and Beyond

Just as Suzuki epitomized the intellectual reach of the Zen boom, it may be possible to capture the more popular facets of the time and continue the story through the 1960s by focusing on a single character: the transplanted Englishman Alan Watts. Watts's eccentric career as a scholar-entertainer travels a ragged arc from the 1930s to the early 1970s, along the way touching most of the important figures and movements in the meeting of Eastern and Western religious thought and practice, particularly as they offered insights that could be used in psychotherapy. The arc described here is drawn with the help of his autobiography, *In My Own Way* (1972), whose punning title suggests the paradox of sustaining a powerful public self to earn a living while discussing the dissolution of the ego, and Monica Furlong's feet-of-clay biography, whose original title, *Genuine Fake* (1986), carries an ambiguous truth.

An intellectually precocious and sensitive religious seeker, Watts spent his early years at King's School, Canterbury, which is next to the ancient cathedral. There, the history-steeped atmosphere and rich liturgical expression cast a spell and created a love of ritual that never left him. In his adolescent years at the school, he developed an interest in Buddhism, which he was able to defend on a very high level in debates with faculty. He wrote to Christmas Humphries, the great promoter of Buddhism and Theosophy and the founder of the Buddhist Lodge in London, who assumed the letters were from a faculty member. When they finally met, Humphries became a mentor, providing guidance for reading and practice, and connecting Watts to other Asian scholars, including D.T. Suzuki. By 1935, having foregone an Oxford University scholarship to study what appealed to him, Watts published his first book, written at age nineteen, *The Spirit of Zen*, which was almost a guidebook to the densities of Suzuki's *Essays on Zen*. Watts' studies expanded, he came to read and write Chinese at a scholarly level, and read deeply in Taoism, as well as Vedanta, Christian mysticism, and Jung's psychology.

Through the Buddhist Lodge, he met a mother and adolescent daughter, Ruth Fuller Everett and Eleanor. Ruth had been a member of the *ashram*-cum-zoo, as Watts called it, of Pierre Bernard — known as Oom the Magnificent — who catered to the New York society ladies by teaching Hatha yoga and tantrism. Through that association, she learned of Zen Buddhism, and, taking Eleanor as a traveling companion, set off for Japan. The two became the first Western women to sit in meditation in a Zen monastery. Years later, Ruth married a Zen teacher and eventually became a teacher herself. Watts and Eleanor courted, in a way, and attended meditation sessions together.

Watts's practice at the time was simply to be in the present moment, learned from the independent spiritual teachers J. Krishnamurti (who called it choiceless awareness) and G. I. Gurdjieff (who called it constant self-remembering). He was becoming frustrated with his inability to concentrate on the present, and discussed this with Eleanor on their walk home from a session at the Buddhist Lodge. Eleanor said, "Why try to concentrate on it? What else *is* there to be aware of? Your memories are all in the present, just as much as the trees over there. Your thoughts about the future are also in the present, and anyhow I just love to think about the future. The present is just a constant flow, like the Tao, and there's simply no way of getting out of it" (Watts, 1972, p. 152–153). That was *it*. He came to think of this as his true way of life, and continued to practice in this way in various guises throughout his lifetime.

The couple married and moved to the United States, just ahead of the war in Europe. After all his resistance and protest, at this point in his development Watts felt drawn to try to fit himself into a vocation that made sense in the West. With his rich Anglican background, the logical choice was the priesthood of the Episcopal Church. Although he had no undergraduate degree, Watts proved the depth of his learning and entered Seabury-Western Seminary in Chicago for a 2-year course of study. In his second year, his standing was so far advanced that he was excused from classes and undertook expansive theological reading in personal tutorials. His researches resulted in the book *Behold the Spirit*, which brought insights from the Eastern religions into profound dialog with a Christianity he painted as in need of refreshment. Reviewers in and outside the church greeted it warmly. Ordained, he was made chaplain of Northwestern University, where his feeling for ritual, his skills as a speaker, and his ability to throw a great party brought quick success. Yet tensions in his growing family and his own tendency for excess ended his career; the church in 1950 did not take affairs and divorce lightly.

With a new wife and no job, Watts's prospects were, indeed, uncertain as he began work on a new book, *The Wisdom of Insecurity* (1951). An influential friend, Joseph Campbell, managed to get Watts a grant from the Bollingen Foundation, funded by one of C. G. Jung's wealthy patients, to support research on myth, psychology, and Oriental philosophy. The book, fueled perhaps by the indigence and indignities of his situation, brought him to the directness and clarity of expression that characterizes work from here on. Here is a description of working with pain by trusting that the mind "... has *give* and can *absorb* shocks like water or a cushion" (p. 96):

> [H]ow does the mind absorb suffering? It discovers that resistance and escape — the "I" process — is a false move. The pain is inescapable, and resistance as a defense only makes it worse; the whole system is jarred by the shock. Seeing the impossibility of this course, it must act according to its nature — remain stable and absorb.
>
> ... Seeing that there is no escape from the pain, the mind yields to it, absorbs it, and becomes conscious of just pain without any "I" feeling it or resisting it. It experiences pain in the same complete, unselfconscious way in which it experiences pleasure. Pain is the nature of this present moment, and I can only live in this moment ....
>
> This, however, is not an experiment to be held in reserve, as a trick, for moments of crisis .... This is not a psychological or spiritual discipline for self-improvement. It is simply being aware of this present experience, and realizing that you can neither define it nor divide yourself from it. There is no rule but "Look!" (pp. 97–99)

In no time, Watts landed on his feet, invited into a position at the founding of the American Academy of Asian Studies in San Francisco, a precursor of today's California Institute of Integral Studies. He also landed in creative ferment. Instead of the business people and government officials learning Asian languages and culture that were the expected students, the Academy drew artists and poets and religious and philosophical thinkers who were open to the kind of exploration for which Watts and his faculty colleagues had prepared their whole lives. Students included the Beat poet Gary Snyder, with whom Watts struck up a deep friendship; Michael Murphy and Richard Price, who would found Esalen; and Locke McCorkle, who would become a force in EST (Erhard Seminars Training). As Watts added administrative duties to his teaching, he brought in an amazing range of guest lecturers: old friends such as D.T. Suzuki; his ex-mother-in-law Ruth Fuller Sasaki who spoke on Zen *koan* practice; Pali scholar G.P. Malalasekera and Theravada Buddhist monks Pannananda and Dharmawara; and the Zen master Asahina Sogen. As the Academy found its place in the community, local connections were made with Chinese and Japanese Buddhists. Through the Academy, the Zen Master Shunryu Suzuki came to understand the need for a Western Zen institution, later creating the San Francisco Zen Center. Watts himself spoke and gave workshops up and down the West Coast, and began a relationship with the Berkeley radio station KPFA, the first community funded station in the United States, broadcasting regularly, and appearing as well on the educational television station KQED. He was stirring what was fermenting, and that would soon distill itself as a kind of renaissance.

The core of the Beat writers coalesced for a moment in 1956 in San Francisco, and Jack Kerouac captured it in his novel, *The Dharma Bums* (1958). Its central character is the poet and Zen student Japhy Ryder (Gary Snyder), whom the narrator Ray Smith (Kerouac) idolizes for his "Zen lunatic" lifestyle, combining Zen discipline and esthetics with freewheeling sensuality. One scene in the novel recounts the Six Gallery poetry reading, at which Snyder, Philip Whalen, Michael McClure, and Philip Lamantia read, and Allen Ginsberg's incantation of *Howl* did, indeed, scream for a generation about the agonies of 1950s' fear and conformity (and fear of conformity). *The Dharma Bums*, coming fast on the heels of Kerouac's best selling *On the Road* (1957), drew a huge readership of the young and aspiring hip, who saw in Ryder/Snyder a new template for living, a chance to go beyond the confines of suburban expectations. This fueled the Zen boom from the popular culture side, prompting complaints from the Western Zen community of practitioners and academics about the authenticity of the Beat's Buddhism. Both the popular and elite outlooks drew a chastening commentary from Watts in his essay "Beat Zen, Square Zen, and Zen" (1958/1960), as he showed that their differences arose from the same fundamental background and impulse:

> [T]he Westerner who is attracted to Zen and who would understand it deeply must have one indispensable qualification: he must understand his own culture so thoroughly that he is no longer swayed by its premises unconsciously. He must really have come to terms with the Lord God Jehovah and with his Hebrew-Christian conscience so that he can take it or leave it without fear or rebellion. He must be free of the itch to justify himself. Lacking this, his Zen will be either "beat" or "square," either a revolt from the culture and social order or a new form of stuffiness and respectability. For Zen is above all the liberation of the mind from conventional thought, and this is something utterly different from rebellion against convention, on the one hand, or adapting to foreign conventions, on the other (p. 90).

Watts, already a friend and admirer of Snyder, whom he exempted from his criticisms due to Snyder's level of Zen scholarship and practice, soon came to count the rest of the beats as friends, and accepted many of them as "serious artists and disciplined yogis" (Watts, 1972, p. 358). He had connections to many seemingly disparate worlds. There were old-guard spiritual seekers, like expatriate friend Aldous Huxley; members of the highest circles of art, music, and literature; Asian meditation teachers from many different traditions and cultures; psychotherapists of every stripe; and the old-guard bohemians, the beats, and the students: all of whom, as the 1960s began, would come together to create a culture into which Watts was not fitted, but built.

The Revolutionary 1960s

The catalyst of the new culture was the beginning of experimentation with lysergic acid diethylamide (LSD) and other psychedelic drugs in the 1950s, and the publicity surrounding it. Aldous Huxley's descriptions of his experiences in *The Doors of Perception* (1954) were illuminating, but for Watts, it was about embodiment — that his once ascetic and severe "Manichean" friend had been transformed into a more sensuous and warm man made the promise real. Watts's own controlled experiments, in which he found his learning and understanding of the world's mystical traditions and meditative practices extremely helpful, resulted in powerful experiences, followed (inevitably) by enthusiastic essays and broadcasts, as well as by a book, *Joyous Cosmology: Adventures in the chemistry of consciousness* (1962). His position as a proponent of the drugs for experienced, disciplined explorers of consciousness helped fan an interest — the more so when Watts coincidentally was given a two-year fellowship at Harvard just as Timothy Leary and Richard Alpert (later Ram Das) were beginning their engagement with psychedelics. The spread of psychedelics beyond the specialists added a key facet to what Roszak (1969) dubbed the counter culture: "It strikes me as obvious beyond dispute, that the interests of our college-age and adolescent young in the psychology of alienation, oriental mysticism, psychedelic drugs, and communitarian experiments comprise a cultural constellation that radically diverges from values and assumptions that have been in the mainstream of our society since at least the Scientific Revolution of the seventeenth century" (Quoted in Furlong, 1986, p. 143). The 1960s, then, mapped directly to Watts's life's work.

Just as the 1950s' Zen boom can be captured in the Fromm — Suzuki meeting in Mexico in 1957, the 1960s can, perhaps, be captured in a meeting — admittedly much larger — the "Human Be-In" in the Polo Field in Golden Gate Park, San Francisco, in 1967. A procession led by Snyder, Ginsberg, and Watts, among others, circumambulated the field as in a Hindu or Buddhist rite to open the day. Tens of thousands found their way there, dressed in colorful finery, raising banners, dropping acid, listening to the Grateful Dead, Jefferson Airplane, and Quicksilver Messenger Service, and digging the mix of the crowd — Timothy Leary and Richard Alpert, political radical Jerry Rubin, Zen Master Shunryu Suzuki, and activist/comedian Dick Gregory suggest the organizers' intention to unify "love and activism." The Be-In became a model for gatherings around the United States and the world. The color, light, and promise of the day were captured by Paul Kantner of Jefferson Airplane in "Won't You Try/Saturday Afternoon" (Kantner, 1967). The soaring harmonies and instrumental arrangement convey a fuller experience; but if you can't listen, try to visualize this stanza:

> Saturday afternoon,
> Yellow clouds rising in the noon,
> acid, incense and balloons;
> Saturday afternoon,
> people dancing everywhere,

Loudly shouting "I don't care!"
It's a time for growing,
and a time for knowing love ...

And another shift had already begun. At the leading edge of cultural change, seekers had learned what was to be learned from psychedelic experience, and were turning toward the practice of meditation. As Watts (1972) put it in his unique blend of the pontifical and the plain: "[W]hen one has received the message, one hangs up the phone" (p. 402). Where an infrastructure for teaching and practice of Zen Buddhism already existed, such as in San Francisco, seekers turned in that direction, following Watts and Snyder. Another infrastructure had also been building, since 1959, using a mass marketing model to encompass much of the Western world: The Maharishi Mahesh Yogi's Transcendental Meditation (TM). This was an adaptation of Hindu mantra meditation for Western practitioners, in which the meditator brought the mind to a single pointed focus by repeating a word or phrase — in TM, the mantra was secret, potently exotic, and specially chosen for the meditator (Mahesh Yogi, 1968; Johnston, 1988). The Beatles, among many other celebrities, discovered (or were "recruited" into) TM in 1967, bringing it to prominence on the world stage. The connection seemed direct. Perhaps the psychedelic experience linked more directly to Hindu meditation than Zen, as well. Watts (1972) describes this from his own experience: "... LSD had brought me into an undeniably mystical state of consciousness. But oddly, considering my absorption in Zen at the time, the flavor of these experiences was Hindu rather than Chinese. Somehow the atmosphere of Hindu mythology slid into them, suggesting at the same time that Hindu philosophy was a local form of a sort of undercover wisdom, inconceivably ancient, which everyone knows at the back of his mind but will not admit" (p. 399). Transcendental Meditation was able aggressively to take advantage of the publicity available to it. In 1965, there were 350 TM meditators in the United States, and by 1968, there were 26,000; by 1972, there were 380,000; and by 1976, there were 826,000. (Later Deepak Chopra was able to vault onto the New York Times bestseller list with appropriated ancient AyurVedic wisdom by asking each of the TM meditators to buy ten copies of his first book.) The marketing strategy targeted specific populations, giving the practice and its benefits a spiritual spin, a political-change spin, or a pragmatic "self help" spin depending on the target. The pragmatic approach, designed to reach the middle-class, middle-management heart of the market, was given impetus through scientific research into TM's physical and psychological outcomes (e.g., Wallace, 1970; Seeman et al., 1972), which subsequently captured the attention of the medical establishment. The result was development of and research on medicalized versions, such as the Relaxation Response (Benson, 1975) and Clinical Standardized Meditation (Carrington, 1998). The factors at work here — translation into Western language and settings, popular recognition, adoption within scientific research in powerful institutions, and the use of sophisticated marketing and public relations techniques — represent a model for success in the building of new social movements (Johnston, 1988).

On both the substantive and popular levels, then, the market for Eastern and Eastern-inflected spiritual practices grew steadily. Looking from 1972 back to himself in 1960, Watts provides perspective on this growth:

> In my work of interpreting Oriental ways to the West I was pressing a button in expectation of a buzz, but instead there was an explosion. Others, of course, were pressing buttons on the same circuit, but I could not have believed — even in 1960 — that [there would be] a national television program on yoga, that numerous colleges would be giving courses on meditation and Oriental philosophy for undergraduates, that this country would be supporting thriving Zen monasteries and Hindu *ashrams*, that the *I Ching* would be selling in hundreds of thousands, and that — wonder of wonders — sections of the Episcopal church would be consulting me about contemplative retreats and the use of mantras in liturgy (p. 359).

At the turn of the decade of the 1960s, through political dislocations, waves of immigration, and economic opportunity seeking, new teachers from many of the Eastern traditions became available to offer instruction in the West. At the same time, Westerners of the post-World War II cohort who studied in the East, or with Eastern teachers in the West, began to find their own approaches and voices for teaching as well.The 1970s was a time of institution building at an unprecedented scale, a time in which, for example, Buddhism in America took its essential shape. Watts only flashed on this; only saw the promised land from afar. He died in 1973, at age 58, of a heart attack. His health had been in decline for some time, due to overwork and problems with alcohol. And in that, his example was again prophetic — foreshadowing the revelations in the 1980s of many spiritual teachers' feet of clay.

Paradox

The West Went a Long Way to Find What It Left at Home

The injunctions to relieve suffering and to live a more integrated, creative life by paying attention to what is arising in the present moment and turning towards discomfort — mindfulness and acceptance — are easily located within the three Abrahamic religions: the ones closest to home. But the encrustation of tradition and the carelessness of familiarity hide them quite well.

In Judaism, there is the marvelous text from Ecclesiastes (3:1–8), here in the King James' Version, which may ring in your ears with the "To everything turn, turn, turn" motion of the chorus of the song by Pete Seeger.

> To every thing there is a season, and a time to every purpose under the heaven: a time to be born, and a time to die; a time to plant, and a time to pluck up that which is planted; a time to kill, and a time to heal; a time to break down, and a time to build up; a time to weep, and a time to laugh; a time to mourn, and a time to dance; a time to cast away stones, and a time to gather stones together; a time to embrace, and a time to refrain from embracing; a time to get, and a time to lose; a time to keep, and a time to cast away; a time to rend, and a time to sew; a time to keep silence, and a time to speak; a time to love, and a time to hate; a time of war, and a time of peace.

There is also the tradition that everything should be blessed. Indeed, when one hears good news, the blessing traditionally said is "Blessed are you G-d, Sovereign of the Universe (who is) good and does good." On hearing bad news such as the death of a friend or relative one says, "Blessed are you G-d, Sovereign of the Universe, true judge." Such blessings acknowledge G-d as the source of everything, good or bad (Kravitz, personal communication), or in Buddhist perspective: "could be good, could be bad."

In Christianity, the natural mode for many is to do for others, to focus outward. This "Letter to a Christian Lady" from C. G. Jung (who had carved over his fireplace in Zurich, "summoned or unsummoned, G-d will be there"), which was made into a text for speaking by Jean Vanier (2005, pp. 63–64), is a refreshing corrective:

I admire Christians,
because when you see someone who is hungry or thirsty,
You see Jesus.
When you welcome a stranger, someone who is "strange,"
you welcome Jesus.
When you clothe someone who is naked, you clothe Jesus.
What I do not understand, however,
is that Christians never seem to recognize Jesus
in their own poverty.
You always want to do good to the poor outside you
and at the same time you deny the poor person
living inside you.
Why can't you see Jesus in your own poverty,
in your own hunger and thirst?
In all that is "strange" inside you:
in the violence and the anguish that are beyond your control!
You are called to welcome all this, not to *deny* its existence,
but to accept that it is there and to meet Jesus *there*.

The Christian contemplative teacher Richard Rohr (1999) suggests that, for him, Jesus' refusal of the drugged wine as he hung on the cross is a model of the radical acceptance of what is happening in the moment.

The Sufi poet Rumi makes the injunction for mindfulness and acceptance come alive in "The Guest House" a poem translated by Coleman Barks (1995, p. 109) that has become a very common teaching text in mindfulness-based interventions:

This being human is a guest house.
Every morning a new arrival.

A joy, a depression, a meanness,
some momentary awareness comes
as an unexpected visitor.

Welcome and entertain them all!
Even if they are a crowd of sorrows,
who violently sweep your house
empty of its furniture,
still, treat each guest honorably.
He may be clearing you out
for some new delight.

The dark thought, the shame, the malice.
meet them at the door laughing and invite them in.

Be grateful for whatever comes.
because each has been sent
as a guide from beyond.

Growth and Definition of Buddhism in America

There was a great variety of teaching and practice available as the turn away from psychedelic culture to more disciplined and thoughtful practice began. There was a range of Eastern and Western teachers in Hindu, Buddhist, Sufi, and the independent and occult traditions. There were new takes on Western traditions such as the Jesus People or Jesus Freak manifestation of Christianity, or the resurgence of interest in the mysticism of Kabbalah in Judaism. Yet, in tracing the discourse of mindfulness, by far the most influential tradition was Buddhism. This turn-of-the-decade moment is a fruitful place to focus, as all of the elements at play today come into view.

This was a time of growth. For example, the San Francisco Zen Center (SFZC), which had been started for Western students under the teaching of Shunryu Suzuki Roshi in 1961, expanded in 1967 to include a country retreat center at Tassajara Hot Springs, for which more than a thousand people had contributed money; and by 1969, SFZC had moved to larger quarters in the city and had established a series of satellite locations. The Zen presence in the United States was the most well established, while Tibetan and Theravada-derived teaching and practice infrastructures were in early developmental stages. It is these three traditions, generalized, that represent the shape that Buddhism in America has taken. The discourse of mindfulness draws from all, so understanding them as a group, and individually, will be helpful.

The task of characterizing and defining something that could be called "American Buddhism" is an enormous task, as it requires the parsing of, at minimum, two phenomena under that title. Prebish (1999) suggests that two divisions called Asian Immigrant Buddhism and American Convert Buddhism can be informative: noting, however, that there is considerable disagreement among researchers about how and if such distinctions can be made. For our purposes, it might reasonably be said that the former group is more interested in preserving religious and community traditions, while the latter is more interested in transforming religious traditions for an elite population.

That American convert Buddhism is the preserve of an elite is indisputable, and is an extremely important factor in the development of the discourse of mindfulness that we are pursuing. The group is highly educated, economically advantaged, politically and socially liberal, and overwhelmingly of European descent. This was as true of the crowd at the World Parliament of Religions in 1893 as it was of the students and intellectuals who made the shift from psychedelic experience to meditative experience, or as it is now of the medical, mental healthcare, and other professionals exploring the roots of mindfulness. Indeed, there is a continuity not just of types but of persons (Coleman, 2001; Nattier, 1998).

The signal characteristic of the American converts is a focus on meditation, almost to the exclusion of other forms of Buddhist practice and expression (Prebish, 1999). It is not surprising, then, that the expressions of world Buddhism they have "imported" for their use (as Nattier, 1998, would characterize it) are the meditation-rich Zen, Tibetan, and Theravada-derived traditions. A quick overview of the development and essential practice of each in the United States may be of value.

Zen was the first wave and the "boom" of Buddhism in America. In keeping with the elite nature of American interest, the highly aristocratic Rinzai sect, represented by Soyen Shaku and D. T. Suzuki, was influential until the 1960s. Rinzai emphasizes *koan* practice leading to *satori* or *kensho* — concentrating on a paradoxical question or story to heighten intensity and anxiety until a breakthrough occurs. This is central in the dialogs of D. T. Suzuki, Fromm, and DeMartino, for example. In the 1960s, however, the more popular Soto Zen sect began to reach out of the Japanese-American communities to American converts. Two of the most important figures in this shift, and in the development of Buddhism in America, are from this community: Shunryu Suzuki and Taizan Maezumi. Maezumi Roshi founded the Zen Center of Los Angeles in 1967 to reach Western students. He was in the Harada — Yasutani lineage, which includes koan practice and significant intensity and push for enlightenment. Two Western teachers were also part of this lineage and began their teaching at this same period: Robert Aitken founded the Diamond Sangha in Hawaii in 1959, and Philip Kapleau founded the Rochester Zen Center in 1966. Shunryu Suzuki Roshi of the SFZC was of a more traditional Soto lineage and presented an approach that must have clashed with what most of his students would have read or known about Zen. His focus was not on enlightenment, but on what he presented as the heart of the matter, just sitting. That is, "Our zazen is just to be ourselves. We should not expect anything — just be ourselves and continue this practice forever" (In Coleman, 2001, p. 71). Zen in its original Chinese form, Chan, as well as Korean (Son) and Vietnamese (Thien) arrived much later in the United States. Yet, teachers such as the Korean Seung Sahn and the Vietnamese Thich Nhat Hahn have had significant influences on Buddhism in America — particularly the genuine witness of "engaged Buddhism" advocate Thich Nhat Hahn, who was nominated for the Nobel Peace Prize by Martin Luther King for his peace work during the Vietnam War.

The foundational teachers mentioned here have authorized others to carry on their lineage of teaching. These teachers have often gone on to found their own centers. Some have hewn closely to their teachers' approaches, while others have continued to make adaptations to bring Zen to more Americans. To suggest the flavor of this process, in the Maezumi line, John Daido Loori founded Zen Mountain Monastery in Mt. Tremper, New York, keeping more towards traditional monastic training, yet creating a highly advanced computer-based communications and marketing infrastructure. Bernard Glassman Roshi, Maezumi's heir, has extended not simply Zen training but a deeply felt social engagement, from highly successful initiatives to bring education and employment opportunities to the homeless in Yonkers to the founding of the Zen Peacemaker Order (Prebish, 1999; Queen, 2002). In Kapleau's line, Toni Packer, who had been his successor in Rochester, became disillusioned by the traditional hierarchy and protocols and left that all behind to form an independent center with a Zen spirit all but devoid of the tradition — including that of lineage (Coleman, 2001; McMahan, 2002).

If it were possible to characterize "typical" Zen practice, one might see most of the following (Coleman, 2001; Prebish, 1999) protocols for meeting teachers and entering and leaving meditation halls, including bowing; chanting, often in the original Asian language; ceremonial marking of changes in status, anniversaries of events, and the like; and a meditative engagement with manual work around the center. Central to Zen is the sitting practice, *zazen*, in which the adherence to correct physical posture is considered extremely important. Initial instruction may be to count one's breaths — say, to ten — and, when the attention has wandered, to just notice that this has happened and begin the count again. When capacity for concentration has grown, one may begin *shikantaza*, "just sitting" with full awareness, without directing the mind (Coleman, 2001; Suzuki, 1970). Retreats, or *sesshins*, are intensely focused on sitting meditation, with short periods of walking meditation in between; retreats are rarely longer than seven days.

Tibetan teachers began to leave Tibet in response to the Chinese repression in the 1950s that killed or drove more than a third of the population into exile. Buddhism's central role in the culture made teachers and monastics a major target. While a few scholars had come to the United States in the 1950s — notably Geshe Wangal, Robert Thurman's first teacher — it was not until 1969 that Tibetan teachers reached out seriously to American students. Tarthang Tulku established the Tibetan Nyingma Meditation Center in Berkeley. The basic approach was very traditional, with students asked to undertake hundreds of thousands of prostrations, vows, and visualizations before receiving meditation instruction. Tarthang Tulku created the Human Development Training Program to teach Buddhist psychology and meditation techniques to a professional healthcare and mental healthcare audience, and create as well the Nyingma Institute to support Buddhist education and study. In 1971, Kalu Rinpoche, who had been asked by the Dalai Lama to teach in North America, came first to Vancouver to start a center, and later created a center in Woodstock, New York (Coleman, 2001; Seager, 2002).

Chogyam Trungpa, who had escaped from Tibet to India in 1959, came to the West to study at Oxford University; during the years he spent in the United Kingdom, he moved away from the traditional monastic teaching role and eventually gave up his vows. In 1970, as a lay teacher, he came to the United States, where he had an instant effect. He had arrived after the "boom," after the beats, but "Beat Zen" described him better than any Zen master. Allen Ginsberg became a student, and many of the original beat contingent taught at the Naropa Institute (now Naropa University) in Boulder, Colorado, which Trungpa founded. The appeal to the counter-culture was swift and far reaching. In a very short time, he created a thoroughgoing infrastructure, including a network of practice centers (now worldwide), and developed a "secular path" called Shambhala Training, to make the benefits of meditation practice and Buddhist psychological insights more available. Trungpa's approach to teaching was not the traditional one, but an amalgam that included much that he had learned from his Oxford education in comparative religion, as well as wide-ranging exposure to Western psychology. He not only powerfully shaped Tibetan Buddhism in the West, but he offered spiritual perceptions that had a much wider reach — particularly the idea of "spiritual materialism," which he defined in this way: "The problem is that ego can convert anything to its own use, even spirituality. Ego is constantly attempting to acquire and apply the teachings of spirituality for its own benefit" (Trungpa, 1973).

Tibetan Buddhist practice in America is richly varied; characterizing it in a paragraph is a hopeless challenge. It is the most exotic and sensual of the three traditions under consideration. The iconography and rituals are complex; the teachers are often Tibetan, rather than Westerners as is common in the other traditions. There is considerable emphasis on textual study. The ritual relationship of student to teacher is hierarchical and devotional. Many of the difficult issues of "belief" that are subdued in the other traditions are right at the surface in Tibetan doctrine and practice — karma, rebirth, realms of supernatural beings. And the practices themselves are guarded, only revealed by initiation, face to face with an authorized teacher. Vajryana or Tantric practice, roughly conceived, includes visualization by the meditator of him/herself with the attributes of a particular enlightened being. Less traditional teachers work differently; Trungpa began his students with sitting meditation much like that of his friend Shunryu Suzuki. The *dzogchen* teachers have an approach that seems easily accessible to Western students, a formless meditation akin to *shikantaza* in Zen. Within the tradition, this is considered a high teaching, available only after years of preparation. In the West, however, it is offered differently. Lama Surya Das, a Westerner, explains: "... one surprise is that people are a lot more prepared than one thinks. Westerners are sophisticated psychologically, but illiterate nomads (as in Tibet) are not" (In Coleman, 2001, p. 109). Retreats in the Tibetan tradition may be adapted for Americans as day long or weeks long, or more traditional lengths such as three months or three years.

Vipassana meditation is the latest tradition to flower in North America. It is drawn from Theravada Buddhist practice, the tradition most directly connected to the historical Buddha, and perhaps the most conservative. Theravada was an early and profound influence on the development of Buddhism in the United Kingdom and Europe, dating back to the nineteenth century, through colonial connections. In the United States, the connection came much later, in the Buddhist Vihara Society of Washington, DC, founded in 1966, with teachers Dickwela Piyananda and Henepola Gunaratana; and also as young Americans in the Peace Corps or traveling in Southern Asia in the 1960s came into contact with Theravada teachers, such as Mahasi Sayadaw, S. N. Goenka, and U Ba Khin. The influential Vipassana or Insight movement in the United States can be said to begin when two of those young Americans, Joseph Goldstein and Jack Kornfield, came together to teach Vipassana at Chogyam Trungpa's request at Naropa Institute in 1974. Their connection, which also included Goldstein's friend Sharon Salzberg, another of the travelers to become a teacher, deepened. In 1975, under their leadership, the Insight Meditation Society (IMS) was founded in rural Barre, Massachusetts. IMS grew quickly into a major retreat center as the Insight approach found broad appeal. In 1984, Jack Kornfield left IMS for California to found Spirit Rock Meditation Center, which quickly became a second wing in American Vipassana practice (Coleman, 2001; Fronsdal, 2002; Prebish, 1999).

The Insight movement is the most egalitarian and least historically conditioned of the three traditions under consideration. Ritual, ceremony, and hierarchy are deemphasized, and meditation is of central importance. In contrast to zen orderliness and Tibetan richness, there is ordinariness and a very American democratic, individualistic atmosphere. Students and teachers alike wear casual clothes and are known by first names. Teachers are less authority figures than "spiritual friends," and language is more psychological than specifically Buddhist. Vipassana is highly psychologized; in fact, many, if not a majority, of Vipassana teachers in the Insight movement are trained psychotherapists.

Meditation practice commonly includes two forms, concentration on the breath, and open awareness (insight) of whatever is arising in the moment. Practices for cultivating loving kindness, as well as compassion, sympathetic joy, and equanimity, are also a part of training. Retreats are commonly 10 days in length, with long days of intense practice in silence. A typical schedule would find retreatants rising at five in the morning and moving through periods of sitting and walking (walking periods are as long as sitting periods, in contrast to the short breaks in Zen) with breaks for meals, until ten in the evening (Coleman, 2001; Fronsdal, 2002; Prebish, 1999).

Perhaps most important for the discourse of mindfulness is not the differences in these three traditions, but rather the essential similarities. Batchelor (1994) neatly summarizes:

> The distinctive goal of any Buddhist contemplative tradition is a state in which inner calm (*samatha*) is *unified* with insight (*vipassana*). Over the centuries, each tradition has developed its own methods for actualizing this state. And it is in these methods that the traditions differ, *not* in their end objective of unified calm and insight.

Passage to Maturity

If the 1960s and 1970s were the period of foundation and growth, the 1980s and 1990s could be seen as the painful passage to maturity. In the many Buddhist centers around the United States, large but intimate communities had grown up, often with charismatic leaders. In most instances, the sharp discipline of Asian monastic practice, with celibacy and renunciation at its core, had been replaced by more casual, worldly, "extended family" types of community. As Suzuki Roshi told SFZC, and Downing (2001) construed as a warning, "You are not monks, and you are not lay people" (p. 70). There was no map, as communities sought ways forward. Perhaps the scandals around sexuality, alcohol, finances, and power that began to plague these institutions could not have been avoided, and were necessary in catalyzing change. By 1988, Jack Kornfield could write, "Already upheavals over teacher behavior and abuse have occurred at dozens (if not the majority) of the major Buddhist and Hindu centers in America" (In Bell, 2002). None of the three traditions was spared. A précis of a scandal from each will help illustrate the commonality of the problems, and the importance of their aftermaths and resolutions.

At the San Francisco Zen Center, Suzuki Roshi appointed Richard Baker his successor, not just as abbot but as principal authority over the entire enterprise, which included associated meditation centers and successful businesses such as

Tassajara Bakery and Greens restaurant. Following Suzuki's death in 1971, Baker held a tight rein over the institution, with little input from board members or other authorized teachers. In 1983, the board called a meeting, and the outcome was Baker taking a leave of absence. This was precipitated by an incident in which it became obvious that Baker, married himself, was having a sexual relationship with a married female student — indeed, the wife of a friend and benefactor. This was not an unprecedented situation; Baker had a considerable history of infidelities with students. There was more: in a community where the residents willingly worked long hours for low wages, Baker spent more than $200,000 in a year, drove a BMW, and had his personal spaces impeccably furnished with antiques and art- work. Further, Baker had surrounded himself with an inner circle of "courtiers" and failed to treat other senior members who had been ordained by Suzuki Roshi as valued peers. The most painful thing for the community was Baker's reaction: he did not comprehend that he had done anything wrong. More than 10 years after "the apocalypse" as it came to be known, he stated, "It is as hard to say what I have learned as it is to say what happened" (In Bell, 2002, p. 236; Downing, 2001).

In Chogyam Trungpa Rinpoche's organization, teachers and students alike flaunted their disregard of contemporary Western mores. Trungpa's sexual liaisons with female students, his heavy drinking, and his aggressive outbursts were well known, generally accepted within the community, and considered as part of his teaching tradition. He was both open and unapologetic about his behavior, helping to avoid scandal (Bell, 2002; Clark, 1980; Coleman, 2001; Hayward, 2008; Mukpo, 2006). In planning the future of the organization, Trungpa named as his heir Osel Tendzin, an American, who was not a universally popular choice. When Trungpa died in 1987, Tendzin became what amounted to supreme ruler of the enterprise, holding untouchable spiritual and executive power (Coleman, 2001; Sanders, 1977). In 1988, after a period of silence and disagreement, members of the board revealed to the community that Tendzin was HIV positive, and that although he had been aware of his condition had continued to have unprotected sex with male and female members. At the urging of the board, senior members of the organization, and a revered Tibetan teacher, Tendzin went into retreat, and died soon thereafter (Bell, 2002; Coleman, 2001). It is interesting to note Tendzin's vagueness and self-delusion, perhaps reminiscent of Baker's. Tendzin stated, "I was fooling myself.... Thinking I had some extraordinary means of protection I went ahead with my busi- ness as if something would take care of it for me" (Fields, 1991, quoted in Coleman, 2001, p. 170). Asked how it happened, Tendzin replied, "It happened....I don't expect anybody to try to conceive it" (Fields, 1991, p. 47).

At the end of an Insight Meditation Society retreat taught by an Asian Theravada teacher, Anagarika Munindra, a woman came forward to say that she had had sex with the teacher during the retreat. The woman had been psychologically troubled, and this had traumatized her further. The IMS guiding teachers were divided as to how to handle the situation — how much to reveal publicly, and how to deal with Munindra, who had returned to India. Kornfield pushed for complete disclosure and an immediate confront- ing of Munindra. As he put it, "If parts of one's life are quite unexamined — which was true for all of us — and something like this comes up about a revered teacher, it throws everything you've been doing for years into doubt. It's threatening to the whole scene" (In Schwartz, 1995, p. 334). Eventually, Kornfield was sent by the board to India to speak directly with Munindra, who agreed to apologize to the community.

In the aftermath and resolution of all of these incidents, American Buddhism lost its idealized self-image and came to the maturity it carries now. In this process, common themes and practices arose. Leadership power moved away from the charismatic models, and was rationalized and distributed more widely, with checks and balances, and boards accountable for oversight. Ethics were addressed formally with statements and policies. The model of teacher-student interaction was scrutinized, and methods for diluting intensity were developed and instituted, as possible. Of course, this remains the most difficult of all relationships to manage, as meditation training carries the teacher-student dyad into areas of intimacy and power differential analogous to those in psychotherapy.

A Universalizing and Secularizing Discourse

The historical narrative we have presented here captures much of the discourse up to the beginnings of the mindfulness-based interventions as described in Chapter 1. It remains now to draw together the overriding themes and to suggest directions forward.

The first theme is the need for an expanded vocabulary of words, images, and ideas with which to express tacit experience. As we have more and more shared language — verbal or nonverbal — the possibilities for teaching expand. The second theme is the drive for a universalizing of the experiences and the language surrounding them. This may emerge as explicitly spiritual language, as with Emerson or D. T. Suzuki, or in more secular language, as in the mindfulness-based interventions. The third theme, more specific, is the discovery/rediscovery of the principle of turning *towards* suffering and taking on an attitude of nonjudgment alloyed with kindness. This is a universal insight that is both spiritual and psychological in nature. As the verbal and nonverbal discourse of mindfulness continues to expand, universalize, and secularize, the potential for teaching will continue to expand as well. But this is only possible if a fourth theme is considered: the fact that this discourse is predominantly a product of an elite social group, with significant socioeconomic advantages and a level of education that is "right off the charts" (Coleman, 2001, p. 193). As professionals and members of an elite, we teach from our own experience, and give voice to it in language that may reflect our own elite position and exclude others. Therefore, we must continually be sensitive to, and learn from, the language of our clients, patients, and students.

One window into the possibilities of expanding discourse is suggested in the work of the postmodern theologian Don Cupitt (1999), who undertook an exercise in "ordinary language" theology. He collected and analyzed more than 150 idiomatic expressions in English that use the term *life*. His hypothesis was that these idioms have arisen to reflect the overall population's reaction to the shifts in religion or spirituality from the mid-nineteenth century onward — the era of the development of the East-West discourse under consideration. He suggests that for a great many people, *life* has become the privileged religious object. Consider, for example, the switch since the mid-twentieth century from funerals oriented towards the deceased's place in the hereafter to a "celebration of the life of" the deceased. It might be said of the deceased that "she loved life." Phrases like "the sanctity of life," "the value of life," and "the quality of life" have become current since the 1950s; in fact, in healthcare, there are scales to measure "quality of life." And then there is the imperative phrase "get a life!" that became so popular in the 1990s: What are its implications as a religious phrase?

The usual rhetoric about religion in contemporary Western culture is that it has been *secularized.* Cupitt suggests just the reverse, that ordinary life has been *sacralized.* We can trace the roots of this shift back again to mid-nineteenth century. Thoreau recorded this new attitude in *Walden,* as he went to the woods to "live deliberately," as he puts it. Says Cupitt (1999):

> It is clear straightaway that Thoreau is not going to live in the wilderness for any of the Old World's traditional reasons. He's not going into the desert like Elijah or Muhammad to listen out for the voice of God; he's not going like Jesus or Anthony to be tempted of the devil; and he's not going, like Wittgenstein or Kerouac, in order to seek relief for his own troubled psychology. He's going to try to find out for himself what it is to be a human being with a life to live … (p. 21).

This attitude is of considerable importance in the discourse of the mindfulness-based interventions. In MBSR, for example, a poem such as Mary Oliver's "The Summer Day," with the last lines "Tell me, what is it you plan to do/With your one wild and precious life?" dropped into the silence of a class creates a sacred space and a sacred pause for reflection. It is secular liturgy. It is the work of teaching mindfulnes as a professional.

Another window into the further possibilities of the discourse of the mindfulness-based interventions is suggested by the sociologist of religion Robert Wuthnow. In *After Heaven: Spirituality in America since the 1950s* (1998), he maps out three approaches to spirituality that may suggest language, images, metaphors, and assumptions that will promote connection of contemporary Americans to mindfulness practice. The approaches he names follow the arc of the narrative of this chapter: the traditional *spirituality of dwelling*, the contemporary *spirituality of seeking,* and the emerging *spirituality of practice.*

Dwelling spirituality dominates in settled times in history, when it is possible to create stable institutions and communities, when sacred spaces for worship can be *inhabited.* The metaphor of this spirituality is a *place.* In the narrative we have been following, the hundred years from mid-nineteenth to mid-twentieth century were dwelling times. In America, the overwhelming majority of the population is identified with Jewish or Christian tradition. Towns were small, church buildings and synagogues were central, and one — and one's entire family — simply *belonged.* Lives were spent from infancy to funeral within a community, a place. The few at the end of the nineteenth century who saw and felt the withdrawal of the tide of the sea of faith — the first Buddhists — were anomalous harbingers.

Seeking spirituality dominates in unsettled times, when meaning must be negotiated, and all that is on offer may be explored. Wuthnow notes that a major shift was beginning in the America of 1950s, as the culture became more fluid, complex, and threatening to individual identities. The opening to new possibilities from the East and from the culture of recovery and self-help brought new products and perspectives into the spiritual marketplace. The seeking of the 1960s and 1970s was pervasive, and continues today, as the market becomes more fragmented and the culture more unstable The metaphor for seeking spirituality is a journey.

Practice spirituality is the new bright edge in the culture. In a profound way, it integrates both dwelling and seeking. It requires setting aside a sacred space/time for the practice, yet that space/time is potentially fluid. Further, practice spirituality begins to reconcile or mediate the split between dwelling and seeking. Practice encourages both discipline and wide-ranging exploration, and can be undertaken within the shelter of an organization and community or pursued independently. There is not a metaphor for practice, but rather an impulse and attitude to "live deliberately," as Thoreau and Cupitt suggest.

It is here, now, in this emerging moment, with a democratic and ethical view of spiritual teacher-student relations, a secular spirituality of life, and a drive for the paradoxical fluidity and stability of spiritual practice that the mindfulness-based interventions are growing and evolving. With one hundred and fifty years of evolving discourse behind and within, it may now be possible to define what mindfulness is — at least for us.

Chapter 3
Defining Mindfulness for the Moment

In the preceding chapters, we have described both the broader discourse of the meditative and contemplative traditions and the specific discourse of the mindfulness-based interventions (MBIs). In the long journey from the nineteenth century Romantic and Transcendentalist discoveries of Asian religious texts and practices to the current flowering of the empirically supported MBIs, a variety of streams of this discourse have been active. At times, one stream has predominated; at other times another has drawn the most attention and found the most utility.

Particularly over the past 60 years or so, such shifts in the discourse have reflected or led the spirit of the times, as we have shown. In the 1950s, a highly intellectual and theoretical form of Zen Buddhism — emphasizing paradox and a sudden overturning of ordinary consciousness — helped to shape esthetic, spiritual, and psychotherapeutic contributions to U.S. culture. The psychotherapeutic manifestation of this trend was reflected in the evolution and expansion of the Humanistic and Existential therapies. In the 1960s, the discourse shifted to greater affectivity — emphasizing ecstatic experiences — with an emphasis on spiritual practice and the place of the guru, reflected in a growth of interest in Hindu and Tibetan Buddhist traditions. The most salient therapeutic expressions of that time were, perhaps, the efflorescence of experiential therapies and the adaptation of mantra meditation for use in medical settings. Most recently, the predominating discourse is of a more democratic, more psychologically and therapeutically focused version of Theravada Buddhism, with *vipassana* — insight — meditation practice at its core. This phenomenon, by distancing itself from many traditional Asian Buddhist features, such as hierarchies of ordained male teachers, elaborate rituals, exclusive vows, esoteric vocabularies, and presumptions about specific beliefs and worldviews, has helped to make mindfulness practice accessible to a broader population than ever before. Its fit with the culture in the United States and other Western countries has been easier, and its acceptance, perhaps, quicker. Adding to this ease and speed has been the willingness of many highly educated practitioners, well placed within the academy and the professions, to submit mindfulness practice and its expected outcomes to the rigors of research and analysis within the modern, scientific paradigm. The result has been the careful development, enthusiastic adoption, and rapid expansion of the MBIs in medicine and psychotherapy described in Chapter 1.

D. McCown et al., *Teaching Mindfulness: A Practical Guide*
for Clinicians and Educators, DOI 10.1007/978-0-387-09484-7_3,
© Springer Science+Business Media, LLC 2010

Given such historical shifts in the dominance of the streams of discourse and the fact that now many streams are flowing concurrently, the task of developing a working definition of mindfulness is challenging. And the first challenge is philosophical. We must be as clear as we can about *how* we are speaking about mindfulness and the *location* from which we are speaking. It will be helpful, therefore, to become more technical and critical in approaching the discourses of mindfulness.

The Trouble with Discourses

Previous chapters have used the term "discourse" in its nontechnical, dictionary denotation of a "formal and orderly expression of ideas" and a "conversation." With the task of defining mindfulness before us now, it will be helpful to apply some of the more technical insights and uses of discourse within cultural and critical theory, and literary theory. The objective here is not to isolate or criticize particular discourses; rather, it is to enrich the resources of the pedagogy of mindfulness by bringing seemingly disparate discourses together.

In cultural and critical theory, the term discourse is perhaps most commonly associated with Michel Foucault. His work identifies sociocultural mechanisms by which discourses are formed and controlled. The major procedure in forming a discourse is exclusion, by making certain subjects taboo, dividing rational from irrational, and willing towards a truth. Discourses are then controlled from inside through generations of commentary on preferred texts, and through the maintenance of specific disciplines (say, medicine or psychology) with rules, definitions, techniques, and instruments that boundary out other ways of knowing and speaking and effectively close down alternatives (Foucault, 1972, 1981; Mills, 1997). In literary theory, the work of Mikhail Bakhtin suggests that competing discourses can be used for profound exploration. Bakhtin (1984) found in Dostoevsky's highly complex novels characters whose differing voices or discourses are independent consciousnesses: "In Dostoevsky's polyphonic novel we are dealing not with ordinary dialogic form, that is, with an unfolding of material within the framework of its own monologic understanding and against the firm background of a unified world of objects. No, here we are dealing with an ultimate dialogicality, that is, a dialogicality of the ultimate whole." This principle of polyphony, of polyvocal dialog, is a model for collaborative practice when discourses are separated and competing. Differing discourses can enter into dialog — not to bring about resolution but to explore options and generate possibilities (e.g., Gergen, 1999).

The suggestion, then, is that in teaching mindfulness as a professional, you must be aware of the discourse in which you are embedded. It may be a difficult — even painful — process to bring those boundaries and assumptions into consciousness; yet, there is an ultimate value. By understanding where you are located, in the moment, you become free to meet others where they are — to explore the polyphonic possibilities of the pedagogy of mindfulness in working with the infinite variety of potential participants, patients, or clients.

That is the suggestion of this chapter, in which a range of definitions of mindfulness from various discourses is presented. When you encounter a definition, you can fully appreciate it within its discourse. More important, you can appreciate the variety of definitions and the possibilities for connections, corrections, and reflections between them. It is not necessary to choose one or to synthesize one from many. Rather, you can allow your teaching to be enriched by all of them. You can allow them to come into dialog, to create a rich polyphony, and to help generate as many "working" definitions as there are teachable moments.

DOMINANT VOICES, SILENCE, AND MINDFULNESS

In any professional discipline, there are a variety of subgroups, each with their own discourse. When one subgroup focuses enough institutional, financial, and personal power in support of their discourse, their language and practices come to predominate. With a dominant voice, then, comes greater access to the popular media and to the ears of decision makers in the public sector. As a result, other subgroups' discourses are effectively, although perhaps unintentionally, silenced, as suggested by Foucault (1972, 1981). This is a process with ideological and political implications and impact, as is clearly evident in the shifts of discourse around meditative and contemplative practice in medicine and mental healthcare over the last 60 or so years. Early domination by psychoanalysis was followed by the humanistic psychotherapies, followed in turn by the current ascendance of the cognitive-behavioral approaches. Whoever the dominant voices have been, the process essentially has been the same, although ideologies and funding sources involved have differed.

As an example, consider the current situation. Researchers with ideologically acceptable credentials, working within politically approved institutions, have secured funding from highly controlled sources in government and the private sector to pursue research in a way that supports the accepted ideology, towards an end that is also ideologically acceptable. Thus, *empirical research* efforts in *clinical trial* format aim to support *evidence-based treatments* for codified *diagnoses* and *disorders* that will prove *cost effective* for the affected *individuals*. (The italics suggest the political and ideological content of this discourse, such as its scientific, quantitative, reductionist, free-market-based, individualist assumptions, as well as some of the content it excludes, for example, postmodern, qualitative, collaborative, collectivist approaches.).

In the MBIs, it is not uncommon for researchers also to be teachers, as is true for us. There is enormous tension between the almost inexorable drive of the discourse of research to exclude and dominate and the indispensable permissiveness of the discourse of teaching to include and empower. In attempting to work with this duality, this paradox, there are times in which the wise choice is to close down for the sake of research, and others, when heart and mind demand to open for the most healing teaching. The crucial question, as always, is "What is this moment asking of me?" The answer can only come through experience of the precision and kindness of mindfulness, or from making "mistakes" and learning from them.

Making Choices for "Working" Definitions

In selecting specific language and concepts to help generate "working" definitions of mindfulness, we have *knowingly* made three decisions that impose limits on this presentation. Our hope is that these decisions simultaneously make this presentation wieldy enough for developing a practical pedagogy and offer access to a rich polyphony of discourse. These decisions are pragmatic and admittedly idiosyncratic. They come from our own experiences and reflections as teachers and researchers. What matters for us is that this polyvocal presentation works for us in the thick of the action (or stillness!) in the group or dyad. Certainly, we also *unknowingly* have made decisions that impose their own limits. What is here is here for the moment; we know it will change through ongoing practice and encounters with others. We invite you into dialog, to edit, expand, and critique what you see — and what you don't see.

The first decision reflects our emphasis on the trouble with words and discourses. We have chosen to adopt a social constructionist perspective (e.g., Gergen, 1999), in which we accept that knowledge is not an "objective" reflection of what is "out there in the world" but rather is co-created within relationships. There is no "true" definition of mindfulness — they are all "working" definitions, shaped by the assumptions, aims, and strategies of those at work in the moment. This is the case inside the professions, say, as the MBIs attempt to define and operationalize mindfulness for research purposes. More important for us, this is the case within each group or dyad; teacher and participants will hold many different "working" definitions throughout their time together, moving from basic shared language to highly nuanced tacit understandings co-constructed in practice and dialog.

The second decision is to privilege secular language, while allowing the religious and spiritual dimensions of experience to have their essential influence. Given its centrality in the MBIs, the Buddhist discourse is presented here, yet professionals teaching mindfulness are encouraged to hold doctrinal concepts and structures lightly. Such lightness is perhaps cultivated by noticing the congruence of Buddhist thought with that of other spiritual traditions, so that the diversity of available concepts and terms suggests the ultimate utility of ordinary language. As the teacher and participants struggle to bring their experiences into ordinary language, the underlying topography of the spiritual can be revealed in a way that opens possibilities for learning and sharing for everyone involved. As noted in Chapter 2, the privileged religious object can be seen as *life* (Cupitt, 1999). And in its broadest form spirituality can be seen as "an individual's struggle to come to terms with his or her humanity" (Isanon, 2001).

The third decision is to promote the productive coexistence of the proven and the proposed. The MBIs are opening new territory inside and across professional disciplines and their discourses. Empirical evidence may not be strong; theories may be speculative. Yet, for teachers (and researchers) there is much that is exciting — and worth rubbing on the touchstone of direct experience to see if it is indeed gold, to paraphrase the Buddha. What we present here has been rubbed already, in our work with groups and dyads. Speculative or not, it has been helpful in our teaching. And, as we have said, we know that both our understanding of mindfulness and our approach to teaching will continue to grow and change.

Paradox

The Definition Dilemma: What's Helped the MBIs Expand May Result in Unintended Limits

There is an effort underway within the discourse of the MBIs to develop a single, scientific account of mindfulness for researchers and clinicians. The undertaking is difficult and complex, as many researchers admit (Allen et al., 2006; Baer, 2003; Bishop et al., 2004; Brody and Park, 2004; Brown and Ryan, 2004; Claxton, 2006; Grossman, 2008; Hayes and Feldman, 2004; Hayes and Shenk, 2004; Hayes and Wilson, 2003; Ivanovski and Malhi, 2007; Rothwell, 2006; Shapiro et al., 2006). The difficulty may arise from efforts to fit mindfulness into the Western biomedical paradigm as a "complementary/alternative" therapeutic modality. These attempts never work well, as the paradigm of the alternatives is broader than that of biomedicine. The specific reasons given for this difficulty include (1) the use of identical terms in significantly different outlooks and discourses, from Buddhist texts and their English translations in a variety of traditions, to humanistic psychotherapy, to scientific psychology, as well as differences in subjective descriptions by more, less, and differently practiced individuals (e.g., Dryden and Still, 2006; Grossman, 2008); (2) a basic confusion as to whether mindfulness is a practice, a process, an outcome, a transient state to be exploited, a way of life to be cultivated, or, indeed, even a single construct (e.g., Grossman, 2008; Hayes and Wilson, 2003); and (3) the group contexts and inclusion of disparate didactic and experiential components in MBIs, which provide many competing mechanisms of action (e.g., Bishop, 2002; Ivanovski and Malhi, 2007; Shapiro et al., 2006). Of course, from outside the effort towards definition, all of these issues or problems may also be seen as resources that enrich the language and perspectives of teachers and participants, broadening understanding of direct experience in the moment.

The tension inherent in definition-building is illustrated in the effort by Baer et al. (2006) to distil individual "facets" of mindfulness. Their program was to synthesize the hodgepodge of self-report instruments independently developed within the scientific discourse of MBI researchers. Through forms of analysis acceptable to scientific discourse, they isolated certain facets that were judged to be common and important. The five most salient facets — observing, describing, acting with awareness, nonjudging of inner experience, and nonreactivity to inner experience — were then proposed as a superior parsing of the facets of mindfulness. The terms of such a de facto definition, when installed in instruments and research methods, can guide and shape what researchers talk about when they talk about mindfulness.

Clearly, there is a powerful pragmatic drive towards this kind of definition within the MBI research community. Such work can help to generate a consensus on usable terms and concepts, and to further the empirical research enterprise. From outside the community, however, such an undertaking and the resulting definition can be seen as self-referential, reductionist, and dismissive of other communities of interest, their languages and perspectives, and their potential contributions to the ultimate clinical aim of reducing suffering. Left uncriticized, the research drive to define, operationalize, and measure mindfulness has the potential ultimately to limit and direct the language and pedagogical practice of professionals teaching mindfulness in the MBIs. This problem is parallel in the general problems inherent with trying to fit "alternative therapeutics," into the biomedical paradigm.

Defining Mindfulness in MBSR

The most commonly quoted definitions of mindfulness in the MBI literature come, not surprisingly, from Jon Kabat-Zinn:

- "...paying attention in a particular way: on purpose, in the present moment, and non-judgmentally" (1994, p. 4).
- "Mindfulness meditation is a consciousness discipline revolving around a particular way of paying attention in one's life. It can be most simply described as the intentional cultivation of nonjudgmental moment-to-moment awareness" (1996).

Three key elements of the definition — intentionality, present-centeredness, absence of judgment — are repeated and reinforced both in the ongoing scientific-research-oriented discussions of MBSR, and through MBSR teachers in hundreds of classes unfolding week by week around the world. These three key elements continue to shape the thinking, practice, and experience of an ever-changing and expanding MBI community.

It is telling that the first attempt at developing an operational definition of mindfulness took place within the greater community of the many mindfulness-based and mindfulness-informed interventions, in which other *ad hoc* definitions are also current. The result was a two-part definition that omitted the element of intention (Bishop et al., 2004). A "second generation" model uses the above-quoted Kabat-Zinn texts as a touchstone (Shapiro et al., 2006). This model, shown graphically in Fig. 3.1, posits three axioms: intention, attention, and attitude (IAA), which are simultaneously manifesting elements of the moment-to-moment practice of mindfulness, whether formal or informal. Each axiom captures a part of the direct experience of a participant. As to the axiom of intention, Shapiro, et al., note that a personal vision or motivation for initiating mindfulness practice is not explicit in the "secular" construct of MBSR in the same way that it is found in its religious corollaries. The vision of each participant, then, is "personal" and has been shown to shift along a continuum "from self-regulation, to self-exploration, and finally to

Model of Mindfulness

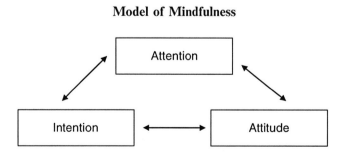

Fig. 3.1 The three axioms of intention, attention, and attitude (IAA) are not sequential, but rather are engaged simultaneously in the process of mindfulness (Shapiro et al., 2006).

self-liberation" (Shapiro et al., 2006). As to the axiom of attention, this captures the different capacities involved in attending to one's moment-to-moment experience. Shapiro et al. (2006) suggest that the essential capacities are sustained focus and flexibility of focus. These are cultivated explicitly in the MBIs through formal mindfulness practices that are introduced in a sequence that emphasizes the capacity to focus first and then opens to emphasize flexibility. As to the axiom of attitude, the nonjudgment that is called for is not an affect-free "bare awareness," but rather an accepting, open, and kind curiosity towards one's own experience (Shapiro et al., 2006) (Fig. 3.1).

In the descriptions of outcomes of mindfulness practice both inside and outside the discourse of the MBIs, a major emphasis is placed on a particular shift in the practitioner's relationship to self and experience — the awareness of an observing consciousness that is both *a part of* and *apart from* the experience. In MBSR classes, in the authors' experiences, such realization may be typically revealed in expressions by participants along the lines of, "I am not my thoughts," or "I am not this pain."

In many scientific accounts across the different investigating disciplines and the different discourses of meditation and mindfulness, this shift has been identified as a central mechanism. McCown (2004) reviewed early studies, pointing out that Deikman (1966) suggested a mechanism of "*de-automatization* of the psychological structures that organize, limit, select and interpret perceptual stimuli;" Linden (1973) and Pelletier (1974) noted the increased *field independence* of practiced meditators, evidenced by their ability to discern the hidden shapes in Embedded Figures Tests; and, in pioneering EEG studies, Kasamatsu and Hirai (1973) noted a *de-habituation* to stimuli in Zen Masters that they described as "constant refreshing of perception of the moment." Martin (1997), reviewing later concepts, notes Deikman's later *observing self* (1982); and Safran and Segal's (1990) contribution of such terms as *deautomization*, in which habitual modes of perception are suspended, and *decentering*, in which a capacity to view experience from "outside" is cultivated. Jon Kabat-Zinn (2005) uses the phrase "orthogonal rotation in consciousness" to describe this shift: "…a rotation in consciousness into another 'dimension' orthogonal to conventional reality," in which the conventional and new "dimensions" co-exist, and "everything old looks different because it is now being seen in a new light — an awareness that is no longer confined by the conventional dimensionality and mindset" (p. 350).

Flowing from their MBI-informed definition of mindfulness, Shapiro et al. (2006) propose a meta-mechanism that they call *reperceiving* and define as "a rotation in consciousness in which what was previously 'subject' becomes 'object.'" They further suggest that this meta-mechanism is basic to human development, and, therefore, that mindfulness practice simply strengthens and accelerates the growth of this capacity. The statements quoted above from participants in our MBSR classes illustrate this capacity to move from a position in which one is completely identified with one's experience to a position in which the experience becomes available for observation. It must be noted here that within MBSR pedagogical practice

(1) reperceiving does not create distance and disconnection from one's experience, but rather enables one to look, feel, and know more deeply; (2) importantly, the "observing self" is not reified, but rather is seen as a temporary platform for observation and questioning.

With one's experience thus available for reflection and inquiry, additional mechanisms may come into play. Shapiro et al. (2006) highlight four. One is *self-regulation and self-management*, where with reperceiving one can gain knowledge about experiences that may previously have been too challenging to explore in depth or over time, and one can identify and then choose to override habitual reactions and respond with more balance and greater skill. Second is *values clarification*, where reperceiving provides an opportunity to reflect on values that may have been adopted unquestioningly and to choose to adapt or adopt values more resonant with our current context. Third is *cognitive, emotional, and behavioral flexibility*, where the "objective" viewpoint inherent in reperceiving allows a clearer view of the thoughts, emotions, and (anticipated) actions of an emergent situation, from which may follow new, situation-specific responses. Fourth is *exposure*, where reperceiving's "objective," nonreactive character provides the space and time for intimate encounters with formerly disturbing emotions, thoughts, and body sensations, in which their capacity for disruption is reduced.

SO, WHERE DOES ONE POINT THE ATTENTION?

In MBSR teaching, a connotative distinction is made between awareness and attention. Awareness is the flow of "data" from the senses, which include the conceptualizing mind. Awareness is continuous and expansive — sight, sound, smell, taste, touch, naming, planning, emoting. Any given instant would

---

Attitude: Nonjudgment as a Pillow

The IAA definition is often the first one we give to participants. The challenging letter of course is the second "A" — the attitude of nonjudgment. It can feel cold; it can convict one, as in "Oh, I'm judging again! I need to stop that." One way we have found to emphasize the kindness and gentleness towards oneself and one's experience that we hope nonjudgment will help establish is to read a very short story — one of Arnold Lobel's *Mouse Tales* (1972):

The Wishing Well.
A mouse once found a wishing well. "Now all of my wishes can come true!" she cried.
She threw a penny into the well and made a wish. "OUCH!" said the wishing well.
The next day the mouse came back to the well. She threw a penny into the well and made a wish. "OUCH!" said the well.
The next day the mouse came back again. She threw a penny into the well. "I wish this well would not say ouch," she said. "OUCH!" said the well. "That hurts!"
"What shall I do?" cried the mouse. "My wishes will never come true this way!"
The mouse ran home. She took the pillow from her bed. "This may help," said the mouse, and she ran back to the well.
The mouse threw the pillow into the well. The she threw a penny into the well and made a wish.
"Ah. That feels much better!" said the well. "Good!" said the mouse. "Now I can start wishing."
After that the mouse made many wishes by the well. And every one of them came true.

And so, with teaching and dialog around this story, a group or dyad begins to co-create a unique understanding and experience of mindfulness practice.

be overwhelming. Choice is necessary. You can choose, for example, to feel the soles of your feet on the floor in this moment, leaving aside many other possibilities in current awareness. That is an act of attention.

In working with attention within awareness, it is good to have a map or grid, some way of sharing coordinates. Some teachers at the University of Massachusetts Medical School's Center for Mindfulness (UMASS CFM) created such a scheme, called the "triangle of awareness" — (1) body sensation, (2) thought, and (3) emotion. With this simple way of navigating, teachers can more easily guide practice, and participants can better locate and describe their direct experiences.

Mindfulness in Buddhism

As noted in chapter two, the ways that people have come to understand and practice Buddhism throughout Asia are amazingly varied. Across the many cultures, different features receive more or less emphasis: practice and "progress" in practice are approached and understood from different perspectives, various branches and schools have elaborated divergent beliefs and rituals, and reform movements have punctuated tradition with change. All of this complexity is compounded as Buddhism comes into the West, where our own cultural conditions — including religious and philosophical traditions, past and current scientific paradigms, and even forms of language — are re-shaping what we receive from the traditions we have chosen to welcome.

It is clear, then, that making a thumbnail sketch of mindfulness in Buddhism is a difficult undertaking, which will, however successful, be only very partial, very "thin." Please read what follows with the understanding that it is not sufficient background for thinking one understands the Buddhist discourse of mindfulness adequately for the purpose of teaching mindfulness in secular settings. That is a life-long exploration. This is only a beginning. In attempting to create a useful thumbnail for the very secular work of teaching mindfulness as a professional, we have leaned on the work of Stephen Batchelor, whose intellectual enterprise for many years has been an attempt to delineate an "agnostic" or "atheist" Buddhism for the West — something of the practical essence, shorn of the religious, philosophical, and cultural trappings of the Asian cultures from which it comes to us, and hewing as closely to the earliest understandings of the historical Buddha's teachings found in the original sources of the Pali canon.

The life of the Buddha is an ancient story, alive in its mythic and psychic resonances, and enchanting in its historical reality. A prince, Siddhattha Gotama, is raised in royal retreat from the pains of the world. His father ensures that he cannot witness suffering or death. Yet the prince intuits that there is more to the life of the world than satisfaction and sensual pleasure.

At last, approaching the age of 30, he comes face to face with reality, in the forms of an old person, a diseased person, and a corpse. He understands that he too must come to this. He sees as well a religious ascetic. And knows what he must do.

On a day of joy, the birth of his son, he leaves the palace to follow the ascetic disciplines in hope of transcendence.

He spends the next six years wandering. He studies every doctrine and system of thought with the wisest of teachers. He practices dramatic austerities that leave his body emaciated and broken. But he comes at last no nearer to the truth of life that he was seeking. It's up to him, alone.

He cleans himself up, eats a little, and sits down under a fig tree to work it out for himself. He does: he wakes up; the light goes on. And then he faces a challenge. How can he explain this to others? In fact, he thinks he may not bother — they'll never understand. After 50 days of sifting through what he realized, he decides that teaching is worth the risk. He begins by finding his most recent ascetic companions and bringing his experience into language for them. He speaks of a "middle path" that led to his awakening, running between his former ways of royal indulgence and extreme renunciation. And he speaks of what he awoke to as four truths (de Bary, 1969; Gethin, 1998).

FREE SOURCES FOR RESOURCES: ACCESS TO INSIGHT

The important original texts for this section are available free on the Internet at accesstonsight.org. Often a number of translations are offered. Reading the *suttas* (the Pali term) or *sutras* (the Sanskrit term) can add to the appreciation of the discourse of Buddhism in the West.

The *Dhammacakkappavatthana Sutta* is the Buddha's first "sermon," setting out the middle way and four ennobling truths. Find it at *http://www.accesstoinsight.org/ tipitaka/sn/sn56/sn56.011.than.html*

The *Maha-satipatthana Sutta* delineates and describes the four foundations of mindfulness. Find it at *http://www.accesstoinsight.org/tipitaka/dn/dn.22.0.than.html*

The *Anapanasati Sutta* provides detailed instructions in the practice of mindfulness specifically working with the breath. Find it at *http://www.accesstoinsight.org/ tipitaka/mn/mn.118.than.html*

The *Brahmavihara Sutta* describes the reasons for and benefits of practicing the four sublime states. Find it at *http://www.accesstoinsight.org/tipitaka/an/an10/ an10.208.than.html*

The Four Ennobling Truths

After more than 2,500 years, it may be difficult to hear with any immediacy the Buddha's struggle to bring his experience into words. Those first pronouncements have become tenets of belief for hundreds of millions of followers today. They are hallowed — or is it *hollowed*? — by time. A dip into the history of our Western discourse, into Dwight Goddard's *A Buddhist Bible* (1938), which translates and formulates the truths in a way that sounds definitive and dogmatic: (1) the Noble Truth of Suffering, (2) the Noble Truth of the Origin of Suffering, (3) the Noble Truth of the Extinction of Suffering, and (4) the Noble Truth of the Path that leads to the Extinction of Suffering.

Stephen Batchelor (1997) helps resuscitate these tenets by making them the answers to a different question: not "What do you believe?" but the "What did you do, and how did you do it?" of the Buddha's first audience. Framed in this way, the Buddha's first teaching is revealed as essentially relational and experiential. It is possible to imagine him actually saying, "Don't take my word for it, check it out for yourself!" Therefore, Batchelor (1997) prefers the term *ennobling* truths. There is activity, here. By testing the Buddha's process, one can realize the outcome oneself, and be awakened, raised up, *ennobled*.

The four truths, then, are a flowchart, a map of territory to be investigated. Thus, the process is one of interdependent steps (Batchelor, 1997, 2004). As suggested in Fig. 3.2, the first two steps state the problem, a diagnosis, while the second two provide the resolution, a prescription. By fully understanding suffering that stems from the mind (1), it becomes clear that it comes from craving. Then this understanding suggests "letting go" of craving (2). Letting go of craving results in a (momentary!) cessation of suffering, or liberation, (3), leading to a desire to cultivate further the path to liberation (4). The path to be cultivated is Buddha's middle way. It is an eightfold group of moral and practical disciplines — right view, right resolve, right speech, right conduct, right livelihood, right effort, right mindfulness, and right concentration. One way in which the ennobling truths can be investigated and the path cultivated is through meditation — the development of mindfulness and concentration.

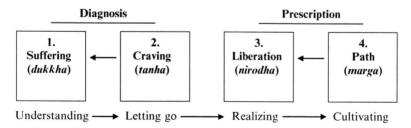

The four ennobling truths as a process (Batchelor, 1997, 2004)

Diagnosis   **Prescription**

| 1. Suffering (*dukkha*) | 2. Craving (*tanha*) | 3. Liberation (*nirodha*) | 4. Path (*marga*) |

Understanding ⟶ Letting go ⟶ Realizing ⟶ Cultivating

Fig. 3.2 Note that the arrows point to cause and effect relationships: (*top, right to left arrows*) craving causes suffering, the path leads to liberation, and (*bottom, left to right arrows*) understanding suffering leads to letting go of craving, which leads to realizing cessation, or liberation, which leads one to cultivate the path. This is not a linear model. These are not stages of progress, but rather an integrated undertaking. The charge to cultivate the path lands one right back at the drive to understand suffering. One does not leave any of the truths behind, as they constantly inform each other.

THE THREE MARKS OF EXISTENCE

These marks are hard to see because we'd rather do just about anything than look for them. If we can bring ourselves to "turn towards" our experience, this is what we might report (more likely in English than in Pali).

1. *Anicca* (impermanence): Everything changes; nothing is *always* there for me. This is true for the things I want to hold onto and the things that I wish away.
2. *Dukkha* (unsatisfactoriness): Whether I want it or don't want it, my relationship with anything — even the most exquisite experience — is ultimately unsatistfying.
3. *Anatta* (non-self): Things are not what I think they are. There's nothing essential, or enduring that makes a chair a chair, or even that makes me, me. There's nothing you can put your finger on; there's just the way it is right now.

(Analayo, 2003, Batchelor, 2004; de Bary, 1969; Goddard, 1938; Wellwood, 2000)

Mindfulness and its Four Foundations

Mindfulness is the translation of the Pali term *sati*, which appears in the eightfold path — *samma-sati*, right mindfulness. It is the practice, the instrument, so to speak, for the process of investigation suggested in the four ennobling truths. It is to be cultivated formally in the practice of meditation and informally at all times. It is the key to awakening. Engagement with Buddhist terms and their possible definitions is part of the current discourse of the MBIs, as shown in the box below titled "Working on a definition."

As an overview of the attitude and practice of mindfulness, the following description of "bare attention," a term used by Nyanaponika Thera (1965) is technical and concise:

> Bare Attention is the clear and single-minded awareness of what actually happens *to* us and *in* us, at the successive moments of perception…. [A]ttention or mindfulness is kept to a bare registering of the facts observed, without reacting to them by deed, speech or by mental comment which may be one of self-reference (like, dislike, etc), judgement or reflection.

Working on a Definition (Cullen, 2008)
Mindfulness has become an increasingly popular term in the west due to the influence of several prominent meditation teachers and authors, including Thich Nhat Hanh, Jon Kabat-Zinn, and Jack Kornfield. Thich Nhat Hanh (1975), world-renowned Vietnamese Zen master, poet and peace activist, defines mindfulness as "the miracle which can call back in a flash our dispersed mind and restore it to wholeness so that we can live each minute of life" (p.14). Jon Kabat-Zinn (2005), author and founder of Mindfulness-Based Stress Reduction, widely taught in secular settings including health care, education and business worldwide, writes, "Mindfulness can be thought of as moment-to-moment, non-judgmental awareness, cultivated by paying attention in a specific way, that is, in the present moment, as non-reactively, and as openheartedly as possible" (p. 108). Jack Kornfield (2005), co-founder of two primary mindfulness meditation centers in the U.S. has described mindfulness as "an innate human capacity to deliberately pay full attention to where we are, to our actual experience, and to learn from it." Nyanaponika Thera (1965), a Buddhist monk, teacher, and scholar in the mid-twentieth century, wrote a book in which he named mindfulness as the heart of Buddhist meditation. All these definitions refer to a quality of mind or way of being which is not only aware in the present, but wholesome insofar as it is "open-hearted", "restores wholeness," and permits learning.

So here is Kabat-Zinn'st definition of paying attention on purpose, in the present, without judging. Then the tradition goes on to prescribe what to pay attention to and how, elaborating four foundations of mindfulness (here and below, Analayo, 2008; Gethin, 1998; Nyanaponika, 1965; Watson, 1998).

The first foundation is *mindfulness of body*, which typically begins with bare attention to the sensations of the breath, bringing the mind and body together and calming them. Then, other body sensations may be observed, in all the potential postures and movements of formal practice and daily living.

The second foundation is *mindfulness of feelings*, in which bare attention is brought to the feeling-tone of the experience of each moment. "Feelings," as the term is used here, are not emotions. Rather, they are an immediate knowing of experience as pleasant, unpleasant, or neutral before reactions such as emotions or attitudes come into play. Feelings are simply observed as they arise, linger, and pass away.

The third foundation is *mindfulness of mind*, which directs bare attention to the quality of the activity of the mind, registering awareness of states or dispositions, such as distraction and concentration, or one of the three roots of suffering — desire, hatred, or delusion. Again, these can be observed as they arise, linger, and pass away.

The fourth foundation is *mindfulness of mind-objects*, in which bare attention is directed towards all that the mind encounters within and without. Here a wonderful characteristic of Buddhism, the making of lists, shapes recommended practice, as the traditional instructions are to observe the arising and passing of the five hindrances (sense-desire, anger,

Historically, the Pali word sati has been translated as mindfulness but, according to Alan Wallace (2006), the root meaning of *sati* is simply that of recollection, of memory. In the Theravadan Abhidhamma [Buddhist psychology], *sati* is precisely defined as one of nineteen "beautiful" mental factors whose function is the "absence of confusion or non-forgetfulness" (Bikkhu Bodhi, 1993, p.86). In the context of the Nikaya [Buddha's Discourse], sati is referred to as a "kind of attentiveness that . . . is good, skillful or right" (Nyanaponika Thera, 1965, p.9) and can become a shorthand for *satipatthana* which is usually translated as the establishment of sati but also refers to the complete methodology in which this establishment is accomplished (Nyanaponika Thera, 1965, p.9). Bikkhu Bodhi, Buddhist monk, scholar and student of Nyanaponika Thera, writes, "we have no word in English that precisely captures what *sati* refers to when it is used in relation to meditation practice" (Nyanaponika Thera, 1965, p.6). Here, then, are at least three contexts in which sati is used a little differently, though the English translation remains fixed as "mindfulness."

Many contemporary Buddhist teachers use the term mindfulness in a more comprehensive way than simply "remembering" or "lacking confusion." According to John Dunne, a Buddhist scholar at Emory University, the components of mindfulness as it is more broadly construed might include not only *sati*, but also *sampajanna* (clear comprehension) and *appamada*, (heedfulness). Clear comprehension includes both the ability to perceive phenomena unclouded by distorting mental states (such as moods and emotions) and the meta-cognitive capacity to monitor the quality of attention. Heedfulness in this context can be understood as bringing to bear, during meditation, what has been learned in the past about which thoughts, choices, and actions lead to happiness and which lead to suffering.

Though the contexts and interpretations of these terms may vary, scholars and meditation teachers would probably agree on the factors of *sati*, *sampajanna*, and *appamada* as foundational to the development of mind. Moreover, as both Buddhist and secular mindfulness programs proliferate in the West, this broader use of mindfulness sloth and torpor, agitation and worry, and doubt), the five aggregates (material form, feeling, perception, mental formations, and consciousness), the six subjective/objective sense factors (eye/form, ear/sound, nose/smell, tongue/taste, body/touch, and mind/concepts), the seven factors of enlightenment (mindfulness, investigation of reality, energy, enthusiasm, tranquility, concentration, and equanimity), and, at last, the four ennobling truths.

Perhaps it helps here to see the connection or reflection of the four foundations of mindfulness in the "triangle of awareness" — body sensation, thought, and emotion — used in the pedagogical discourse of the MBIs.

has become a culturally meaningful and accessible "umbrella" term for the vast majority of practitioners unversed in the intricacies of translating Sanskrit or Pali.

Bikkhu Bodhi, ed. (1993). *A comprehensive manual of abhidhamma: The abhidhammattha sangaha.* Kandy, Sri Lanka: Buddhist Publication Society.

Hanh, T.N. (1975). *The Miracle of Mindfulness. Boston:* Beacon Press.

Inquiring Mind. (2006). "Mindfulness: The heart of Buddhist meditation? A conversation with Jan Chozen Bays, Joseph Goldstein, Jon Kabat-Zinn, and Alan Wallace," *Inquiring Mind,* 22(2): 5.

Kabat-Zinn, J. (2005). *Coming to Our Senses.* London: Piaticus Books.

Kornfield, J. (2005). "Finding my religion," *San Francisco Chronicle,* November 28.

Nyanaponika Thera. (1965). *The Heart of Buddhist Meditation.* York Beach, Maine: Weiser Books.

TWO FORMS OF MEDITATION

There are two main forms of meditation. Concentrative meditation, *samatha* in Pali, focuses the attention on an object such as the breath or sound to the exclusion of other mental activity. This can lead to a calmness and tranquility of mind, which is measured by levels of absorption. For example, Transcendental Meditation is a concentrative form. In Buddhist practice, *samatha* is often seen as training that will allow more effective use of the other form of meditation, *vipassana*. *Vipassana* practice is opening to the fullness of direct experience. This offers the opportunity for seeing into the way one's world and self are constructed and interrelated, that is, for insight. *Vipassana*, or the cultivation of mindfulness, is the characteristic form of meditation in Buddhism — central to all its meditative streams.

The Four Sublime States

In the description of the seventh stage of the eightfold path, right mindfulness, the Buddha exhorts his followers to cultivate the four *Brahmaviharas,* variously translated as the cardinal virtues, sublime states, divine abodes, the immeasurables or illimitables — each translation sheds a bit of light on the whole meaning (de Bary, 1969; Narada, 1980). They are conceived as parallel to a set of negative states, which could just as easily arise. Thus, cultivating the sublime state of *metta,* often translated as loving-kindness, makes it more difficult for *dosa,* anger, to grow; *karuna,* or compassion, counterbalances *himsa,* cruelty; *mudita,* or sympathetic joy, opposes *issa,* jealousy; and *upekkha,* or equanimity, undermines the anxiety of attachment and aversion.

The practices for cultivating these sublime states can be seen as complementary to the practice of mindfulness. Traditionally, they can be used to cultivate concentration. Rather than simply registering whatever arises with "bare attention," the meditator inclines the mind towards the chosen state.

Loving-kindness can be thought of as a softness of heart or an unconditional friendliness. It is the most important of the four and can be seen as fundamental to the other three (Nyanaponika, 1965). When it is practiced, it is often directed first to oneself, then extended outward to those one loves, then to those one is neutral to, then to those where the relationship is difficult, and finally towards all beings without limit. The practice is to incline one's heart towards loving-kindness, often using phrases or verses that offer wishes of peace and happiness, and freedom from suffering, disease, worry, and anger.

Compassion is the wish to take away the suffering of others, whatever that suffering might be. The practice is to extend compassion without limit to all who suffer — the poor, the sick, the helpless, and the lonely, as well as the ignorant, the vicious, the impure, and the undisciplined (de Bary, 1969).

Sympathetic joy is rejoicing in another's good fortune. Just as compassion is a positive way of addressing the suffering of the world, this is a positive way of addressing those who are thriving. Simple enough with loved ones, but the practice is, again, to extend this outward to others without limit.

Equanimity is the most difficult of all, as it means to embrace whatever arises, pleasant or unpleasant, good or bad. It is easily misinterpreted as a kind of passivity. There is a story of the Buddha that suggests its greater dimensions and utility. The Buddha and his followers are out seeking alms. A man, a Brahmin, in fact, invites him to his home and then begins berating the Buddha with every epithet in his seemingly endless repertoire. The Buddha is not moved. As the man finishes, Buddha asks, "What do you usually do when you invite guests to your home?" The man replies, "Why, we prepare a feast for them." Buddha inquires what he would do if the guests refused to eat. The man replies, "Eat it ourselves, of course." The Buddha tells him, "Well, you have invited me to your home and offered me a feast of insults. I will not eat it; it is yours" (retold from Narada, 1980).

The Western Discourse of Mindlessness — Mindfulness

There's a stream of discourse in Western psychology that came to a concept of mindfulness through a different route than the engagement with Asian spiritual thought and practice. In fact, it started not from mindfulness, but from its opposite, mindlessness. Ellen Langer (1989) was drawn into study of this duality through experiments that suggested the ultimate costs of mindlessness. Seniors in a nursing home were either offered a choice of houseplants for which they had to care and were expected to make other decisions about their daily lives as well, or they simply were given a plant that staff cared for and were not expected to make the decisions. After 18 months, the group with responsibilities and decision-making expectations were not only in better physical, mental, and emotional shape than the others, but, fewer than half as many had died compared to the other group. From many perspectives, the suggestion is that mindfulness enhances life, mindlessness reduces it.

What is most "Western" about Langer's conception is its dominant orientation towards the cognitive, the active, and the external. One overcomes the tendency to be mindless by actively changing one's ways of thinking, particularly about the information coming from the outside world — one's perceptions.

Langer sees the essence of mindlessness as "premature cognitive commitment" (1989); that is, thinking and acting from a position in which we *already* know. She points to three basic ways in which this is problematic. First, as you grow, mature, and become "educated," you create or learn categories with which to order the world, and then they begin to order you. Auden (1970) has great fun with this in his commonplace book, capturing the suggestion that if you were served coffee in a wine glass, you would be slightly disturbed, and if your place at the table for a steak dinner was set with scissors instead of a knife, you would be horrified. Second, while new information is essential, it is easy to miss the the small changes because you already know what to expect. (Did you catch the repeated *the* in that last sentence?) Third, your view of the world is from a particular perspective, yours, which it seems right and logical to accept as the only one. Coming to realize that there are others can be a shock. Say, you agree to meet a colleague for breakfast at 7:00 am. You rise at 5:30 to a series of mini-catastrophes — the cat threw up, your underwear is still in the dryer, the dog runs out of the yard, and you have to stop for gas and directions on the way.

MINDLESSNESS, NOVELTY, AND THE ROOTS OF WESTERN PSYCHOLOGY

In the first half of the nineteenth century, many of the academic and clinical disciplines and discourses we know today were just coalescing. In Germany, the interests of E. H. Weber, a physiologist, and Gustav Fechner, a physicist, were sympathetic. Weber's work on the perceptual systems helped Fechner to figure out how to measure sensations. Fechner defined a unit of measurement, the *just noticeable difference (JND)*, which was tied to the psychological experience of sensation to a measurable stimulus. Thus, threshold values could be established for perception, such as, charmingly "the tick of a wristwatch at 6 m in a quiet room" for hearing, or "an insect falling on your cheek from a height of one centimeter" for touch (in Schwartz, 1986, p. 50). The next JND would begin to construct a scale. Such measures allowed for "psychophysical" experimentation — and Fechner's status as a founder of quantitative psychology. From his experiments, Fechner derived his *psychophysical law*, that magnitude of sensation is proportional to the logarithm of the threshold value. More simply, as a stimulus increases, equal increments appear to be smaller and smaller — as they are perceived against the growing basis of comparison. It's the basis for the decibel scale. A clear and homely illustration is a three-way light bulb (Dossey, 2004); from darkness to 50 watts of light is a dramatic, easily perceptible change; the next click, from 50 to 100 watts is an equal increment, but is much less dramatic; the third click to 150 watts is again an equal increment, but it might easily pass unnoticed, so embedded are we in the 100 watts of background. It's the same with the crème brulee you're anticipating at your favorite restaurant. The first spoonful is rapture of the highest order, the second is awesome, and the third goes down unattended as you return to your table talk. You are embedded in crème brulee.

Fechner's law may not have held up well to increasingly sophisticated critiques and methodologies, yet it has a ring of truth. And it offers metaphorical possibilities for the culture in which we are all embedded. As Langer notes, the experience of *novelty* changes us, brings us out of our embeddedness and into the present moment. Westerners seem to

You stride (short of breath) heroically into the restaurant at 7:10 to be greeted with, "I thought we said seven?"

To overcome mindlessness, Langer (1989) prescribes active modes of retooling one's thinking and even physical approaches to the world, for learning, problem solving, and creativity. To overcome the tendency towards premature cognitive commitments, the active use of strategies to create or sustain five psychological states is encouraged. The cultivation of mindfulness can be seen to comprise "(1) openness to novelty; (2) alertness to distinction; (3) sensitivity to different contexts; (4) implicit, if not explicit, awareness of multiple perspectives; and (5) orientation in the present" (1997, p. 23). These states, then, constantly inform one another, becoming one another, and engaging the whole person. An example may help: Movingly, Langer (1989) suggests that strong emotions toward someone may be tied to globaliz-

depend on new and powerful experiences coming from *outside us,* to *bring* us to mindfulness — to force us to experience our world. Our relationship to the new is complex, however. Consider, for example, the history of Western art from the Renaissance through Modernism, in which each successive development brought a new and not always comfortable way of seeing the world, which came to be seen and acted on as a narrative of emergence — each succeeding movement brings novelty, a new perspective, a change of context, and a distinct new category (e.g., Danto, 1993). The same drive for and resistance to novelty can be seen in all the histories of all the compositional and performing arts in the modern West. In the same vein, the advertising industry relies on novelty, judging successful advertising as that which lifts a message out of sameness. This is an explanation of both the increasing use of special effects and the increasing vulgarity of the media.

It seems entirely sensible that those of us teaching mindfulness as professionals would consider the Western perspective as well as the Asian in our pedagogy. If we do it well, we can bring participants into the present moment from *outside* with novelty and from *inside* with the novelty of beginner's mind.

ing categories. If I feel enmity towards a coworker, I see him as all one thing — bad. Putting forth the effort to view and describe him in detail, however, may reveal characteristics that strike me as new thoughts. Now I must make distinctions about what my coworker is like, seeing that some of his characteristics may actually be positive in different contexts. Such an insight can suggest that he may be different with others, and others might have a different perspective on him. My feeling may soften, and in my next encounter, I will be present to him in the moment — and even more open to novelty. Langer's Western concept of mindfulness is aligned with our active culture, is psychologically available, and can move one further on a path of transformation.

This concept of mindfulness offers important insights for the teaching of any subject matter, and may be especially applicable to pedagogy within the MBIs. Langer (1997) notes that ordinary culturally sanctioned approaches to learning emphasize top-down or bottom-up learning of skills, with practice targeting the "overlearning" of the skill so that it becomes conditioned — a mind*less,* context-independent skill. She opposes this with a way of teaching that is "based on an appreciation of both the conditional, or context-dependent, nature of the world and the value of uncertainty" (p. 15). When we teach conditionally, with a continual awareness of and reference to what is required in each moment, participants remain engaged, and make creative use of the material for their personal contexts, moment by moment, day after day. It is stunning how deeply ingrained this is in the pedagogy of the MBIs, as will become quite clear in the character of the skills of the teacher described in Chapter 5.

A (Tentative) Discourse of Intersubjectivity and Mindfulness

This definition or model of mindfulness is our own, and has been developed with the challenges of teaching in the foreground. Our central goal is to create a "clinically" useful scheme that can be remembered easily and accessed quickly to help guide decision making in the emergent moment in a group or dyad.

Despite the insights of Buddhist thought, postmodern philosophy, and the study of infant attachment and human development, which have resulted in serious questioning if not rejection of the idea of isolated, individual minds (Gergen and Hosking, 2006; Tronick, 2007), the vast majority of the studies of mindfulness have been limited by scientific discourses that privilege the experience of the individual. As a result, in many areas we must extrapolate from data developed with subjects studied in supposed isolation and considered to be practicing an objectively defined mindfulness meditation, rather than subjects considered in relationship, practicing a mindfulness meditation that was co-created within a relationship.

What we present here is both provisional and pragmatic. It views the experience of mindfulness in the classroom and therapy room from our first-person perspectives of what we've seen help participants to "get it"; from third-person perspectives in discourses of empirical research in the MBIs, of emerging understandings in social neurobiology, and of ongoing research in infant — adult interaction and attachment; and from systems theory, philosophy, and anthropology.

Two Intriguing Starting Points

The possibilities of an intersubjective discourse of mindfulness are manifest on both the experiential and empirical levels. It can be felt as important, and it has been (tentatively) quantified, too.

In the realm of experience, here's a story from our teaching that may resonate with you. *Before ringing the bell to end the final meditation session of a daylong retreat, I open my eyes and gaze around the circle of 60 other participants. Aware of the stillness of the postures, hard fought or simply surrendered. Aware of a softness in the faces holding everything from subtle amusement to deepening grief. Aware of an incessant silence interweaving with the HVAC hum, the voices in the lobby, and the traffic in the street. Aware of a peace descending within my being. And simultaneously aware of a desire arising to hold on to this moment, to keep it unbroken, to dwell in it forever. I ring the bell.*

I ring the bell, and the other participants come to their own awarenesses of the group environment. Perhaps peace descends on us all as the bell sound fades. Certainly, we sit together in a quiet all seem loath to disturb. Curious, finally, I ask, "What are you noticing? What is the energy like in the room right now?"

Tentative answers come back. "I'm noticing I don't want this to end." Quiet. "The energy is full...good...balanced." Quiet again. "I'm feeling awake, but there's no pressure, no anxiety about what's next." Nodding and murmurs of assent. "My

*grandmother always said that when a group gets quiet an angel is passing over."
Rustles of agreement and deeper breathing in and out.*

*I float an image. "I'm feeling a 'companionable silence.'" Met with noddings and
a few head tiltings. "Like when you're on a long drive with someone you know really
well, and there's just no need to talk." More nodding. "But there are sixty of us here.
So, maybe we're on a companionable tour bus ride..." Slowly, gently, gear-by-gear,
as participants begin to speak, we move deeper into shared territory.*

From an empirical perspective, it took almost 30 years to happen, but the first
significant study of group effects in MBSR was completed (Imel, Baldwin, Bonus,
and MacCoon, 2008). Working with data from nearly 60 groups, accounting for
more than 600 individual subjects, researchers used multilevel statistical models to
find how much group participants differed in symptom change from pre- to post
intervention, adjusted for preintervention severity.

The results are aligned with what a teacher would predict from the felt experience
of group mindfulness. The group effect (whatever it is!) accounted for 7% of the
variability in psychological symptom outcomes. To put that 7% in perspective, in
individual psychotherapy, the therapeutic alliance, long considered the most important predictor of outcomes, accounts for about 5% of variability (Horvath and Bedi,
2002). In interpreting the findings, Imel and colleagues (2008) suggest:

"(a) that something about the group impacts the ability of an individual to learn
and practice specific mindfulness techniques, (b) that something about [the] group
influences outcome through 'non-mindfulness' pathways (e.g., expectation of change,
provision of support, group cohesion), or (c) a combination of these" (p. 741), with
the last the most probable.

Back to experience: There is indeed *something about the group*. Regularly in our
classes, participants will make statements such as, "I have trouble doing the practice
at home but can do it in class," or "I don't know why, but practice is much more
profound in some way when I'm in the group." Let's put some things together.

An intrasubjective neurobiology of mindfulness practice: Let's start with a
microscopic view of a single brain cell. Researchers working with monkeys
found that the same motor neuron that fired when the monkey grasped or tore an
object *also* fired when the monkey watched a researcher do the same things

GROUP ACCEPTANCE AND COHESION

The contribution of shared mindfulness practice to the group experience could be
cast in the traditional group therapy terms of *acceptance* or *cohesiveness* (Block
and Crouch, 1985; Yalom, 1985), or, as Yalom (1985) suggests, it could be cast in
Rogers's individual psychotherapy term as a collective form of *unconditional positive regard*. Yalom (1985) notes that acceptance by the group actually may be more
powerful for its members than acceptance by the therapist. In fact, a review of
empirical evidence of the relationship of group cohesiveness to patient improvement (Burlingame et al., 2002) states that cohesion is a powerful predictor of outcome, and that the *group itself*, rather than any individual member or the leader, is
most important in creating and maintaining cohesion.

(Gallese et al., 1996). Dubbed *mirror neurons*, the existence of such cells was posited in humans and their function was extrapolated to a simulation theory of mind reading — in which these mirror neurons are part of a system that helps us inwardly represent, feel, and track the actions and even intentions of another (Gallese and Goldman, 1998). These mechanisms may have evolved to optimize such crucial group behaviors as hunting, gathering, and collective protection from predators or aggression from other groups (Cozolino, 2006). As Siegel (2007, p. 166) puts it, "This is big news: Mirror neurons demonstrate the profoundly social nature of our brains."

Humans are built from the ground up to attune to and resonate with one another. The common term is *empathy*. Reflect for just a moment on what happens in your body if you see a friend (or even a stranger!) catch their finger in a door or a drawer. You've just touched a live wire in what Daniel Siegel (2007) named the "resonance circuit." In this circuit, described by Carr, Iacoboni, Dubeau, Maziotta, and Lenzi (2003), the mirror neuron system takes in and processes the movement of, say, finger-in-drawer, which is sent to the superior temporal cortex where the sensory consequences are predicted (sharp pain!). Then, this information is communicated through the insula to the limbic regions for processing of the emotional content (surprise, anger). This is fed back through the insula to the prefrontal cortex where it is interpreted and, finally, attributed to your friend. The circuit is complete. Your somatic and emotional states are now attuned to your friend: You tense your hand, cringe, and maybe even say "Ouch." The empathy you feel is based on perceiving your friend's experience — with/in your own body. When you say, "I feel for you," you really mean it. This example uses obvious and powerful images and sensations that are easy to conjure in the imagination, so that you can "get" the feelings — and the concept — with the very "thin" layer of information available through reading. More important for our purposes is the subtlety with which this works when you're actually in the presence of someone else, and "thick" layers of information from facial expression, posture, vocal tone, prosody, gesture, and other nonverbal communication are available. Someone smiles, and your mirror neurons fire for that facial expression too. Through the resonance circuit you "try on" their face — implicitly or explicitly imitating it — so that you share the other's embodied emotional experience of the moment.

Siegel (2007) proposes a possible connection of the social brain and the resonance circuit with the intra-subjective process of mindfulness meditation. It starts with intention. The resonance system lets you predict, even map, the intended actions of others. It feeds the information that lets fencers parry and riposte, and dancers anticipate and respond to each other in flowing movements. The idea, then, is that the resonance system also can be reflexive, can allow you to predict not only others' but your own intentional states — however concrete or abstract — and attune to those states in the present moment.

Let's start with the concrete, a meditation on awareness of the breath. You notice the in-breath. Your resonance circuitry predicts that an out breath is coming. It happens! And happens again. As you coincide repeatedly with your own intention, breath by breath you begin to resonate with yourself. This is a primal experience, like infant and caregiver attuning in ways that help create secure attachment, as we'll explore further in the next section. And this same pattern is true for more abstract intentions, such as the one in a meditation practice like choiceless awareness, notes Siegel (2007). In this case, the intention is to be open to whatever comes. While we cannot map the "whatever comes" with the resonance system, we can, however, easily map the intention to be open. When our experience coincides with the map of being open, intrasubjective resonance begins.

So, this capacity we're describing through which we resonate with ourselves and others suggests a link from the individual meditator to the group, from the experience of one passenger to that of a busload. Adding just two more layers of ideas will help to build a model of group mindfulness that mindfulness teachers may find useful in the moment in the classroom. The first new layer of ideas involves mostly conscious, explicit regulation of our internal experience, while the second new layer involves mostly unconscious, implicit self-regulation. Both reflect the evolutionary, phylogenetic principle that newer, more complex structures of the nervous system can control older, less complex ones.

First, in the description of the intrasubjective resonance circuit above, the prefrontal cortex (PFC), a newer and complex structure, is involved in interpreting and attributing feelings. Its inclusion in the circuit may be of great significance (Siegel, 2007, 2009). Mindfulness practice seems to harness the capacity of the PFC — particularly the medial and ventrolateral areas — to regulate the reactivity of the limbic system, particularly the amygdala, an older, less complex structure. For example, recent studies (Creswell, Baldwin, Way, Eisenberger, & Lieberman, 2007; Lieberman, Eisenberger, Crockett, Tom, Pfiefer, & Way, 2007) suggest that the mindfulness task of labeling emotion activates these areas of the PFC in a way that inhibits activity in the right amygdala, helping reduce negative affect and reactivity. Such a "dampening down" of reactivity has long been remarked in research on meditation (e.g., Davidson, R., Schwartz, G., and Rothman, L., 1976; Schwartz, G., 1975; see McCown, 2004, for a review).

Thus, mindfulness practice offers a way of being in which limbic reactivity is reduced, which expands the possibility of observing, approaching, and even exploring in detail difficult emotional experiences, and being receptive to what is happening in the moment with self and others. Further, this is not just a state of mindfulness practitioners during practice. It seems that this can become a trait, a capacity in our everyday walking through the world. Mindfulness practice changes the brain, as studies are showing. For instance, the brains of long-term mindfuness practitioners, compared to controls, were found to have increased thickness in cortical areas responsible for sensory, cognitive, and emotional processing (Lazar, Kerr, Wasserman, Gray, Greve, Treadway, et al., 2005). Mindfulness training, even of short duration such as the 8-week MBSR curriculum, has been shown to reduce both state and trait levels of anxiety and negative affect, and to increase positive affect (Davidson, Kabat-Zinn, Schumacher, Rosenkranz, Muller, Santorelli, et al., 2003). Recently, MBSR has been associated with changes of brain structures of particular interest: Reduced levels of perceived stress in MBSR participants correlated positively with reduced gray matter in the right amygdala, (Hölzel, Carmody, Evans, Hoge, Dusek,

Morgan, et al., 2009), the area in which negative affect and reactivity are inhibited through mindful awareness and labeling, according to the Creswell et al., and Lieberman et al., studies cited above.

The next layer of information involves a subconscious system for detecting and reacting to threat or safety, described by Stephen Porges (1995, 2004). Porges's "polyvagal theory" of regulation of the autonomic nervous system (ANS) has significant explanatory power for understanding the mindfulness group. The theory is grounded in the evolution of the ANS in vertebrates, in which three phylogenetic stages are expressed in mammals as three subsystems. These three subsystems are linked to three behavioral strategies that help us adapt to the full range of potential environmental situations, from catastrophic and life-threatening, to dangerous or challenging, to, at last, safe and caring. (For the following description, see Porges, 1995, 2001, 2003, 2004, 2007, 2009.) First is immobilization or feigned death — "freezing" — a reptilian strategy associated with the subsystem of a primitive, unmylenated vagus nerve that reacts to threat by significantly slowing the metabolism. Second is mobilization — "fight or flight" — a strategy associated with the sympathetic nervous system and the hypothalamic-pituitary-adrenal (HPA) axis, which react to threat by tuning the metabolism for combat or active avoidance. Third is social engagement — calm and communication — associated with the myelinated vagus that responds to a sense of safety by slowing the heart, inhibiting sympathetic nervous system reactivity, and dampening the HPA axis response. In addition, this third subsystem also regulates the muscles of the face and head for social engagement: Eyelid opening allows eye contact, and the same neural pathway for that also helps tune the inner ear to the range of the human voice; the muscles of the face provide expressive potential; laryngeal and pharyngeal muscles offer subtleties of sound and speech; and muscles for tilting the head allow telling gestures.

The social engagement subsystem may be particularly useful as we consider the intersubjective resonance of the mindfulness group. The polyvagal reaction to perceived safety is transformative. It inhibits the defensive strategies of fight, flight, and freeze. It gives tone to the muscles of face and head required for prosocial communication. And it prompts release of the neuropeptide oxytocin (the "love" hormone released during birthing, nursing, and pair bonding), creating what Porges refers to as "immobilization without fear" (2004, p. 21) — an openness to approach and embrace. This transformation can only happen when we perceive safety. So, how does that perception happen implicitly, below our conscious experience? Porges (see 2003, 2004, 2009) suggests that we are continually scanning the environment for risk and safety through "neuroception," which is so named to highlight that it is associated with subcortical processes rather than conscious perception. Neuroception of familiar or friendly faces, voices, gestures, and postures can trigger the social engagement strategy, which in turn promotes a sense of safety. Thus, a sense of safety and the unconscious polyvagal response to it within a group is potentially recursive and self-reinforcing. However, neuroception can also be colored or compromised by intrasubjective visceral states. That is, when fight, flight, or freeze strategies are underway, it is more difficult to detect the prosocial signals that help dampen reactivity and begin the social engagement strategy. Both self-regulation and social support may be required to re-establish the calm of the social engagement response.

It seems that the neuroception process and the resonance circuit may share neural structures, particularly in the temporal cortex, involved in visual input to the mirror neuron system for detecting movements, facial expressions, and vocal features (Porges, 2003, 2009; Thompson, Thompson, & Reid, 2009). Porges (2003) notes the connections between temporal cortex and amygdala and the potential for top-down inhibition of fight, flight, and freeze strategies at an automatic, implicit level of consciousness. The Creswell, et al., (2007) and Lieberman, et al., (2007) studies, on the other hand, describe how mindfulness, particularly the activity of labeling emotions, relies on the prefrontal cortex and inhibits limbic reactivity at an intentional, explicit level of consciousness.

So far, we've been describing intrasubjective resonance and self-regulation; considering experience from an individualist perspective. Now, we can turn to a shared perspective, to see how the group is affected through mindfulness practice. We can focus on intersubjective resonance. The "in-house philosopher" of mirror neuron theory, Vittorio Gallese (2003, 2006), proposes that the capacity of mirror neuron activity to produce "like me" or "as if" experiences of the sensory, intentional, or emotional state of the other depends upon the existence of a shared, "we-centric" space. This space is created through a process of embodied simulation that is automatically triggered by observing the other. We have used this space and process since birth to understand our social environment. Gallese describes it: "When we observe other acting individuals, and face the full range of their expressive power (the way they act, the emotions and feelings they display), a meaningful embodied interpersonal link is automatically established" (2003, p. 519). Now, let's talk about the companionable silence on the mindfulness group "tour bus." We can even propose a model that should prove useful in group situations in the MBIs generally (Fig. 3.3). So, let's go back to the daylong retreat. Just consider the moment the bell rang to end the meditation session. Certainly, across the 60 people in the room, there were many different experiences. Some, perhaps a majority, were intrasubjectively resonant, and were more disposed to approach, rather than avoid, their experience in the moment. Others, perhaps, were struggling in their meditations, or anxious about what was to come, or dozing. As the group began to reconnect in the stillness and silence, they encountered each other — the full range of their expressive power — and were affected. For the many experiencing intrasubjective resonance, their experience was met, matched, and reinforced. For some who had struggled, the faces and postures of the surrounding resonant folks provided an object for embodied simulation that automatically shifted their experience. And for any in highly reactive fight, flight, or freeze states, the signals of safety available to neuroception saturated the room, providing an optimum environment for the social engagement strategy. In short, we could say, with Gallese, that the group created a shared, meaningful, we-centric space — as the invited comments arising from the silence wrote a kind of poem:

"I'm noticing I don't want this to end."
"The energy is full... good... balanced."
"I'm feeling awake, but there's no pressure,
no anxiety about what's next."

The actions that created this poem could be described as an intersubjective resonance circuit. The intrasubjective resonance circuit is situated in each participant's mirror neuron system, limbic system, and insula; it is easily locatable. The intersubjective resonance circuit, in contrast, is harder to pinpoint. Certainly, on a neurophysiological level, it comprises the same structures as the former; yet its location is not discrete. Rather, it is distributed among participants and throughout the shared space. On the most concrete level, its components include the thick layers of nonverbal and verbal communication of each participant — facial expression, eye contact, posture, breath rate, gesture, vocal tone, prosody, silence, scent, even social signifiers. Less concrete, of course, are components such as the sensations, affects, and intelligible understandings conveyed (and contained) by the group. The intersubjective resonance circuit pulses with this energy and information, as participants share and simulate the embodied experience of the moment, both unconsciously and consciously, through neuroception and perception.

Figure 3.3 is now workable for teaching. As a prescriptive model, the starting point on the diagram is anywhere. For example, to develop a workable environment, the teacher can begin class with a mindfulness practice session. This may shift many of the participants towards intrasubjective resonance (A), resulting in affect supporting receptivity and approach towards the experience of the present moment (B1). Then, at the end of the practice session, the full expressivity of the participants is available for automatic simulation, and intersubjective resonance may be possible (C). Here's a second scenario and use of the model. A contentious moment between two participants during a class session could begin to disrupt the intersubjective resonance (C), as neuroception detects reduced safety and the affect of other participants shifts towards reactivity and withdrawal (D2). A call by the teacher for the contentious pair and the entire group to "drop in" for a few minutes of mindfulness practice can bring participants back to their own moment-to-moment experience, potentially creating intrasubjective resonance (A), inhibiting reactivity, and making receptivity and approach more likely in a group of participants (B1). When group relations are reestablished (i.e., the bell rings), the expressions, attitudes and intentions of the resonant participants are available to all the members, so that neuroception of safety and embodied simulation of affect may restore intersubjective resonance and a more workable group environment (C). As a third and final example, in an intersubjectively resonant group (C), one participant could have an intrasubjective experience, such as a sudden recollection of a traumatic incident, in which her affect moves towards reactivity and withdrawal (D2). The teacher could bring that person's attention back to the intersubjective resonance/empathy of the group (C), saying, "Look around the room at who is here with you," thus making the empathic faces and body postures available for neuroception of safety, with a potential inhibition of fight, flight and freeze reactivity, and a possibility for the social engagement strategy to allow the participant to approach intersubjective resonance again.

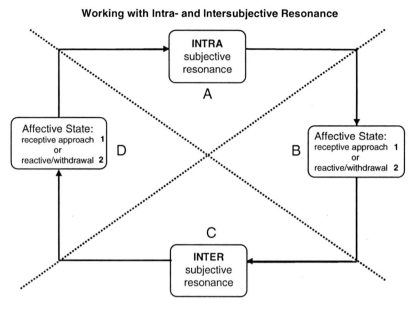

Working with Intra- and Intersubjective Resonance

Fig. 3.3 This model suggests how mindfulness practice may create intrasubjctive resonance (A), which may shift participants' affective states towards receptivity and a willingness to approach even aversive experiences in the moment (B1). The fully embodied affective state of each participant, with its facial expressions, body postures, and other verbal and nonverbal information is then available to the whole group for neuroception of safety and embodied simulation. This may bring group members into intersubjective resonance (C) which is sustained by the ongoing neuroception and simulation of partcipants' affective states (D1), depending on their capacity for self-regulation and intrasubjective resonance (A). The model also prescribes how the teacher may use the components of intra- and intersubjective resonance to intervene and help maintain a workable group environment.

Conceptualizing Mutually Expanded States of Consciousness

The dimension of change must be examined within the intra and intersubjective resonance aspects of the group. One perspective comes through a model of dyadically expanded states of consciousness (Tronick and Members of the Boston Change Process Study Group, 1998). Developed in the context of human development research, this model can be applied as well to many forms of interpersonally mediated learning.

It is based in systems theory, seeing each individual as a self-organizing system moving towards greater complexity and coherence by taking in and incorporating novel information to make new meaning. There is a further understanding that such intrapersonal states of consciousness are limited in their capacity to make meaning. By connecting with another self-organizing system, that capacity can be increase. So, when a dyadic state of consciousness is formed — say, between an infant and caregiver — the interplay expands each person's sense of the world and its possibilities (Tronick, 2007).

Much of the new information that is available to each member of the dyad is "implicit, unconscious, and out of awareness" (Tronick, 2007, p. 505). Here's a deceptively simple illustration from Tronick's work with infants and caregivers:

> Gestural communication is a complex action somewhat beyond the non-self-sitting young infant's ability because the infant is not yet able to control his posture to "free" his arms for communicative purposes. However, the caregiver, by giving the infant postural support in response to the infant's communicative expressions of frustration scaffolds the infant's ability to use gestural communication. The scaffolding "controls" the infant's head and frees the infant to control her arms and hands. Through this process, of providing the regulatory input the now-sitting infant's brain organization takes on a new and different organization with greater coherence and complexity, which is much beyond the infant's endogenous capacities to organize. (Tronick, et al., 1998, p. 295)

In the infant and mother dyad, then, the infant's gestures are "an emergent property of the dyadic system" (p. 296). The action could not take place without the mutual expansion of the states of consciousness of both. This same process allows a dyad to mutually regulate affective states — providing a perspective on the encounter of *the one* with *the other* (described in the side bar Transformation in the "silent land"), so the "breaking of the seven iron bands" can be seen as an emergent property of the dyad sitting on the "common seat." Going back to our "tour bus," we can begin to consider the sense of peace available after the bell rings as an emergent property of the group.

Dyadic expansion of states of consciousness extends relatively easily to adult relationships, such as that between client and therapist. Tronick (2003, 2007) suggests that such dyads differ

---

TRANSFORMATION IN THE "SILENT LAND"

The effect we can have upon one another, considered neurobiologically, is mysterious and powerful — a dialog in the "silent land" of nonverbal communication and knowing that allows transformation or, perhaps, *is* transformation itself. The following description of what appears to be a similar process to that in Fig. 3.3, but in a dyad, brings an additional sense of transformation or expansion of consciousness, It comes from Martin Buber's 1929 essay, "Dialog" (in Buber, 1947).

> Imagine two men sitting beside one another in any kind of solitude in the world. They do not speak with one another, they do not look at one another, not once have they turned to one another. They are not in one another's confidence, the one knows nothing of the other's career, early that morning they got to know one another in the course of their travels. In this moment neither is thinking of the other; we do not need to know what their thoughts are. The one is sitting on the common seat, obviously after his usual manner, calm, hospitably disposed to everything that may come. His being seems to say it is too little to be ready, one must also be really *there*.

So, *the one* is intrasubjectively resonant, mindful, fully present in the moment, and is physically disposed in a way that communicates an ease of well-being, nonreactivity, and an openness to approach himself or the other.

> The other, whose attitude does not betray him, is a man who holds himself in reserve, withholds himself. But if we know about him we know that a childhood's spell is laid on him, that his withholding of himself is something other than an attitude, behind all attitude is entrenched the impenetrable inability to communicate himself.

And *the other* is in a reactive/withdrawal state; indeed it seems that this is a trait, a way of being for the other. He is withdrawn, yet he is in the presence of a resonating being.

> And now — let us imagine that this is one of the hours which succeed in bursting asunder the seven iron bands about our heart — imperceptibly the spell is lifted. But even now the man

from the infant — caregiver type mainly in that they can access an increased repertoire of "age-possible" meanings and meaning-making tools and processes. These include the sophisticated language and symbolic systems of the culture in which the dyad exists; yet they also include all the richness of the more primal nonverbal realms that carry so much information about conscious and unconscious motivation, intention, and action. The interplay is a co-creation, rather than a co-construction; that is, there is no blueprint or rules for the making of meaning, and the meaning is unique to the dyad (Tronick, 2003, 2007), and Stern (2004) argues that it always occurs in the present moment. Further, the co-creation of meaning is a "messy" process: states of consciousness expand and new meaning is created bit by bit through a series of failures and repairs, and through repetitions with inevitable small variations. Looking at infant — caregiver dyads,

> does not speak a word, does not stir a finger. Yet he does something. The lifting of the spell has happened to him — no matter from where — without his doing. But this is what he does now; he releases in himself a reserve over which only he himself has power. Unreservedly communication streams from him, and the silence bears it to his neighbour.
>
> Implicit in this moment of the story is the sense of an *exchange*; the other has come to know a new way of going on in the world, and it is not coincidental that *the one* is present.
>
> Indeed it was intended for him, and he receives it unreservedly as he receives all genuine destiny that meets him. He will be able to tell no one, not even himself, what he has experienced. What does he now "know" of the other? No more knowing is needed. For where unreserve has ruled, even wordlessly, between men, the word of dialogue has happened sacramentally.
>
> Both *the one* and *the other* have come to a new, non-cognitive knowing. Both have been changed, and the change would not have been possible for either in isolation.

Tronick (2003) suggests, "[O]ut of the recurrence of reparations the infant and another person come to share the implicit knowledge that 'we can move into a mutual positive state even when we have been in a mutual negative state' or 'we can transform negative into positive affect'" (p. 478).

This co-created, messy, unique, arising-in-the-moment, reiterative process maps with a powerful congruence to the mindfulness group's toggling back and forth between receptivity and reactivity as intra- and intersubjective resonances are cultivated through mindfulness practice or destabilized by intra- or interpersonal conflict. It seems as if both the group and its individual members, through something very like the dyadically expanded states of consciousness model, come to an implicit knowledge that *"we can transform negative into positive affect."* What is missing in this description, however, is a way of re-conceiving the dyadic expansion of consciousness in group dynamics terms.

Integrating the Theory of Living Human Systems

Agazarian's (1997) theory of living human systems provides the basic insights that allow a view of group expansion of states of consciousness. The theory focuses on the hierarchy and isomorphy of the different systems that make up

Hierarchy of systems (based on Gannt and Agazarian, 2005)

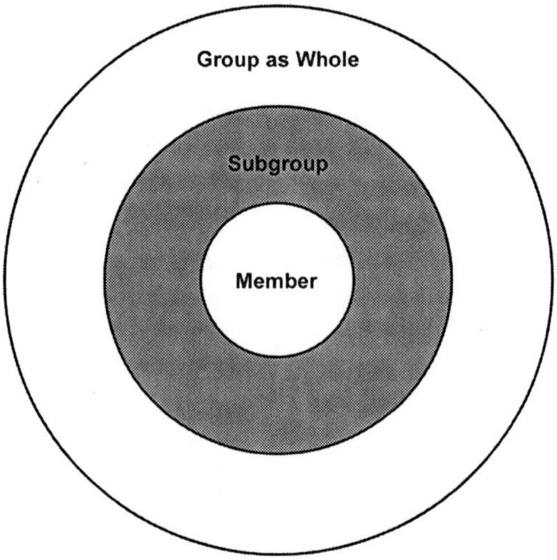

Fig. 3.4 A system hierarchy view of a mindfulness-based group increases the intelligibility of the processes shown in Fig. 3.3. Consider the second vignette in the discussion of Fig. 3.3. The two contentious members, when seen as a subgroup, are influencing both the individual members and the group as a whole, destabilizing members' intrasubjective resonance, and simultaneously weakening the intersubjective resonance of the group as a whole, through shifts in affect, disposition, and non-verbal communication. The call by the teacher to "drop in" to mindfulness practice potentially affects a significantly large number of members who are resonating intrasubjectively; the bell rings and they connect with each other, beginning to resonate intersubjectively. They are then a subgroup that is positioned to influence simultaneously the intra subjective and intersubjective resonance of other members and the group as a whole.

the group. The hierarchical view states that a system acts as context for the one below it and lies within the context of the one above it. A simple graphic (Fig. 3.4) demonstrates these positions. The middle system in the hierarchy then becomes the logical focus when intervening in the entire nested system. It's easily seen that the middle system is contiguous with both the lower and higher system and can therefore affect each of them simultaneously (Agazarian, 1997; Gantt and Agazarian, 2005).

Agazarian's (1997) very valuable tool of functional subgrouping is applied here in the "silent land" of nonverbal or preverbal experience; in Chapter 5, it will be suggested as a way of shaping verbal interventions. To introduce the concept quickly, there is a basic tendency of the human mind — and human groups — to dichotomize, to choose sides and create conflict between two views. By exploring only one subgroup's position at a time, exploring similarities before exploring differences, functional subgrouping subverts this tendency (Ladden, 2007). Here's an intervention using subgrouping in a way appropriate to this discussion: a member of the group speaks of a sadness arising within her during the meditation. The teacher can ask "How many of you have been sitting with sadness?"

— gesturing for a show of hands. Hands go up, and a subgroup identifies itself; they come into direct and peripheral visual contact (and other nonverbal modes of contact) with each other, and connections that generate interpersonal resonance, analogous to dyadically expanded states of consciousness, are created. The subgroup co-creates its own meaning nonverbally, which simultaneously influences the individual members and the group as a whole.

For the teacher, in the moment, in the flow of the class or group, the models of resonance circuits and system hierarchy offer simple, mutually informing ways to organize experience and respond to dynamics of the environment of the group as a whole.

As we look into the pedagogy of mindfulness in Parts 2 and 3, these various discourses will be salient, along with others — our attempt is not to be exclusive or exhaustive, but to use what works. The process is one of acknowledged reduction and oversimplification. Trying to find and hold up for examination the motions, gestures, and felt senses of how teaching and learning (or better yet, just call it learning) happen. Theory doesn't come helpfully into the classroom as theory, it simply arises as a move, an attempt, a drawing out, an elaboration of what is there in the moment of arising — a moment of genuine encounter.

PASSENGERS IN THE BUS SHARE A COMMON SEAT
Van Gennep (1909, in Turner, 1969) first defined *rites of passage*, the rituals that attend the changes of status in society. Van Gennep had transitions of social status, particularly political or religious offices and positions, in mind, but Turner expanded this to include more existential states such as illness (Beels, 2007). Rites of passage comprise three phases, in which the subjects, or *passengers*, first separate from their fixed social position, then enter a threshold, or *liminal*, period in which identity is ambiguous, and at the end of the period are reincorporated in the society with a new identity. This liminal period and the collective experiences of the passengers during that period are helpful in thinking about the mindfulness-based group environment.

Many people come into mindfulness-based groups as the result of a crisis — a difficult life transition, an illness, a loss — for which they do not feel they have sufficient internal resources or even compensatory social support. They are suffering, and are met with the promise of transformation if they will engage with the curriculum. They become passengers, taking their seat in a group where the main shared characteristic is the willingness (however tentative!) to examine one's own experience. The group is liminal, as Turner (1969) describes it. Members have no special roles or positions to distinguish them from their fellows; in fact, much of a group's early work is in exploring the similarities of their suffering. As Turner notes (p. 95), they "tend to develop an intense comradeship and egalitarianism."

This *comradeship* is characteristic of what Turner (1969) calls *comradeship*, in which the group exists in a "'moment in and out of time,' and in and out of the social structure" (p. 96). As Beels (2001, p. 123), adapting this concept to thinking about psychotherapy, explains, "In communitas, the structures and functions of the daily community are suspended in favor of ritual recognition that some members... have not yet come into their powers, are sick and in need of healing, or are not yet ready to function in the next stage of life."

Part II
Authenticity, Authority, and Friendship

Chapter 4
The Person of the Teacher

It's a very old story, told all around the world. A stranger comes to a little community that's been under great stress, where food is scarce, and where people have drawn away from each other and are looking out for themselves. The stranger manages to borrow a cooking pot and starts making soup. He begins with a "magic" ingredient, a stone, maybe a button, or even a nail. The community members become interested in what he's doing, and each secretly comes for a look at the pot. The stranger stirs and tastes. "Ah, it's coming along nicely," he says. "But it would be really wonderful if it had just a little something extra, like a potato, maybe...," he says to one visitor in just the way she needs to hear it. She goes off inspired to find something to offer. "...like a carrot," he says in his just-right way to another. Later, "... a cabbage," and then "...some beans." And soon there's a shy parade of community folks bringing ingredients and standing around a pot that's now aswim with good things — enough for everyone. They share a meal. There's even a little music. Someone sings; another finds his fiddle; there's dancing into the night. And the stranger has already gone, picking up a new "magic" stone on his way to the next community.

Although this story is usually called "stone soup" or maybe "button borscht," nothing in the story happens because of the "magic" ingredient. It happens because of the stranger's presence — more, his ability to *be present* to everyone. That is the marvel and mystery attending co-creation. The stranger simply coaxes out what is already in the individuals and community. The stranger does not require much to do his work: a pot, a fire, a stone; faith, knowledge, and caring: faith that the people of the community always have what is needed; knowledge of how the world (meaning people) works; and caring in a way that supports and inspires others.

So, in teaching mindfulness as a professional, you are the stranger. The work ultimately depends on you, on who you are as a person. You enter the little community of participants with nothing, not even a pot. You meet them just as they are, just as you are. Your faith is exposed, as is your knowledge, and your caring, because to teach mindfulness is to practice it, and to practice means to bring all that you are to every moment. And all that you are is all that is needed; the real you really *is* sufficient.

This definition of the teacher is the most committing of those current in the Mindfulness-Based Interventions (MBIs). It is what drives Mindfulness-Based Stress Reduction (MBSR) and Mindfulness-Based Cognitive Therapy (MBCT) training to

D. McCown et al., *Teaching Mindfulness: A Practical Guide for Clinicians and Educators*, DOI 10.1007/978-0-387-09484-7_4,
© Springer Science+Business Media, LLC 2010

focus so strongly on the teacher's own commitment to the practice and life of mindfulness. As Jon Kabat-Zinn (1999) characterizes it, "The attitude that the teacher brings into the room...ultimately influences absolutely everything in the world. Once you make the commitment, as Kabir (Bly, 1971) put it, 'To stand firm in that which you are,' to hold the central axis of your being human, the entire universe is different."

This chapter begins with this most committing definition for two reasons: first, because it is most congruent with the co-creation of mindfulness, which is at the core of the pedagogical concepts presented in this book; second, because it can be helpful to aspire to a vision — like that of Kabir or Kabat-Zinn.

This chapter, then, is the most important in the book. It is also the shortest and simplest — not because there is so little material, but because there is so much. This chapter is about you: not because you need to be fixed or improved, but because your only option in becoming a teacher of mindfulness is to become more of who you are. This is not so much a chapter for reading as for exploring moment by moment. You'll learn far more from your responses to the practices and suggestions found here than you could from reading a book — this one or any one. Work through. Savor. Come back again. And again.

Authenticity, Authority, and Friendship

Not because it is right or true but because it is useful, we have identified a three-part scheme for talking about the person of the teacher. This allows us to point to ways of exploring who you are or may be as a professional teaching mindfulness, to offer a few broad insights and some practices that we have found helpful in developing ourselves and other teachers.

To put this scheme in the context of the teacher as the stranger, *authenticity* is where the faith arises, the faith that knows that everyone can turn towards whatever is arising — good, bad, or ugly — and discover something within himself/herself. It is the practice dimension of teaching. It is a very pragmatic way of knowing that the practice of mindfulness will reveal what is necessary for each participant and the group. *Authority* is the knowledge of how the world works that gives the stranger the confidence to borrow a pot and start cooking. It is what you know; it is your success in the world. Finally, *friendship* is caring; it is the just-right way of meeting each person.

Authenticity: What You Know

While self-disclosure in the MBIs is not about telling your "story," it is very much about being the person whose story you've lived. For that reason, a good place to start in getting to know who you are in this dimension of authenticity is with how you came to the wish to teach mindfulness as a professional. It may be helpful to you to be able to trace, and to describe the journey that brought you to who you are now. Or, to stick with the soup analogy, it may be useful to be able to share the unique ingredients in the recipe that is you.

This journey or recipe may include psychological work that you have done. It may include your spiritual life, whether within a particular tradition, or more in Don Cupitt's scope of your "life" as the religious object. Certainly it includes your mindfulness and meditation practice, in all contexts, as it has manifested throughout your life: and especially as you may be practicing now.

You are reading this book. That is a fact of the moment. Take some time now, if you would, to explore what that fact means to you, using the practice that follows.

PRACTICE 1: A MEDITATIVE INQUIRY ON YOUR AUTHENTICITY

Sitting in a comfortable position.
Bringing your attention to your body.
Feeling the support beneath you.
Noticing your breath wherever you feel it most vividly in the moment.
Simply following your breath moment to moment.
And when you find your mind settling, beginning mindful inquiry by dropping this question into the silence...
"What brings you to this book?"
And noticing what answer or answers come to you.
Sitting in silence and listening.
And when you are ready asking the question again...
"What brings you to this book"
Sitting in silence and continuing to listen.
Repeating the question and allowing answers to reveal themselves to you from a deeper and deeper place within...
"What brings you to this book?"

Were You on an Ancient Path to This Moment?

It is surprising how often those who are drawn to the healing potential of mindfulness have stories that are evocative of the journeys of healers among indigenous peoples. Did your reflection suggest any of the eight traditional pathways to the healer's role defined by Landy (1977)?

1. Inheritance — did a relative play a part?
2. Selection by others — was it suggested by those who know you in a close way; other healers, elders?
3. Self-selection — being so drawn to it that you would apprentice yourself to learn what another knows?
4. Undergoing a profound emotional experience — a feeling of awe and a sense of true calling?
5. Self-dedication to a healing cult — this sounds a bit intense, but how about the contemporary version of having recovered from an illness with a desire to help others with that illness?

6. Miraculous self-recovery — getting a "new lease on life" and wishing to use it for helping others?
7. Genetic, congenital, or acquired physical disability — or any sense of difference from others?
8. Exceptional personal traits — gifts that cry out to be used?

If you made connections to this list, what does that mean to you? Do you feel more, or less, interested in teaching mindfulness as a professional?

Who are the Teachers Within You?

As you sat with your journey, your soup recipe, perhaps you became aware of people who had powerful influence on you at one point or another in your life. These we might call teachers. They may actually have had that role, or they may have engaged you in some other way — a relative, friend, or colleague who embodied some quality or qualities that have great appeal. It may be that such teachers are from a different generation or century — this can include authors, artists, figures from history (or even fiction) that have left a lasting impression. Because you aspire to be a teacher that participants will allow to live inside of them, it is helpful to know who lives in you. This sounds dramatic, yet you can test its truth. Do the teachers within you respond when you need them? Are you ever comforted by recalling what someone important to you said? Have you ever told someone "…and then I heard your voice telling me…" Spend some time investigating these questions. Learn about your teachers, who they are, how they came to be within you, and how they may help you become more of who you are.

PRACTICE 2: TEACHERS WITHIN

Sitting in a comfortable position.
Taking a few full breaths.
Bringing to mind/heart a teacher who has inspired you.
What qualities does this teacher embody that inspire you?
What truth (about yourself) has this teacher helped to reveal?
When you think of this teacher what feelings are evoked inside you?
Then allowing the image and felt sense of this teacher to fade.
Continue with other teachers, or take a few minutes after each to write about what you discovered.

That was history. The question is, who are your mindfulness teachers now? As we've suggested, mindfulness is a co-creation. You learn it with others — at least one other. That teacher is with you as you practice; there's a voice in which you hear those first instructions that keeps coming back to you. It may be a spoken voice or a written one; it is a voice nonetheless.

With whom are you studying? If your major contact is through books and recordings, how deeply have you explored? Who does (did) your favorite teacher admire? Find, read, listen. Broaden your exposure. You'll be teaching many different types of people, and not all of them will respond to the same kinds of language and imagery. Get to know how other teachers teach — even ones that you don't think will appeal to you — you may make some surprising connections.

Given the challenges of *embodied* teaching that a professional teaching mindfulness faces in the dyad or group, we believe that a teacher needs to have an ongoing one-to-one relationship with someone who can hold her accountable for practice and can assist her when questions arise. This need not be some highly accomplished, enlightened being in an Asian practice lineage. In fact, it may be more helpful if this person is much like yourself: perhaps a local teacher in the MBIs; perhaps a member of a local Buddhist organization who offers to work with others; perhaps a spiritual director from your own religious tradition — or from a different one! A useful resource for locating such a person anywhere in the United States and around the world is the *Seek and Find Guide* of Spiritual Directors International, which you can access online at http://www.sdiworld.org/.

Practice, Practice, Practice

Commitment to regular formal mindfulness meditation practice is defined at minimum as practicing with the frequency and duration expected of participants (Kabat-Zinn, 2003). This means six days a week, 45 min a day in the case of the Center for Mindfulness (CFM) program; frequency remains the same, but duration may differ in other programs.

If you are just developing a practice, as you commit to such a regimen, you will find a way to "build it in" to your schedule rather than "fit it in." With the best intentions in the world, the "fit in" model does not work with consistency. Many who have ongoing practices have found that practicing first thing in the morning ensures that it happens: nothing else can come between you and the practice.

What is your practice? This may be another useful question. If you are teaching MBSR or one of the MBIs that uses its basic structure, you'll be teaching body scan, sitting meditation, Hatha Yoga or some other form of movement, walking meditation, loving kindness meditation, and mountain or lake meditation. If you have not done so, you should spend significant time — perhaps 90 days — with each of these as your daily practice. It is essential in teaching that you understand any practice from the inside out before attempting to guide others in it or work with their direct experience.

PRACTICE 3: KEEPING A PRACTICE JOURNAL

The practice of keeping a meditation journal can be invaluable in bringing increased awareness to what happens when we meditate and to tracking our growth. Aspects of our meditative experience that may go unnoticed or be forgotten can come to light by writing in a journal after we meditate.

It is best to have a journal designated specifically for the purpose of writing about your meditative experiences. It is also best to write your reflections as soon after meditating as you can.

As you reflect, write about body sensations, feelings, and thoughts that you experienced during meditation. Were there predominant feelings, thoughts? What discoveries, surprises, insights, and challenges did you have during meditation? Are there any new insights arising as you write? What do you notice after writing?

Reviewing your journal entries can help you gain insight on themes and patterns that are emerging and allow you to see your areas of strength and areas that need further development or cultivation.

Prolonged periods of practice can provide developing teachers with opportunities for greater insight into the mind — body complex and into the practices themselves. Ideally, then, you might undertake a regular pattern of silent retreats of five days or more, say, one or two per year. This is required of teachers working in the CFM MBSR program (Santorelli, 2001), and of candidates for training beyond the foundational level through the Center for Mindfulness in Medicine, Health Care and Society (2007).

Retreats are not extensions of daily practice, not just "more of the same." There is a qualitative as well as a quantitative difference between what is revealed by formally cultivating mindfulness for, say, one hour, and seamless formal and informal practice for one's waking hours over, say, ten consecutive days. The arising and dissolution of sensations, emotions, and thought in an hour might be considered metaphorically as a photograph of a natural scene, while the metaphor for a 10-day retreat might be a time-lapse movie of the same scene as seasons change: both are dense with potential for experience and insight, yet the movie reveals and opens for exploration dimensions only hinted at in the photo.

A useful way to begin to understand the power and value of longer term intensive practice is to engage in a self-retreat at home for a day or perhaps a weekend. This can be an introduction and is also an easy method to keep you in touch with this dimension of practice between longer retreats.

A listing of retreat centers offering the silent, teacher-led *Vipassana* style retreats that are preferred by teachers in the MBIs can be found in the Appendix. As many of the retreats are led by teachers, this is also a good way to find new teachers and hear new approaches to language and practice.

PRACTICE 4: A SELF-RETREAT

Choose a day or weekend when you can be on your own without any interruption. Inform your family and friends that you will not be available, that you are taking time for self-reflection and self-nurturing. Sylvia Boorstein (1996), in her book, *Don't Just Do Something, Sit There,* says retreat practice starts before the retreat. It begins with the decision to practice, with the intention to be mindful.

Plan in advance and prepare what you will need for your retreat, whether you are doing a self-retreat at home or away from home (a cottage, a retreat center, a natural setting). What food you will have? What clothes you will wear? What meditation supplies you will be using (cushion, chair, yoga mat, shawl, blanket)? Create your daily schedule before going on retreat and keep your schedule with you, along with a clock and timer. It is best to start with the intention to keep as close to the formal schedule as possible.

Start your retreat by turning off your phone, computer, TV, radio. Slow down, breathe, relax...

Creating a Retreat Schedule. This is one possibility for a day's schedule, based on the type of schedule used in *Vipassana* style retreat centers:

6:30 am	Wake, wash, and dress mindfully, and sit until breakfast
7:15	Prepare and eat breakfast; clean up
8:00	Walk
8:45	Sit
9:30	Mindful Movement-yoga, tai chi, qigong
10:15	Sit
11:00	Walk
11:45	Sit until lunch
12:00 pm	Prepare and eat lunch; clean up; rest
2:00	Sit
2:45	Walk
3:30	Sit
4:15	Walk
5:00	Prepare and eat dinner; clean up
6:00	Listen to a recording of a talk by a teacher who inspires you; read something by a favorite teacher
7:00	Walk
7:45	Sit
8:30	Tea, retire, or continue to sit

The schedule could also be designed in MBI style, to include body scans, Hatha Yoga or other body-based practices, and even expressive practices such as writing, drawing, or painting.

Authority: What You Have Learned

The term *authority* is meant to evoke the Latin *auctoritas*, suggesting power derived from legal authorship, rather than power granted by some outside agency. The indication of authority is that you know what you know so well that you could be the author of it. In other words, you have lived it and loved it, conferring both intellectual and moral authority.

This authority may be demonstrated in an MBI curriculum or a particular way of working with others using mindfulness practices. It is a competence that comes from *learning* deeply and well, unlike authenticity, which comes from *knowing* deeply and well. The most pristine example of such authority is the confidence that a clinician has with a curriculum of an MBI that she has developed on her own. She moves smoothly within it, trusting it, trusting herself as it unfolds in the session and through its duration.

Authority also includes the professional training you have that is useful in understanding "how the world works," as the stranger might say. Perhaps your training is in medicine, or occupational therapy, or psychology, or education. There are profundities within your particular professional discourse that you have learned as truths. Many of them are useful in helping people become more themselves; it is work you know how to do and you are good at. Don't leave it behind. How can you incorporate it in your undertaking of teaching mindfulness? There may be other truths from your authority that are not so helpful, that draw people away from their own experience of the moment to some place where they need to be fixed or changed — by you. It may be that such learning is authoritative, because it has historically given you the confidence to move towards or work with particular people. It may also be that such learning is worth questioning, because it no longer fits your more mindful way of working. Your authenticity — your own mindfulness practice — may be showing you that people have what they need already inside them, that they just need the space to become more of what they are. At this point, it is time to take stock. To see when what you *know* is more important than what you've *learned*.

PRACTICE 5: LEARNING AND UNLEARNING

This is a practice that explores the sometimes one-sided nature of our thinking and learning. It is adapted from Jack Kornfield's (1993), *The Wise Heart*.

Contemplate an area in your life where you hold strong beliefs — perhaps your professional life or your spiritual life; maybe beliefs about your role in a relationship or at work; or beliefs about the future, the past.

As you sit quietly, bring to mind the key thoughts/stories you tell yourself about yourself, another, a situation, an institution… "I am _____." They are_____." It is _____."

After you have clearly identified these beliefs, begin to inquire closely. Are these beliefs completely true? Are they true at all times? Are they one-sided? What if some of the opposite is true?

What is your experience if you stay open to possibility, if you let go of the thoughts and beliefs? As much as you are able, let go of the thoughts/stories, and rest in an open awareness of not knowing. How does that feel in the body, in the mind? How does this affect your relationship to self… and other?

Friendship: Offering All That You Are

This is a term gleaned from the contemporary Buddhist theologian, Stephen Batchelor (1997). His description of friendship in the world of Buddhist practice and study fits the mindfulness teacher's role with a participant:

> We are participatory beings who inhabit a participatory reality, seeking relationships that enhance our sense of what it means to be alive... [A] true friend is more than just someone with whom we share common values and who accepts us for what we are. Such a friend is someone whom we can trust to refine our understanding of what it means to live, who can guide us when we're lost and help us find our way along a path, who can assuage our anguish [Batchelor's term for what is usually translated as "suffering"] through the reassurance of his or her presence.

This same non-hierarchical, non-pathologizing, deeply humane sensibility is found in the other spiritual traditions as they approach friendship. Consider the basic position assumed in Christian spiritual direction. As described by Aelred of Rievaulx, a twelfth century Cistercian abbot, in his *Spiritual Friendship* (in Neufelder and Coelho, 1982):

> What happiness, what confidence, what joy to have a person to whom you dare speak on terms of equality as to another self. You can also without shame make known whatever advances you have made in your spiritual life. You can entrust all the secrets of your heart to him and before him you can lay out all your plans. What, therefore, is more pleasant than to unite your spirit to that of another person and of two to form one. No bragging is to be feared after this and no suspicion need be feared. No correction of one by the other will cause pain; no praise on the part of one will bring a charge of excessive flattery from the other...

So friendship begins with the intention of meeting people "where they are," of coming to any encounter *without* an agenda or intention to fix or improve the other, and *with* a willingness to allow relationships and situations to unfold in a fresh way.

What are You Bringing to the Meeting?

As we have spoken of self-disclosure, the teacher has no choice, but is exposed completely in each moment of being. There is, however, a choice of what is disclosed through talk and trading stories. It may be that your personal experience could be valuable to participants. The discernment is about what do you share, and when? If the answer would help the other in the sense of friendship we've described, the only question is, then, "Is it still too raw, or can I speak from it helpfully?" Thus, knowing how it is with you in your own areas of growth and challenge is not a sometime thing for a teacher; it's a necessary discipline. Knowing what's too raw to speak of can keep you out of difficulties. And tracking that rawness over time can help with your own capacity for self-acceptance and forgiveness.

PRACTICE 6: WHAT'S RAW IN ME?

Write journal responses to this question. A technique offered by writer Natalie Goldberg involves setting aside a specific length of time to write (setting a timer for 10 min), picking up a pen, and keeping your hand moving on the paper for the duration of the time. In this case, begin the practice by writing the question "What's raw in me?" or writing "What's raw in me is...," and then continue to write without taking your pen off the paper. If the writing slows down or stops, simply rewrite the question or statement again, "What's raw in me?" or "What's raw in me is...," and continue writing your response.

Sharing Direct Experience with the Other

In teaching in any population, the teacher is asked to meet participants' suffering: to meet them with friendship where they are. This can feel daunting, especially when we feel that the suffering is outside our experience. In working with those in extreme or chronic pain and emotional suffering, the teacher needs a place to work from — a sense that everything can be worked with mindfully. The teacher needs to trust the practice and the participant to have just what is needed. This tall order is closer to being filled when you have done significant experimentation with your own physical and emotional pain. Following are two practices that help you allow your own experience and see just how trustworthy you and mindfulness practice really are.

PRACTICE 7: BEING WITH PHYSICAL DISCOMFORT

Scanning your body with a gentle awareness. Notice any area or areas of holding or discomfort in your body.

Turning your attention toward an area of discomfort; allowing your mind to rest in this region of the body.

Noticing sensations as they arise. Are the sensations subtle or strong? Is there tightness or pressure or heat? Do the sensations stay the same or do they change? Noticing the nuances of sensation.

If the mind wanders to thought, noticing if there are any thoughts or stories associated with this discomfort: "I don't like this," "I hate this," "This is killing me..."

As much as possible letting thoughts come and go, not attaching to thoughts, rather allowing sensations in the body to be the primary focus of attention.

Noticing if there is a tendency to want the sensations to be different, if you are struggling in the moment.

As much as you are able, bringing a receptive presence to what is arising moment to moment.

PRACTICE 8: BEING WITH DIFFICULTY

Sitting in a comfortable position. Bringing your attention to your body. Feeling the support beneath you. Noticing your breath wherever you fell it most vividly. Simply following your breath moment to moment.

And when you are ready, calling to mind a situation that you are struggling with. It may be a conflict in a relationship, or financial concerns, or difficulty at work.

After you have called this situation to mind, bring your attention to your body and notice what you are feeling. Notice what body sensations are arising, what mood states are arising. Is there tightness or pressure in the body?

Is there a word that describes your experience? Afraid, sad, restless? Simply name what is arising — tightness, heaviness, anger, sadness... Noting or naming with a whisper what is arising moment to moment. Not straining to find the "right" word, just noting what is most prominent.

After naming your experience, gently inquire while paying attention to sensations in the body: "Does this word or these words describe what I am feeling right now? If not, is there another word or words? Continue to mentally note what unfolds in your experience moment to moment.

At times you may get lost in thoughts. When you notice this, simply note "thinking," or "planning," or "worrying..." and bring your attention back to your body. Continue to note what you are sensing in your body. Naming what is true moment to moment (adapted from Tara Brach's (2003) meditation, "Naming what is true in difficulty.")

It All Amounts to Spiritual Maturity

This sense of the teacher as the stranger, this looking into the depths of your own authenticity, authority, and friendship, is a way of describing the teacher of mindfulness. This is not the same as your identity as a professional, but it can become part of it. The key is the development of some level of spiritual maturity — not some idealized, "enlightened" position, but a down-to-earth possibility. A useful definition, perhaps, comes from Fowler's (1981) elaboration of six "stages of faith": Stage 5 of the 6 is characterized by *dialogical knowing*, in which knower and known enter an I — Thou relationship. This is much of what you're exploring in this chapter, through mindfulness and self-reflection. Fowler makes the important point nicely: "What the mystics call 'detachment' characterizes Stage 5's willingness to let reality speak its word, regardless of the impact of that word on the security or self-esteem of the knower" (p. 185). In the MBIs, detachment might be rendered as "non-attachment," to emphasize that there is no sense of dissociation or distance, just clarity and perspective. The value of such mature spirituality for a teacher working with her participants is clear in Fowler's (p.198) statement that, "...this stage is ready to spend and be spent for the cause of conserving and cultivating the possibility of others' generating identity and meaning."

Chapter 5
The Skills of the Teacher

In teaching mindfulness as a professional, the teacher works from her or his own unique authenticity, authority, and friendship. That means, of course, that all individual teachers are different, with singular ways of integrating and embodying mindfulness. In fact, for this purpose, integrating and embodying are the same thing. Teachers know what they know, and can do what they do, based on the fruits of their practice and on the skills they have developed along the paths of their own professional and personal development. As a result, the skills each teacher possesses may be a *mélange* of ideas, which is not so much integrated theoretically in the thinking, but, rather, more directly in the body of the teacher. Even at the Center for Mindfulness at the University of Massachusetts, the programs of teacher training comprise such a mélange. Pragmatic and eclectic, these trainings make use of a wide range of insights and practices from medicine, psychotherapy, education, anthropology–sociology, and world wisdom traditions. Again, the integration of all of this substance is not in theory but in the body of each teacher. Yet, at the same time, we also believe that there are general skills that teachers share; that is, we believe each teacher uses comparable skills to work with participants in her own inimitable way.

We have discerned a scheme for parsing and elaborating the skills of teaching mindfulness as a professional that is helpful for us in our own development as teachers, in working with other new teachers and those aspiring to teach, and — most important — in continuously improving the experiences of the participants in our programs.

WE HAVE IDENTIFIED FOUR SKILL SETS THAT SEEM TO BE SHARED AMONG TEACHERS IN THE MBIS

1. *Stewardship* of the group;
2. *Homiletics,* or the delivery of didactic material;
3. *Guidance* of formal practices and informal group experiences;
4. *Inquiry* into participants' direct experience.

D. McCown et al., *Teaching Mindfulness: A Practical Guide for Clinicians and Educators*, DOI 10.1007/978-0-387-09484-7_5, © Springer Science+Business Media, LLC 2010

The four skill sets are interrelated. For example, stewardship of the group involves a broad set of skills that, as will become apparent, may be seen to include the other three. Further, the development of voice and body for communication most closely associated with the skills of homiletics are also significant for guidance and inquiry, while the forms of language used in guidance influence all other verbal communication, and the dialogical understandings developed in the group through inquiry inform homiletics and guidance. Of course, all four are dependent completely upon the teacher's authenticity, authority and friendship — her or his capacity to remain present and to respond thoughtfully and compassionately to whatever is arising in the moment.

Stewardship of the Group

Working with mindfulness is not group therapy. It is not psychoeducation. And it is not classroom teaching. All the "group-work skills" can be seen, rather, as rooted in the co-creation of mindfulness among teacher and participants. From this perspective, the distinctive features of the mindfulness-based group and its demands on the teacher become evident. First, because it is a *co*-creation in which the teacher may be a catalyst, but in which *every* participant contributes, a nonhierarchical, non-pathologizing ethos develops. Everyone involved, teacher and participant alike, shares the sufferings and joys of the human condition. Second, all share the intention, explicit or implicit, to explore his or her own direct experience. Such explorations have the potential of revealing one's authenticity in the moment to the group. Third, every participant has the opportunity to be supported by the group in his or her exploration, and to offer support as well. Finally, all are contributors to the maintenance of the mindfulness, the inter-subjective resonance, of the group.

Stewards of the Group's Three Treasures

Our response to these features is to define the teacher's overarching group-work skill with the term *stewardship*. The word itself, in its derivation from Old English words suggesting a guardian of the meeting hall, captures the most basic sense of the teacher's duties in the group — that is, holding the space in which participants can work. It also highlights the ordinariness, the humility, and the service that are implied in such a position. Further, current connotations of the term suggest diligent care of treasures or powers of great value held in trust for others, as in environmental stewardship.

In a way, then, the teacher holds the treasures of the group in trust for the participants as they grow into the ability to care for those treasures by themselves — that is, as they firmly establish mindfulness and inter-subjective resonance. These three treasures reflect the distinctive features of mindfulness-based groups.

The first is *freedom*. This is the permission for the participant to become who she or he is, to come more fully into her or his experience. Participants are continuously offered the possibility of surrender to how they are in the moment — not to how they think they should be or how the teacher or any teaching point may suggest. The teacher's role in this, while the group's capacity to hold each other in freedom grows, is in the nonverbal expression of authenticity and friendship, as well as the more verbal expressions represented in the other major skill sets described in this chapter.

The second treasure is *belonging*. This is the ongoing opportunity for the participant more and more to understand and feel his or her influence on the life of the group in the moment, and to experience both the offer of care and the demand for restraint inherent in being a participant. This feature of the group is a participant's natural or inevitable accountability to others. Through the teacher's skill in keeping the tensions of belonging active in the life of the group, participants find ways to integrate freedom and belonging in themselves — a self-regulation that is integral to the co-created mindfulness of the group.

The third treasure is *resonance*. This is the co-created inter-subjective resonance of the group from moment to moment. This gift of the group touches and helps to optimize the freedom and belonging of each of the participants. The teacher ensures this as the group's capacity increases — and beyond — by gently intervening in ways that generate both rifts and repairs, thus deepening resonance.

These three treasures of freedom, belonging, and resonance are interdependent: a shift in the quality of one in a participant or the group will almost inevitably result in concurrent shifts in the others. For example, in an inquiry dialog with the teacher, if anxiety increases for a participant while exploring his present moment experience, his capacity for freedom may deteriorate and sense of belonging diminish. Through his withdrawal and through emotional contagion, the group's inter-subjective resonance may also decline. Intervention by the teacher or group to restore the participant's sense of freedom or belonging, can, in turn, reestablish balance among the three treasures and effect deeper resonance in which to continue the work. This will be described in further detail later in this section.

GROUP-WORK SKILLS AND "UNLEARNING"

There are suggestions in the literature that prior training in leading groups is valuable for one teaching mindfulness as a professional. Certainly, this statement is true, in that the core skill sets defined in this chapter are incorporated in many other types of group-work; but they are shaped by a significantly different context — co-created mindfulness. We suggest, therefore, that prospective teachers place skills developed in other group contexts under scrutiny, and adopt a sense of "unknowing" that may lead to the "unlearning" that the Melbourne Academic Interest Group (2006) identifies in its review of the MBIs: "[P]reviously learned group-work skills are likely to require modification, and indeed some unlearning may be necessary for the mindfulness model of practice" (p. 292).

Roundness: Shaping the Group From the Start

Participants come into a circle to sit together at the beginning of each session (Fig. 5.1). Across cultures and around the world, the circle is a symbol of completion, fullness, perfection. Certainly, it has layer upon layer of meaning, from the Zen *enso,* suggesting the totality of the universe and enlightenment; to the *ouroboros,* the serpent biting (or devouring) its tail of the Western occult sciences (and of Kundalini Yoga), suggesting the endless round of life and the reconciliation of opposites; to the *mandala,* the Eastern tool for spiritual exploration, which C. G. Jung explored as a vehicle for individuation. Indigenous peoples, who sit in circles as communities, have a marvelous grasp of the circle's ubiquity and symbolic power, as suggested in these observations by Black Elk (Neihardt, 1961):

> You have noticed that everything an Indian does is in a circle, and that is because the Power of the World always works in circles, and everything tries to be round.... The sky is round, and I have heard that the earth is round like a ball, and so are all the stars. The wind, in its greatest power, whirls. Birds make their nests in circles, for theirs is the same religion as ours. The sun comes forth and goes down again in a circle. The moon does the same, and both are round. Even the seasons form a great circle for their changing, and always come back again to where they were. The life of a man is a circle from childhood to childhood, and so it is in everything where power moves. (p. 198).

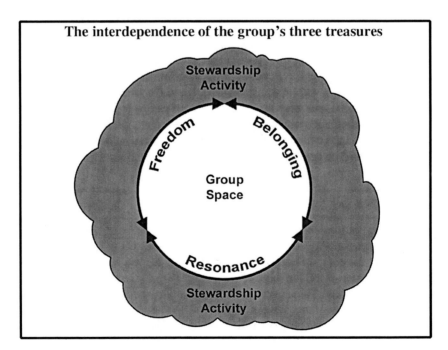

Fig. 5.1 This illustration shows the relationship of freedom, belonging, and resonance. As revealed in the meeting of arrow points, each one touches and potentially influences the other two. As one is built up, all may be built up, and as one diminishes, all may diminish. The teacher's stewardship activities are shown as taking place on the "outside" of the group space, because they are protective of the co-created group space that is formed and sustained by the interrelationship of the three treasures.

Gaston Bachelard, in *The Poetics of Space* (1964), is struck by the consistent intuition in great thinkers that "being is round." He attempts to consider roundness without filters of philosophy or culture — as a pure phenomenological experience. He notes, "…images of full roundness help us to collect ourselves, permit us to confer an initial constitution on ourselves, and to confirm our being intimately, inside. For when it is experienced intimately from the inside, devoid of all exterior features, being cannot be otherwise than round" (p. 234).

Making a circle also sets a boundary. It creates order within from chaos. It divides outside and inside. It excludes and includes. It can alienate and ignore or hold and nurture. And so, we ask participants to "come *into*" a circle, a phrase and action that emphasizes inclusion, holding, and nurturing, as well as the symbolism of fulfillment. For instance, after a long session of Hatha yoga practice, participants were spread out through the room and chairs and cushions were distributed and disrupted. The teacher asked that everyone "come into" a circle for dialog. With pushing and pulling and jockeying around, a shape took form — not like one marked by a compass, but like one co-created in the moment to accommodate a need. One participant noted, "Well, this isn't much of a circle." No teacher could ask for a better straight line. The reply was, "On the contrary, as long as everyone's inside, it's a perfect circle." In this sense, then, what is important is the *inside* of the circle. That is where participants find themselves. That is where the group comes together.

So, stewardship begins with tending the circle. The teacher's actions as guardian of the meeting hall, as servant-leader, are often very concrete and domestic. When you teach mindfulness as a professional, chances are you are going to get your hands dirty and do some heavy lifting to get the environment right for participants: setting or adjusting the chairs in a circle in a way that will work for the group; ensuring the same number of chairs as participants, to enhance the sense and symbol of fulfillment; making sure that empty chairs are removed when participants are absent. And accommodating both the chairs and the circle to those who use wheelchairs or who are challenged physically to come into a close circle.

The teacher also cares for the site of the circle, doing what is possible to reduce discomfort and distraction. Adjusting lights and temperature, and doing what you can to prevent noisy interruption of the group — by custodial workers or members of the next class, for example. There is, however, no need to ask for quiet, as the ordinary (and even extraordinary) sounds and events in and outside the space are part of the fabric of practice, guidance, and inquiry, as will be discussed. This is not a perfect world and stewardship does not attempt to make one. It makes instead a place where participants can feel reasonably safe, secure, supported, and connected.

The circle is an embodied expression of timeless symbolism in the present moment. There is a fullness and completion that is potentially available to participants who glance around the circle. There is an undermining of hierarchy and status and an affirmation of equality; think of King Arthur's Round Table. There is available, as well, a suggestion of being fellow passengers in a rite of passage, a waiting together for whatever comes next, as described in Chapter 3. The teacher can make as much or as little of this suggestion explicit in starting the group as fits her or his style and aids in teaching.

There are, of course, natural limits to the use of circles. A circle of 10–30 participants supplies all its own logistical needs — participants can all see and hear each other easily. From 30 to 50 participants, in our experience, the circle still works, provided the teacher and group maintain attentiveness to the required voice levels. Beyond 50, our preferences are to set one circle within another when using chairs, or to have a circle of chairs and a group seated on the floor within the circle. This does, however, begin to erode the nonhierarchical nature of the group and focuses more attention on the teacher. The use of such larger groups is, therefore, best restricted to applications where delivery of didactic information is a significant proportion of the session — such as introductions, orientations, and short professional trainings.

Responsibility: Turning Towards Each Other

In the first session, particularly, the nonhierarchical nature of the circle is hidden beneath what we might call the *MacDonald effect*. In a much told and much varied folk story from Scotland, the chief of the MacDonald clan arrives late at a gathering and sits in an open seat. He is then invited to come to the head of the table. In response, he proclaims, "Where the MacDonald sits *is* the head of the table." So participants may inevitably see the teacher's seat as the head of the circle, and rest their attention and expectation there. Certainly this effect is useful and flattering in the early moments of the session. Yet, as sessions move on, and mindfulness and intra-subjective resonance are co-created, a continual focus on the teacher becomes counterproductive. It keeps the teacher's status elevated, suggesting this is where to look for answers. Diffusing the focus through the group suggests that the answers lie within the participants.

It is also true that if participants are too much oriented to the teacher's seat, when eyes open after (or during!) mindfulness practice, the resonance of the group is more deeply and directly influenced by *mirror neuron responses to the teacher's nonverbal disposition* than any other factors. Again, this is perhaps of some value in early sessions, but it is best to work to spread out this "responsibility" for group resonance to all participants. As they turn towards each other, the potential of mindfulness and inter-subjective resonance comes to belong less to the teacher (or to the more extroverted participants) and more to the entire group, helping to protect each participant's freedom and belonging.

The teacher can turn participants towards each other directly and indirectly. The direct mode is most applicable in the initial group dialogs. The teacher can simply ask that participants speak to the whole circle, not just to the teacher. The teacher can reinforce this indirectly in the early sessions — and throughout all sessions, as needed — with nonverbal cues. The teacher can acknowledge but then avoid sustained eye contact with the participant who is speaking directly rather than to the group. And the teacher can allow her eyes to continually rove around the circle; embodying the broader focus that is useful in keeping the group together.

The teacher will also help the participants become more comfortable with the shared experience by using dyads and small groups as methods of dialogic exploration whenever possible. Each teacher will develop her own style and rhythm of such usages, yet there are some basic moves. We often ask that participants speak to a dyad partner — a different one each time — for a preliminary dialog on the experience of each mindfulness practice introduced, before bringing the larger group together to continue the dialog. This approach has a number of benefits besides simply "mixing up" the participants, helping them to get to know each other and make personal connections. It also allows participants to bring their nonverbal experience into words in a preliminary way before exploring in the larger group, making that dialog perhaps richer. Further, it provides a platform for those who are reticent to talk in the larger group to have the benefits of bringing their experience into words.

Rifts and Repairs: Working with Reactivity and Aggression

The stewardship of the circle is stewardship of the co-created mindfulness, the inter-subjective resonance of the group. The teacher's skills in this arena are to build it and help the group stay within it to do their work — inner and shared. The resonance is not fragile, yet it can easily be tested, and may diminish considerably under pressure. Such pressures may come from the environment, through dramatic distractions, or from within the group itself, where expansive emotion or conflict may draw attention and undermine resonance.

In working with full or potential rifts in the group resonance, the teacher's tool of stewardship is mindfulness itself. Relying on techniques or tools from outside sends a signal to the group that mindfulness practice is only useful to a point. Therefore, the teacher's "only recourse" is simple: to trust the practice and to use the group.

In the event of an outside distraction, the teacher can call participants' attention to the distraction, reinforcing the essential move of "turning towards" aversive experience. If the distraction is continuing — say, a series of fire engines passing with sirens in the street — the teacher can (in good voice) ask the group to "drop in" to practice and to notice what is arising for them in the moment: then, by making space in which to watch the arising. When the distraction has passed, the group can be engaged in dialog around the experience. In effect, this is "normalizing" the experience by making it simply a part of mindfulness practice.

In working with large emotions arising for an individual in inquiry, or independent of outside stimulus, there is the possibility of many in the group being caught up in emotional contagion and being unable to maintain the resonance that sustains everyone's freedom and belonging. The teacher must, at this point, hold the group, acknowledging what is arising in the moment not just for the individual but for the entire group, and embodying nonjudgment towards the individual and confidence in the practice. The teacher has a number of directions in which she can move — all of which emphasize the workability of the situation and mindfulness. First, she can use the basic physiology of the breath to effect a shift from the stress reaction into the parasympathetic response, by instructing the individual, and those in the group who wish to, to take several deep breaths and release them with a relaxing sigh (see sidebar).

With such a reduction in reactivity, it may then be possible to move to explore the experience in the body, which places the central "turning towards" motion in a venue that is less aversive, and possibly more interesting than directly encountering the emotions or associated thoughts. Working within the body, a dialogic exploration invokes several factors that help to potentiate intra- and inter-subjective resonance and restore the co-created mindfulness of the group. As the teacher inquires with the individual, the movement from aversion to curiosity, reflecting the movement from withdrawal to approach affect associated with mindfulness, can be set in motion. Further, the other participants, some of whom may be practicing with their own emotions and responding to what is happening in the moment for themselves as well, are making that same shift, creating an inter-subjective resonance that supports further turning towards and further exploration. The teacher must also check in from time to time with the other participants, during such work. This, again, helps both the individual and the group, as the individual benefits from comments by the others and the others have a chance to connect with the (we hope!) renewing resonance of the group.

This resonance is illustrated in an exchange in a mindfulness-based stress reduction (MBSR) class (see below), which was stimulated by the teacher simply describing a dyad practice in which participants would each narrate their present moment experience to another — for a minute or two. Note the choices made and directions pursued by the teacher, to repair the rift through mindfulness and to protect the treasures of the group.

THREE PRACTICES FOR WORKING WITH REACTIVITY
In using these three practices during a group session, even if the reactivity resides in one participant, all participants are invited into the practice. This may help sustain or potentiate a deeper inter-subjective resonance, with potential effects on the participant with whom the teacher is working.

Practice 1: Relaxing Sighs. Inhaling through your nose and exhaling through your mouth, making a quiet, relaxing sigh as you exhale. Taking long, slow, gentle breaths that raise and lower your abdomen as you inhale and exhale. Focusing on the sound and feeling of the breath.

This practice is useful when stress reactivity begins — or when it is anticipated. It is also possible to use cues throughout the day to take three to six relaxing sighs, such as red lights while driving, telephone sounds, waiting for elevators, or waiting in line, which helps maintain lowered reactivity.

Practice 2: The Soles of the Feet. In a stressful situation or anticipating a stressful situation, this short practice helps one to come into the present moment in the body, and thereby into a space in which it is possible to make considered choices. This practice was freely adapted from Singh et al. (2003).

The steps

1. If you are sitting, make yourself comfortable, with the soles of both feet on the floor. If you are standing, stand in a natural posture, allowing the weight of the arms to pull the shoulders down, and bending the knees slightly. If you are walking, slow your pace and, again, allow the arms to help relax the shoulders.
2. Allow your breath to flow naturally. And allow yourself to feel the emotions of the moment, being aware of whatever thoughts and body sensations are arising, without restricting or attempting to change them. Simply observe.
3. Then move your attention to the soles of your feet. Feel your heels on the floor or inside your shoes; feel the curves of the arches, the balls of the feet, and the toes — perhaps moving the toes to make them more present in sensation.
4. After a moment or two, notice again the quality of thoughts and body sensations.

The rifts and repairs in the fabric of the inter-subjective resonance help to knit the group more tightly. As noted in Chapter 3, this circumstance is much like the "dyadically expanded states of consciousness" that Tronick (2003, 2007) describes in infant — caregiver dyads and client — therapist dyads. This situation represents the messy process of the co-creation of meaning. As Tronick (2003) suggests, "[O]ut of the recurrence of reparations the infant and another person come to share the implicit knowledge that 'we can move into a mutual positive state even when we have been in a mutual negative state' or 'we can transform negative into positive affect'" (p. 478). This experience of expansion and new meaning is shared not only with the teacher and one individual, but, potentially, equally among participants.

ATTENDING TO RESONANCE

Participant: *I'm confused, I'm anxious…*
Teacher: *Is anything else arising?*

A nonjudgmental, matter-of-fact, and curious response, giving freedom to explore.

P: *Embarrassment… feeling exposed…*

T: *Feeling exposed just thinking about doing this practice — a practice about speaking about what's true for you in the moment.*

Acknowledging the actuality of the participant's situation.

P: *Yes… Feeling sad right now (participant is crying)… I'm feeling confused about why I'm crying so much.*

5. When you feel as if you can respond and not react, remember that you can choose to disengage, or choose to respond with clarity and creativity.

Special considerations in teaching this practice

1. Everyone feels stress and strong emotions. The object of this practice is not to stamp them out but to work with them creatively.
2. In context, the feelings of the moment may hold valuable information that can be used for a positive solution or helpful response.
3. This practice can be rehearsed to gain more confidence in its use by playing scenarios from the past (or the future!) in imagination and working with the emotions and body sensations that are generated just by thought.

Practice 3: The Three-Minute Breathing Space. In stress or anticipating stress, or simply at regular intervals through the day, this practice, freely adapted from Mindfulness-Based Cognitive Therapy (Segal et al., 2002), can be of use.

Minute 1: Awareness. Taking a pause. If you care to, closing your eyes. Bringing your attention to your body: noticing bodily sensations (e.g., heaviness, lightness, temperature, breath rate, heart rate, etc.); then attending to thoughts: is your mind calm? Or are thoughts racing? What's the quality of thought? (e.g., dense, light, fleeting, sticky, etc.); and attending to mood states: how do you feel in the moment? (e.g., peaceful, anxious, joyful, sad, etc.) Acknowledge and register your experience, even if it is unwanted.

Minute 2: Gathering. Then, gently bring your attention to your breathing, to each in-breath and to each out-breath as they follow, one after the other. When your attention is drawn away, noticing that, and gently bringing it back to the breath.

Minute 3: Expanding. Expanding the field of your awareness beyond the breath, back to the sensations in the body, then to thoughts, and then to mood state. Checking in to how it is with you now.

T: *(Opens to the group) Can the rest of you notice what is arising for you in the moment? And is it possible to hold your own place, your own truth?*

Protecting the freedom and belonging of the other participants. Allowing them to have experiences that are the same or very different from the one that is being inquired into.

T: *(To participant, after a pause) What's happening for you now?*

Genuine curiosity.

P: *I'm trying to get control.*

T: *How does that feel?*

With curiosity: potentiating approach emotion, turning towards experience.

P: *Feels like a fight. I'm trying to hold everything back.*

T: *How does that feel in the body?*

Making the exploration easier, more possible, by bringing it out of the abstract and into body sensation.

P: *I'm so tight I can barely breathe.*

T: *In this moment, can you let yourself be with what is here, put down the fight a bit — the fight to hold everything back?*

Offering an exploration. Offering a small step — "a bit" — that may be more possible.

T: *(After a long pause as participant explores.) So, checking in now... what are you noticing?*

P: *I'm calming down.*

T: *How is that in the body?*

Maintaining the body focus to explore the shift taking place with continuity of sensation and expression for both the participant and others.

P: *I can breathe better... and I'm not as tense.*

T: *Anything else?*

As at the start, a nonjudgmental, matter-of-fact, and curious response, giving freedom to explore.

P: *I'm sad about how much I worry about what others think... I've done so many things in my life based on what others may think... (Pausing)*

T: *And now, what's happening?*

Responding to nonverbal cues of further reduction in reactivity.

P: *I'm letting go of some of my fear about being judged. I'm more calm and open. I'm starting to accept what is.*

T: *Interesting that the very thing you were afraid of, voicing your moment to moment experience to another person, you just did with the whole group... I honor your courage...*

Looking around the circle to check in with others and nonverbally prompt them to meet the participant's eyes or respond in some way, reinforcing the reestablished inter-subjective resonance.

Reducing Reactivity: Models for Group Dialog

The core model for group dialog in the MBIs is based not on speaking, but rather on listening. Again, this emphasizes the stewardship and service attributes of the teacher — and of all participants. From the start, they can be invited to listen mindfully to the one who is speaking, watching the state of reactivity within themselves — particularly urges to comment, contradict, "one-up" the other, or "fix" the other with advice or consolation. They are urged to listen first, and speak as much as possible from their own direct experience. The teacher will explain, and participants will come to understand, that this listening, watching, and authentic speaking provides the ideal dialogic environment for exploration. This is also, however, a difficult task. Depending upon the type of group and its unique membership, participants may need help in maintaining such a nonjudgmental, permissive stance.

We have found that the use of a very simple structure that can be remembered (or prompted!) in the moment can be extremely helpful. We have identified, distilled, and successfully use two such models in our work: (1) *subgrouping* as used in Systems Centered Therapy (SCT) (Agazarian, 1999); (2) *council circle,* an adaptation of the models used in indigenous communities, as described, for example, by Zimmerman and Coyle (1996). Both models are complex. There is a committing path of training for SCT, which has a highly elaborated theoretical base, and a number of trainings in the Way of Council as well. Our distilled usage here is meant solely for the context of an MBI group in which participants may benefit from more structure to help them sit with their own reactivity. For pedagogical purposes, we have borrowed the minimum of language and theory from these other models, preferring overwhelmingly to reiterate and reinforce the language and practice of mindfulness as captured in the practice and exploration in which it is co-created for the group. What is most important is that both these models provide a more explicit focus than the "ideal" model, and both allow the teacher to "remind" the participants of the objective "rules," that all must follow. This maintains the nonhierarchical status of the teacher, and reduces the sense of aggression from any necessary interventions.

Subgrouping

The borrowing made from SCT for helping with reactivity has proven both simple and effective. It is based on the theory of human systems premise that as system, a group can only take in a certain level of difference at a time; that too much contradiction or opposition will cause it to lose energy or resonance. This is true, as well, of resonance as we define it. Therefore, it is helpful to the group to explore similarities, to link one participant's experience of the moment with another's, so that their large samenesses and small differences are appreciated and integrated in the process. The participants exploring their similarities form a subgroup, which resonates together and affects both the plenary group and individuals, as described in Chapter 3. Participants who are noticing differences are asked to hold those differences for a time. Then, when the links to similarities have been played out, a difference may be introduced, and the subgrouping around those new similarities may begin. This way, all positions may be explored, while reactivity is contained; the three treasures of freedom, belonging, and resonance are held gently and protected as much as possible.

The directions to the group can be quite simple, and simply need to be reinforced if they are breached. While SCT supplies the discipline of subgrouping, the rest of the instructions are linked directly to mindfulness practice. The three-point instructions to the group might sound like this, beginning with mindfulness practice:

1. As we begin a dialog together, let's work as mindfully as we can, speaking from what is true in the moment, and, as much as possible, communicating your direct experience as you feel the body.
2. When someone brings in their experience, see if it is possible for you to connect with what is said. If you are having a similar experience *in the moment*, you may choose to share your experience too.
3. If you find that your experience is different than the one being explored, simply notice that, and hold your truth while the others explore. Be assured that we will explore different experiences in turn.

Council Circle

Again, this is a minimal borrowing, in which the purpose is to keep the group resonant and workable, and to reinforce the pedagogical intention around mindfulness rather than around technique. To that end, council circle "intentions" can be introduced quickly, summarily, and then reviewed and reinforced on the fly, during practice, with language that is congruent with the co-creation of mindfulness.

The control mechanism for council circle is the talking piece, which is passed from person to person in the circle. It is passed around the circle, and the person who holds it holds all attention. He speaks, the others listen. It is also traditional that the person with the talking piece may "offer silence" to the group; there is never pressure to speak. We emphasize this point to protect participant's freedom. The piece itself can be just about anything; however, our preference is for the teacher's bell.

The four "intentions" of council circle are simple and clear in the few words it takes to name them (Zimmerman and Coyle, 1996). They can then be described in greater detail, using the language of mindfulness teaching. They are:

1. *Speaking from the heart:* That is, speaking the truth of your present-moment experience. This is embodied talk about what you are noticing in the triangle of awareness — body sensations, thinking, and emotion. This is not speculating or trying to "figure out" what is happening, this is reporting mindfully how it is for you now.
2. *Listening from the heart:* This means being present for what is spoken by the other; listening not just with ears and thinking, but with your whole being. Allowing what is said to "sound" within you. Noticing any reactions and responses in body, thought, and emotion. Not to judge (although you probably will!) but simply to know,
3. *Being of "lean expression":* Of course, there's common sense in this of making sure that everyone gets a turn to speak, and that the session can move along. Yet there is also the sense of approaching the experience you're reporting as *new* —

bringing beginner's mind to it. So the discipline is simply to seek what is true for you, without the story or analysis that might stretch it out.

4. *[Trusting] spontaneity:* This follows directly from the other three intentions. Perhaps the most important relationship is to *listening.* Although you may find yourself drawn to rehearse what you are going to say — especially as the talking piece gets close to you! — if you keep returning your attention to the speaker and listen from the heart, your turn will come and you will be in a place to speak from the heart about your direct experience of the moment. What you need to say (or not say) will be there — that is the trust.

Neither SCT nor council circle must be invoked for all dialogs within the group. As the teacher develops a sense of the group and its needs, decisions can be made to introduce one or the other, or some other model of the teacher's choice, for particular purposes and in particular sessions only.

FOR MORE INFORMATION ABOUT SCT AND THE WAY OF COUNCIL

- For descriptions and schedules for training in Systems Centered Theory, visit the Systems Centered Training and Research Institute: http://www.systemscentered.com.
- For descriptions and schedules for training in the Way of Council, visit the Ojai Foundation: http://www.ojaifoundation.org.

Homiletics: Talking *with* the Group

We have chosen to call the skill set associated with delivering important information to participants' *homiletics.* Just as with stewardship, the choice is based on the power of the word's derivation and connotations to convey principles of the pedagogy of mindfulness. The intent is to see beyond the specialized liturgical use of the word — which does set up a certain expectation of speaking of profound truths. The Greek root and related terms, such as *homiletikos,* which means "of conversation, affable," suggest dialog within a group that has assembled for that purpose. So, the teacher's skills in homiletics are not those of a lecturer, but those of one who engages and responds to those assembled together.

At the heart of the pedagogy of mindfulness is co-creation. This co-creation highlights the preference for drawing as much as possible of the material to be used in making teaching points to the group out of the group itself. As Santorelli (2001) describes it from the influential MBSR perspective: "Importantly, rather than 'lecturing' to program participants, the attention and skill of the teacher should be directed towards listening to the rich, information laden insights and examples provided by program participants and then, in turn, to use as much as possible these participant-generated experiences as a starting point for 'weaving' the more didactic material into the structure and fabric of each class." Thus, participant experiences, as they use their creative faculties to bring them into *their own* language, become "texts" in which teacher and participants can in this conversation of homiletics find meaning.

The use of poetic texts, and stories, and children's books has been remarked upon by those who have closely observed homiletics within the context of MBSR (e.g., Baer and Krietemeyer, 2003; Segal, et al., 2002). In fact, such material circulates like currency through the community of teachers. These texts are often a medium of choice for introducing or reinforcing important teaching points. For example, in an early session, a teacher may choose to help to define mindfulness by pointing to the habitual ways of perceiving the world that might be seen as mind*less*ness, and the dramatic shift of focus in mind*ful*ness. This can become much more clear by telling or reading a story, such as this very short one from children's television icon Fred Rogers (2004, p. 187):

> When I was a boy and I would see scary things in the news, my mother would say to me, "Look for the helpers. You will always find people who are helping." To this day, especially in times of "disaster," I remember my mother's words, and I am always comforted by realizing that there are still so many helpers — so many caring people in this world.

The person of the narrator, the intimacy of the mother — child scene, the content of the story and its social and historical resonances, and its radical shift of focus, all contribute to an experience — and a knowing — that engages participants as whole persons.

When the teacher possesses these two types of "texts" — participant experiences and poems or writings that act like a poem — the potential for generating a homily is available. What the teacher says, then, will arise from her authenticity and authority, moderated by friendship.

The authenticity is in the immediate recognition and connection with the participant's experience; the teacher has been there, known it, and may have worked through or may be working through it herself. She has sat with her own loss, her own pain, her own anger, and can speak from those truths. What she offers will be shaped by friendship: it will not be coming from the place of "I know more and I can fix you"; rather it will be a gentle invitation to turn towards experience. Any reassurance will not come from, "It will be all right"; rather it will be the reassurance of her presence — and the resonant presence of the others in the group.

The authority is in the deep understanding of the matter at hand; the teacher knows her curriculum and its dimensions and layers intimately, as if she had created it from whole cloth — which indeed she may have done. Such knowing informs her total experience of the world. As she encounters a poem, a song, a joke, she may find it shining in a way that pulls her — as a practitioner, as a teacher. She becomes a collector of shiny things, for purposes she understands and purposes that are less clear. Yet, in the moment, the opportunity may arise to use such a text in a homily — pithy and from a unique mastery of her own material. Such usages are very much shaped by friendship. Use of these "shiny things" is not a stunt, not meant to show the teacher's erudition; rather it is highly specific and designed to meet participants where they are. It is meant to help catalyze an event for further exploration, or distill it so intensely that it becomes part of the participant's own authority. For example, in workshops or courses for business and professional people, there are two very shiny lines from the first of Wendell Berry's *Sabbath Poems* (1998) that

become part of the co-construction of mindfulness in the group. They are rel-
ished, rolled on the tongue, and carried off into life by many. They are the last two
of the first stanza; perhaps the effect is there for you, too:

> I go among trees and sit still.
> All my stirring becomes quiet
> around me like circles on water.
> My tasks lie in their places
> where I left them, asleep like cattle.

Three Kinds of Homiletic Tasks

Throughout a course or workshop, the teacher responds by speaking from one or
another of these two kinds of texts, depending on the task she is facing.

The first task is actually the least common but the largest in scope. Within the
curricula of the MBIs, there are modules that require a teacher to provide infor-
mational content that cannot be drawn easily from the group — say, the principles
of stress physiology. Such homiletic tasks require significant authority. The
details of the stress reaction are in a sense a major text in MBSR, as are the details
of depressive relapse in mindfulness-based cognitive therapy (MBCT). The teacher
must master these details in order that she or he may work in the free-est of conversational styles.

New and developing teachers should see this requirement as aspirational
rather than an immediate demand. One very helpful way of moving towards the
ultimately free ways of working through engagement is to first develop brief,
clear, and memorable presentations that engage the triangle of awareness — sensation, thought, and emotion, and delivering them to the group as interactively
as possible. It may be helpful at this early stage to use very basic speaker support
— such as a prepared flipchart or, if the space is technologically equipped, a
simple, concise computer slide presentation. As the teacher practices and refines
the presentation, the material becomes more and more her or his own — it thus
becomes authoritative. This authority is much less about memorization and
developing turns of phrase, and much more about becoming comfortable with
content and principles. Then, with such "broken in" knowledge and material, the
teacher may choose to work in freer and freer ways.

The second task is more common, happening at least once in every session. It
is, however, no less challenging to the teacher, as it requires organization and presentation of material not always available within the group. This task is the introduction of a new practice, or an introduction meant to expand participants'
understandings of an established practice. The teacher must approach the practice
with beginner's mind, to discern what participants most need to know in order to
make their experience valuable for them, not simply in session but over time. The
information to be delivered may best be offered in conversation, yet, this means
the teacher must have all teaching points at her or his command at every moment

— to respond to participant comments and questions, but also to come back to what has been forgotten or overlooked.

Here again, this undertaking requires significant time and effort. The new or developing teacher can make a start by offering brief, well-organized, prepared talks touching on the most important points. Such a talk can be supported by sparse notes that can be read from a distance — in the lap, on the floor. An optimum format is a single sheet of paper or index card that merely provides keyword prompts. Use of such a system ensures organization and completeness, while ensuring as well a fresh, improvised quality of language. Repeated use of such a system will allow the teacher to get free of the support — the key words or concepts are easily available for use in more conversational style. How this might work for a teacher is demonstrated in this short talk below, aimed to introduce the practice of sitting meditation at the most concrete level. The keywords in bold type would be the total support for the teacher. Note how the entire structure is captured in the three words that generate the first paragraph.

AN INTRODUCTION TO SITTING MEDITATION

Place, time, and attitude.
As you begin a personal practice of mindfulness meditation, there are three essential factors that can support it... place... time... and attitude. Working together, these three can help establish and maintain a regular connection with the practice — and with yourself...
Place: Comfortable, just yours, furnished for support.
Choosing a comfortable place where you will not be interrupted by other people, the telephone, or even pets. A space that can be just yours for the time of your practice; a place furnished in a way that makes you comfortable, including a straight backed chair or cushions on the floor that will support you sitting still ...
Time: Built in, not fit in. For being, not doing.
Finding a regular time... a time that can be "built into" rather than "fit into" the day... perhaps it can even be put on your calendar... yet it's a different kind of time... not a time to take on a role or act in a particular way... rather it's a time set aside for not doing, for simply being...
Attitude: Commitment and kindness. Motivation and patience. Serious and gentle.
Assuming an attitude that balances deep commitment to the practice with a deep kindness toward yourself... that balances motivation and patience... put another way, be serious about showing up, and be gentle when you get there...
Remember nonjudgment!
Remembering that mindfulness is paying attention on purpose, in the present moment, and without judgment...

Working with the poetic type of text also provides many benefits for new and developing teachers in these introductory homiletic tasks. Just as the deliberate organization of material in the talk above assists the teacher over time in making it part of her authority and allowing greater capacity for improvisation, so the use of poetic texts offers a platform for internalization, perhaps even memorization of the text, to enhance spontaneity and conversational talk. And there is a further benefit in that the page on which the text is printed can hold the keywords for your talk. The short example talk in italics below might be used in an early session to help participants connect more gently and solidly to the breath in practice.

The practice of awareness of the breath is actually very subtle and tender. You are connecting to something both simple and profound. It is a force that touches all who live — and all who have lived and all who will live. The poet Rilke captures this force in one of his Sonnets to Orpheus:

Breathing: you invisible poem! Complete interchange of our own
essence with world-space. You counterweight
in which I rhythmically happen.

Single wave-motion whose
gradual sea I am:
you, most inclusive of all our possible seas —
space has grown warm.

How many regions in space have already been inside me. There are winds that seem like my wandering son.

Do you recognize me, air, full of places I once absorbed?
You who were the smooth bark,
roundness, and leaf of my words.

(Rilke/Mitchell, 1923/1985)

So, as you practice, is it possible just to allow that connection to the breath? Without struggle, without need to change or improve the experience... Can the breath simply take you and hold you? Can you just rhythmically happen?

Of course, the teacher may also offer the text with no direction or commentary. She can rely on the teaching potential of the text and her own intuition in its choice to touch participants, trusting in their freedom to derive what benefit they can from it.

The third homiletic task is the most common, arising many times during a session. This task is the most clearly conversational, and the most challenging of the tasks. As participants bring their experience into language, the

BEING HEARD: THE DEVELOPMENT AND CARE OF THE TEACHER'S VOICE

The voice is one of the teacher's most important tools. Control of volume, tone, and articulation make a difference in homiletics, guidance, and inquiry, whether speaking to ten participants or fifty around the circle. In many different circumstances, much would be required of the new teacher to develop vocal capacity. In the MBIs, however, teachers have a head start.

The platform for the voice is the breath. Attending to breath, being intimate with breath, is central to the teacher's practice of mindfulness. In vocal training (e.g., Linklater, 1976; Rodenburg, 2000), being centered in the body and allowing the breath to flow easily is a key to working with the voice; gaining flexibility, volume, and resonance. The many exercises include lying on the back on the floor and observing the breath, or learning to sit and stand with easy alignment of the spine with gravity, so that the breath is unimpeded. Perhaps that sounds familiar?

The teacher's body-centered practices are also highly congruent with the physical exercises of vocal training. The standing yoga stretches of MBSR are of a piece with an actor's warm up. In fact, the rolling up and rolling down of the spine — bending from the waist, hanging down, and coming again to vertical — by itself makes a good warm up before speaking to a large group. All the body-centered disciplines — Hatha Yoga, Tai Chi, Qi Gong, etc. — in their joining of breath to movement help develop the breath as platform for the voice.

What is often missing in the mindfulness practices, of course, is production of sound. It is, however, possible to add just one simple sound to the teacher may choose to respond by drawing out a teaching point that may be directed to the group. Thus, a general talk arises from a specific encounter. This is significantly dependent on the teacher's authenticity, her capacity to recognize what is important and generalizable in a participant's experience, and to make something from it that has appeal and potential impact for the other participants. In this task, there is no possibility of sketching, organizing, writing down key words; no possibility of learning for later. The teacher simply responds from her authenticity, with a friendship that makes her want to share some point or insight with the entire group.

The example below is a straightforward demonstration of the shift from an individual conversation to general information and direct engagement with the entire group. It comes from

work you may already be doing — humming — and through that to find gains in vocal ability. In the sensory awareness tradition, a Western mindfulness practice, humming is recommended as a way of experimenting with the breath (Speads, 1992). Humming on the out breath: letting the breath out through the nostrils, with lips closed, and vibrating the vocal folds (vocal cords) in a steady *mmmmmmm* sound. No forcing, no pressing, just allowing the breath to take its course and the hum to end with the breath. Then checking in to see its effect on the breaths that follow. As breathing settles again, add another hum. Gently, reflectively, working with sound. When this way of working becomes more comfortable, vowel sounds can me added: *mmmaaa, mmmeee, mmmooo, mmmuuu*, and the like. Pitch can be shifted as well, to explore further. Carola Speads notes (1992, p. 96), "Teachers, actors, singers, and musicians have greatly profited from these experiments. Your ordinary speaking voice will markedly improve. Voices tend to become fuller, more resonant, carry better, and are often considerably deeper in pitch."

the second session of an MBSR course, at the completion of a sitting meditation. In session two, participants are beginning to grasp the power of turning towards, and are also sensing the profound shift that nonjudging and beginner's mind can bring to experience.

A TALK ARISES FROM AN ENCOUNTER

Participant: *I hated every minute of sitting there. Well, not every minute, because when you said to not react immediately to discomfort, my foot was just starting to fall asleep. So I didn't move. And it actually feels really good when your foot starts to go to sleep. It's very warm and nice.*

Teacher: *Wow. You just turned right towards what was happening. And you found out something you would never have learned any other way than by observing mindfully... (Broadly) This takes us right back to the definition of mindfulness as paying attention, on purpose, in the present moment, without judgment... So much can come out of our willingness to just be with what is happening now. Things may be very different than what we anticipate or what they seem when we've named them and "dealt with" them — that is, dismissed them. Tom might have said, "Oh, I know what this feeling is, and where it's going." He could have missed that nice warm feeling in his foot. Maybe it could interest you to use this as a metaphor for your informal practice this week. How often do you* think *you know what's happening or what's about to happen? If you do, what are you missing out on? Could you leave just a little space open this week to see what your experience might really be?*

Guidance: Not Performance but Connection

Teachers guide meditations "live" in the room where participants often have their eyes closed, and via audio recordings supplied to participants for home practice. This suggests just how much the skill of guidance is dependent on communication in the verbal realm. Effective meditation guidance requires control of four interdependent dimensions: languaging, allowing, orienting, and embodying.

Languaging

This is concerned with the impact that word choice and syntactic structures can have on participants' experiences of mindfulness practice. There are several ways of considering this, and each generates a certain style.

In MBSR, teachers are trained through the Center for Mindfulness to guide meditation. Kabat-Zinn (2004) has analyzed the use of language in guidance and developed a particular style meant to support mindfulness teaching and to get around resistances — particularly to authority — that many participants may have. He identifies four problems that can be introduced through verbal and nonverbal communication, and that can "generate resistance" in participants, or "create more waves in the thought structure": (1) striving, as in "if you did this long enough, you'd be better"; (2) idealizing, as in "I know how to do this and I'm going to teach you"; (3) fixing, as in the implication that something is wrong with you that meditation is addressing; and (4) dualism, as in language that suggests that there is an observed and an observer. As to what kind of language to use, specifically, Kabat-Zinn notes that nobody likes a command — that the teacher should instead make suggestions. For example, rather than say "Breathe in," which can lead to a "who-are-you-to-tell-me-what-to-do" reaction, one could say, "When you're ready, *breathing* in..." The use of the present participle rather than the imperative minimizes the teacher–participant hierarchy, eliminates the subject-object distinction, emphasizes the present-moment experience, and possibly elicits inquiry into just who or what is breathing. The teacher can also create space for exploration and reflection by using the definitive article rather than a possessive pronoun, saying, for example, "lifting *the* right leg" rather than "lifting *your* right leg." Kabat-Zinn (2004) advises that such rules should not be held too tightly, however, as too much use of the present participle can become distracting, while too much distancing through the definitive article may result in a he's-not-talking-to-me reaction.

Following is the beginning of an awareness of breath meditation using the MBSR style of languaging. Noting specifically the use of the present participle, the definitive article, and the balance struck.

AN INTRODUCTION TO SITTING MEDITATION

Beginning by taking a seat... bringing the body to an upright and dignified posture in a chair or on a cushion on the floor...

Aware of the weight distributed in a stable base... on the feet and the thighs and buttocks if you're sitting on a chair... or on the buttocks on a cushion and legs, knees, and feet on the floor...

Allowing the torso to rest on this base, without effort... not straining against gravity... aligned with gravity... letting the earth hold you... Perhaps rocking back and forth and side to side slightly to find that point of comfort, that sense of being centered...

Feeling the sense of the body sitting, noticing perhaps pressure, or temperature, the sensation of air moving, or clothes against the skin... noticing the feeling of the hands, wherever they rest on your thighs or in your lap... aware of the face, relaxing tension, allowing the jaw to drop down in an easy way, the teeth apart, the lips closed...

Bringing the attention to breathing... to the breath entering the body and leaving the body... aware of sensations at the nostrils, in the sinuses, the mouth and throat... maybe noticing the motions of the chest, expansion and contraction... or the rising and falling of the abdomen... you may be aware as well of other, subtle sensations in other parts of the body... Wherever the sensation of the breath is most vivid for you in the body, focusing your attention there...

Another approach to languaging that supports or impels mindfulness is heard in sensory awareness (e.g., Littlewood and Roche, 2004). There are two essential elements to it: permissiveness and questioning. That is, there is a radical freedom granted to explore and find whatever might be available in the realm of sensory experience. Nothing is certain; anything might be discovered. The other feature is a questioning that is not meant to find answers but to spur attention, to catalyze curiosity. A question during walking such as "Can you feel the floor beneath you?" does not so much pull participants into their heads as take them closer to their feet. A question such as "How is the breath responding to this moment?" has as many answers as hearers, and often results in a deepening of attention.

There are precise physical sensations associated with the breath... can you be curious about how the breath actually feels in this moment?... not some thought or idea about breathing, but the experience of the breath itself...

Maybe it's possible to be aware of the breath from the very beginning of an in-breath to the shift, the change, the pause as it turns around and becomes an out-breath... and can you follow from the very beginning of the out-breath to the moment it turns around to become an in-breath again?...

Just sensing the breath in its simple cycle... can you give up the need to control it, change it, or even think about it?... just let in-breath follow out-breath follow in-breath... the breath breathing the body, breathing itself... a process worthy of our trust... and of our attention... (Long pause)

Certainly, these styles can be used together, to provide greater variety and to fit the specific needs of the practice in the moment. That blend might look something like this continuation of the same meditation.

Is it possible to connect with your attention right now? Perhaps it's on the breath, or it may have wandered off following some chain of thought, some story, some emotion, or some other sensation elsewhere in the body... If it has wandered off, knowing that this is quite normal... So with a sense of kindness towards yourself, gently, yet firmly, turning your attention back towards the breath... towards the in-breath or out-breath as it is in this moment... Maybe allowing the breath to be the center of your attention, and letting thoughts, emotions, other sensations be at the outside of your awareness... on the margins... (Long pause)

Where is your attention now? If it's wandered, gently bringing it back to the breath...

Allowing

Of central concern in the pedagogy of mindfulness is ensuring that each participant feels free to have his or her own experience, not some "required" experience specified by the teacher or the group. Allowing is critical, because it encompasses a paradox for the teacher: when one can bring detail and specificity moment by moment into the guidance, participants connect well with the practice, yet each person will be having a unique experience. Teachers find balance by offering a range of choices, and by couching suggestions in tentative phrases. For instance, in guiding a body scan, the teacher may ask participants to focus on the forehead by saying, "Noticing any tightness or softness in the muscles...perhaps there's tingling, or maybe the sensation of the air moving in the room is available to you... or maybe there's no sensation available at all — and that's OK; that's simply your experience in this moment...." Such a construction offers permission for whatever arises, encouragement for exploration beyond habitual responses, and unconditional acceptance of any outcome.

Orienting

Here, again, the teacher faces a paradox. Mindfulness practice makes all of one's experience available as it arises moment by moment, which suggests that the search for organizing concepts or narrative runs counter to practice. Participants are urged to "drop the story" and return the attention to what is arising in the moment. And yet, as they are guided in mindfulness practices, particularly in the early classes, participants need to sense coherence and direction to feel enough safety and security to go on with a practice that is so very different from the ways they typically experience themselves and the world.

PREFERRED PRACTICES: TEACHERS AND PARTICIPANTS ARE NOT LOOK-ALIKES

In thinking about *allowing*, it is important to remember that not all participants will connect to the same practices. Indeed, some will have great difficulty connecting at all. More important still is to remember that teachers have different preferences and needs from their participant groups. Some preliminary work done in this area (McCown et al., 2007), with cohorts of 25 MBSR teachers and 100 participants, suggests that the differences could be significant to pedagogy, if teachers are not aware of them. Teachers may tend particularly to underestimate the attraction of the body scan, or overestimate the appeal of yoga for participants (Fig. 5.2). In the figure, "Love" refers to loving kindness meditation, and "Mtn" refers to mountain meditation.

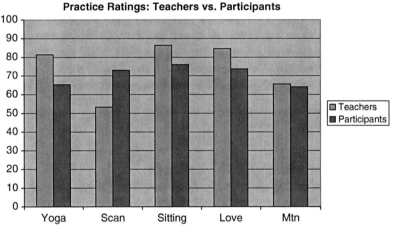

Fig. 5.2 *Preferred practices: teachers and participants are not look-alikes.*

This means the teacher needs to use some form of organizing principle for the guidance to be acceptable. Some practices have an inherent narrative shape. For example, the body scan journeys through sensations of the body sequentially, from head to foot or vice versa. Mindful movement practices such as Hatha Yoga or Qi Gong have inherent structures, both in the individual postures, and in potential sequencing. Sitting meditations may have a "narrative arc," as in an expanding awareness meditation that sequentially opens to experience in the domains of breath, body sensation, sound, thought, and emotion, leading to choiceless awareness of what arises in the present moment in any domain.

Other meditations may have no inherent organizing principle, such as a single focus on awareness of breathing, or the practice of choiceless awareness. Guiding such meditations requires an approach to language that has coherence and integrity. It is an essential skill for a teacher to be able to create purely verbal constructions that provide a secure base from which participants may explore. There are three basic strategies that can create this kind of coherence and safety, and that can be used to help integrate guidance of any type of practice.

First is a simple refrain, a recurring construction that suggests some stability in the flow of experience. For example, in a choiceless awareness meditation, the repeated question "Where is your attention in this moment?" will bring participants back to their direct experience.

Second is the ongoing elaboration or blossoming of a concept. The teacher may introduce a useful principle for practice and then, as the meditation continues, expand its definition and describe different times and reasons for bringing it into one's practice. For example, in an awareness of breath meditation, the teacher could introduce the principle of kindness towards oneself, and then elaborate the practice of cultivating a loving response towards one's own distractions throughout the guidance — working with coming back gently, without struggle or self-blame, when the mind wanders from the breath.

Third is the incorporation of moment-to-moment events in the environment into the flow of the guidance. For example, in the large city, large institution context in which the authors teach, street-level tumult such as sirens or jackhammers, hallway happenings from rumbling carts to whispered conversations, even the undependability of heating and air conditioning can be noted and offered to the group — "What's happening within you as that siren sounds nearer and nearer?" These basic strategies can be combined creatively to improve guidance for any specific practice, for any specific group.

Embodying

This is the most critical dimension of guidance: the connection of the teacher to her own practice while speaking. Guiding a meditation is not an empty performance; the teacher herself is engaged with the practice from moment to moment as she speaks. The verbal constructions she creates are thereby rooted in her experience. Her strategies of orienting are not abstract, but arise from experience; the blossoming of a term or concept is a description of the teacher's own observations, both immediate and remembered. She incorporates what arises in the shared environment, using herself as a sensing instrument, yet allowing for the infinite range of potential subjective experiences of the participants. The importance of embodying to effective guidance cannot be overstressed. In training and development of new teachers, it is quite easy to perceive whether a teacher is "dropped in" to the practice she is guiding; the listener will have a felt sense of authenticity when the connection is there. Word choice, tone of voice, and confidence of expression, all reflect authenticity when the teacher is embodying the practice, and all help to shape participants' experiences.

Recorded Guidance

Audio recordings of mindfulness practices are significantly different from the practices led in session. Much more depends on the languaging, and there is no influence of context and inter-subjective resonance (except what each participant may carry with them in their co-created mindfulness). This means that recordings need to be scripted (in a sense), reviewed, and revised before they are completed and produced. Languaging must be distilled and clear. Because each practice will be heard many times, the information may be "thicker" than in a session guidance, so that participants may hear things that seem new to them at different times.

Allowing is intensified, too, as the practice will be repeated many times. It must be clear that the participant is free to have whatever experience is arising, this day, this moment.

Options for orienting are reduced, in that connecting to the present moment in the environment is not possible. Further, there is a sense in which the recording, heard many times, actually becomes the narrative arc, by default. This is important to take into account, and to ensure the greatest level of allowing language, to help participants stay fresh.

Embodiment is of utmost importance, because context is reduced. The nonverbal dimensions of the teacher's vocal delivery must carry the context, co-creation of mindfulness, and the sense of inter-subjective resonance. All are more likely to be perceived by the participant when the teacher is actually doing the practice — rather than recording a script.

So, the script must be tight and planned through, as can be seen in the sample scripts in Chapter 8. Once scripting is complete, it must be let go of in the moment of recording to follow what is alive in the moment. Note that the teacher actually does the practices as they are recorded. The body scan may be recorded from a lying down posture, while microphone placement for body-centered practice like Hatha Yoga or Qi Gong may require the teacher to connect to the practice in imagination more than in actual motion — although motion can be helpful in maintaining connection.

For the recording process, a professional studio would provide the highest possible quality. However, with a minimal investment in equipment and software, good-quality recordings may be made in any quiet space. What's required is a computer with a sound-recording program (it can be simple and inexpensive; only one track is necessary), a good-quality vocal microphone (visit a music store and be prepared to spend from $100 to $300), a microphone stand (preferably one that allows many different adjustments of angle), and a microphone preamplifier and computer interface.

CDs can be duplicated professionally from such recordings. It is useful to ask the duplication company to balance sound levels from practice to practice. This is easily done, provided recordings are made on a single track.

SCRIPTS FOR RECORDING: TIME AND RHYTHM

A big challenge in preparing scripts for recording is to get the timing right. If you're targeting a 45-minute or a 20-minute length, how can you be sure you'll hit it, especially as much, if not most, of the recording is silent? Like scoring music, for our own use, we developed a punctuation and notation system, based on the breath, that creates a sense of structure and timing. A breath is measured as the full cycle of in and out breath when the teacher is "dropped in" to the practice he is guiding. So the notation looks like this:

(…) = one breath
Paragraph break = two breaths
(pause) = three breaths
(long pause) = six breaths

Anything longer can be noted in combinations or multiples of these. In this usage, each breath has a time value of about 10 seconds, which makes a *pause* 30 seconds and a *long pause* one minute. Knowing this, it is possible to estimate the length of a script and to adjust timing without having to perform and time the entire script a number of times. As noted already, the fresher the reading can be, the better. Bob Dylan often sang his lyrics for the first time at the recording session, which gave the phrasing an uncertain but energetic quality, and preferred to use the first take.

Inquiring: Curiosity About Participants' Experiences

Much of the transformative effect of the MBIs may be potentiated by dialogic encounters with participants in the group. Santorelli (2001) states: "It is recommended that a significant amount of time in each class be dedicated to an exploration of the participants' experience of the formal and informal mindfulness practices and other weekly home assignments." This is an extremely important and dynamic element in participants' experiences in the MBIs that has not been adequately addressed as part of the process in empirical research.

Such dialog between participant and teacher in the group space can assist especially in potentiating the teaching intentions of "cultivating observation" and "moving towards acceptance" as described in Chapters 6 and 7. Teacher-participant dialog is an "inquiry" into the participant's subjective experience — his or her pre-semantic knowing in the moment — with an intention to make more conscious meanings that are then available for further investigation. The skill of the teacher in such an undertaking is directly tied to stewardship of the three treasures. The teacher needs to ensure the participant's freedom, by simply being available and genuinely interested in the participant's experience. She needs to protect the participant's sense of belonging by making sure he sees that he is not "on the hot seat" but rather is helping others do their own exploration. And she needs to be attentive to the inter-subjective resonance of the group, maintaining it to support the inquiry process.

Inquiry, from the teacher's perspective, is a meeting of two subjectivities in which neither assumes an expert position and both are able to work from a "not knowing" position to explore the fullness of possibilities for meaning. To be most helpful in inquiry with participants, a teacher works from (1) a philosophical approach to inquiry that supports a "not knowing" position, (2) an awareness of the cultural and individual resistances to inquiry that may be present, (3) a willingness to abandon language and return to experience and tacit knowing when dialog ceases to generate meaning, and (4) a capacity to remain open to the outcome of any exchange with a participant or the group.

Philosophical Approaches

Batchelor's (1997) attempt to re-imagine the Buddhist teacher for the contemporary West in terms of "friendship" provides a telling parallel to the role of the adult educator as described by Mezirow (2000). Both Buddhist thought and the discipline of transformative education have been major influences on the philosophy of MBSR pedagogy. Batchelor, from the student's perspective, imagines teachers this way (1997, pp. 50–51):

> These friends are teachers in the sense that they are skilled in the art of learning from every situation. We do not seek perfection in these friends but rather heartfelt acceptance of human imperfection. Nor omniscience but an ironic admission of ignorance.... For true friends seek not to coerce us, even gently and reasonably, into believing what we are unsure

of. These friends are like midwives, who draw forth what is waiting to be born. Their task is not to make themselves indispensable but redundant.

Mezirow (2000, pp. 26–27), speaking from the teacher's perspective, uses the term "discourse" in much the same way we are using "inquiry" here:

> Discourse is the process in which we have an active dialogue with others to better understand the meaning of an experience…. Fostering discourse, with a determined effort to free participation from distortions by power and influence, is a long established priority of adult educators. The generally accepted model of adult education involves a transfer of authority from the educator to the learners; the successful educator works herself out of a job as educator and becomes a collaborative learner.

Both assert the importance of a nonhierarchical relationship, the necessity of a shared stance of not-knowing, the power of the action of "drawing out" the tacit knowing of the participant, and the measurement of the teacher's success as found, ultimately, in the diminishment of her status.

Cultural and Individual Resistances

Given the dominant "banking" model of education, in which students are waiting for teachers to deposit knowledge into them, the initial encounters of inquiry may frustrate participants. There is security in the teacher as expert; there is fear in being one's own authority. Overcoming the attendant resistance to inquiry becomes an informal mindfulness practice for participants: they must become aware of, and transform, the lifetime habits of the banking model — working at staying open to their own insights. The teacher's role in this is to bring compassionate curiosity and nonjudgment to the encounter, particularly a capacity to withstand the urges to "fix" or give advice and instead to stand with the participant in a space where meaning may unfold. As is so often true, what is required of the teacher is an embodiment of mindfulness. The teacher's authentic presence reciprocally supports participants' capacities to not know, to not fix, and to stand with/in their own experiences, which may lead to insights.

Language and Experience

It is often the case that an inquiry dialog can help a participant bring their pre-semantic experience of formal or informal mindfulness practice increasingly into consciousness through language. The teacher's genuine curiosity and unassuming presence (that is, being present with no assumptions) may be expressed in very simple questions about an experience, such as "What was it like for you?" This may generate a tentative response. Further open-ended exploration — "Can you say more about that?" or "Is there more that you've noticed?" — requires reflection and an engagement with language that helps the participant towards greater understanding. For example, a participant described his experience with the body scan by saying, "I feel more connected somehow." The question from the teacher, "More connected to what?", provided the impetus and the space for deeper recognition: "More connected to myself and my family and other people," and then a long pause, followed by, "But mostly to myself. That's what's really different." In one way, perhaps that's simply a new shade of meaning; in another way, though, it is a profound recognition of a gulf of experience never before bridged. During such an exchange, the other participants in the group are both witnesses to one person's changing perspective and participants in their own reflections and recognitions. Inquiry is shared work supported by inter-subjective resonance.

Often an inquiry dialog can lead to confusion rather than clarity. At such a point the teacher may suggest that the participant move back into a formal mindfulness practice for further pre-semantic exploration of sensation, thought, and emotion. Such re-visiting often opens again to greater emotional intensity and dialog about direct experience. Therefore, teachers proceed cautiously with the participant and the rest of the group, asking if the participant would like to work more in this way, and inviting the group both to witness the inquiry and participate in their own "inner" dialog if that seems potentially useful for them. The toggling back and forth between pre-semantic experience and open dialog with the teacher can clarify an experience and its meaning. What is required of the teacher in such encounters is simply stewardship, manifested as a willingness to go only where the participant is willing to go, and a sensitivity to the needs of both the participant and the rest of the group.

CATALYZING CURIOSITY TO DEEPEN AN INQUIRY

Curiosity is the key to inquiry. At one level, it more deeply engages the participant with her or his direct experience. At another, it actually helps to shift reactivity — moving away from the withdrawal mode of fear or the stress reaction, and into the approach emotions in which much more experience is available for exploration.

Although the teacher and participant are free to move in any direction at any time, the teacher does have two directions that can be quite useful in the inquiry process. First is to refer the participant directly to the embodied experience of the moment. This referral makes a significant amount of data available for the exploration and in itself deepens the inquiry. Whether the inquiry is about physical pain, uncomfortable thoughts, or difficult emotions, the direction to explore body sensation is often a counter movement to what the participant is hoping for — inquiry is a turning-towards. The question the teacher asks is something like, "Would you be willing to work with this in the body?", which preserves the participant's freedom.

As this type of exploration often rubs against the grain of a participant's desired experience, the teacher can help to further catalyze curiosity and make approach easier by asking specific questions that require turning towards the experience and looking again. Thus, a direct question about a pain — "What is it like for you?" — may yield general information as the participant looks and turns away. "How would you describe it — is it sharp, dull, hot, pulsing?" requires further encounter and yields more data for inquiry. Such questioning can be used to keep the participant turned in the direction of his experience — "Does it have a color?" "A shape?" "Is it always the same?" — each exploration and answer brings more data to the inquiry, shaping and reshaping it.

The intention is not resolution, not relief, but knowledge — of what the experience is like in the moment, and, most important, knowledge that the participant *can* turn towards his experience and be with and in it. The teacher might note: "So it was hard to go there, hard to look at your pain at first, and yet, look how long you were able to explore it without moving away."

Openness to outcome

Inquiry is an invitation to the innate wisdom of the other to show itself, to be known in experience and language. When this spirit of invitation is embodied by the teacher, and supported in the group, it also may become a way of being for the participant (and many in the group). Valuable dialog may take place, yet the value is not simply in the particular insight or construction of experience in language. The value is in loosening the grip of habits of thought, patterns of reaction, and rigid self-concepts.

The potential of inquiry is a new capacity for freedom that is well described in Carse's (1986) metaphor of finite and infinite games. Finite games have specific rules, so that we know what the game is and how to win by defeating others. Infinite games have ever-changing rules, so that we can continue play indefinitely without zero-sum outcomes. At its best, inquiry takes the teacher, participant, and class into the realm of continual play, which can result in epiphanies that may be ongoing, or in planting seeds that may grow in later classes (or years), or in simply going nowhere while maintaining play. No one fails, everyone benefits.

Further, the teacher has no fixed role in the infinite version of the inquiry game. Particularly as participants come to own their co-created mindfulness and resonance, it may be possible for them to inquire on their own, either in "internal" dialog, or with one another.

The following transcript of an inquiry dialog comes from the sixth session of an MBSR course, so the participants have developed a capacity to work individually in internal and/or external dialog. The class has some experience in holding its resonance to support the participant who is engaged in inquiry. This moment comes during the check-in after the opening meditation practice.

PARTICIPANT: *I have had this pain in my jaw for eight or nine years now. My pain doesn't go away. I feel like I can't stand it. I cannot say just let it be there, be kind to it. It requires so much patience. I don't know if I can do it. I doubt that I can be mindful.*

TEACHER: *Are you noticing pain as you sit here?*

Referring the participant to the experience of the present moment, moving away from the eight or nine years of story.

P: *Yes. It's not too bad but it is there, it's constantly there and it gets worse and becomes unbearable. Even when I try not to clench my muscles, somehow they clench. It hurts a lot.*

More data has become available; still entwined in the story of the years.

T: *So what's arising now is pain in your jaw that is not too bad in this moment, and doubt that you can be with this mindfully. Doubting that you have patience to be with the pain. But you have managed somehow with this for years.*

Pointing to present moment experience first, then acknowledging the story of "managing" the pain.

P: *A miserable managing...*

T: *Are you willing to go within and notice what is happening in this moment, to work with this a bit right now, turn toward what is here, and explore mindfully?*

Making the invitation; tending to the participant's freedom.

P: *Yes...*

T: (to class) *I invite each of you, if you care to, to be present with Hope as she explores her experience... to include in your awareness whatever is arising for you moment to moment.*

Extending the invitation: stewardship of the group's three treasures — freedom, belonging, and resonance.

T: (to Hope) *What do you notice now as you check into your body — sensations in the body?*

Turning towards the experience.

P: *My jaw hurts.*

The general information of a tentative "peek" at the experience.

T: *Can you describe the sensation?*

Asking for more specificity; catalyzing curiosity.

P: *It's like a warm penetrating circle. There are times when it gets so unbearable.*

Moving from looking closely to pulling away into the story.

T: *There are times when it gets unbearable but right now are the sensations unbearable?*

Directing back to the moment, the body.

P: *I think the longevity of this situation is so unbearable I can't help feeling aggravated by it. I can't stand it. I try to notice, not to judge, but it doesn't matter... It's always there.*

Staying with the story; staying away from the bodily experience.

T: *So you have certain thoughts about this pain: "It is unbearable," "I can't stand it," "It's always there"...(pausing) Feeling the area of the jaw now, in this moment what do you notice?*

Acknowledging the story, the thoughts, then redirecting to the body.

P: *It's warm... I feel like it may grow (hands tightening, face tightening)*

T: *So the sensation is warm and the thought is that it may grow — a thought about the future, the possibility that the pain may worsen...*

Acknowledging the turning towards and the shift into story.

P: *I'm scared...*

T: *So you are noticing that you are scared... (long pause)... Where do you feel fear in the body in the moment?*

Acknowledging the fear and being present with the participant before redirecting to the experience in the body.

P: *In my shoulders, they are squeezed... I feel tension, the pain may grow bigger...*

Moving onto the body for information, then away.

T: *So you are feeling tension in the shoulders, feeling squeezed and you are thinking about the future, worrying that the pain may get worse... See if you can bring your attention directly into the body, being with sensations...*

Acknowledging; pointing out the difference between feeling and thought. Protecting freedom (see if you can) while directing attention into the body.

P: *My shoulders are tight.*

Data without a story.

T: *Anything else?*

Gently working with the curiosity in the moment.

P: *My face is tight... The pain in my jaw is more intense.*

T: *What has happened to the warm spot?*

Genuine curiosity.

P: *It is sharper, a sharp pain, more intense...*

T: *Can you stay with it?*

Tending freedom; encouraging.

P: *I am wondering if my posture makes it worse.*

Moving into thought and story once again.

T: *Tension may contribute to your pain. It's very natural to want to know what makes pain better or worse. For now can you stay with body sensations?*

Acknowledging the interest, yet encouraging the turning towards.

P: *The pain moved down, it's moving and shifting.*

T: *So it does not stay the same? It's not static? It changes... Is it possible for you to make space for this pain to move and shift?*

Offering an expanded area for exploration.

P: *NO!*

T: *What does that "NO" feel like in the body?*

Acknowledging; tending freedom; offering continued exploration.

P: *(Crossing hands over chest, making fists, crouching inward) Contracted and tight...*
T: *What is happening in your jaw as you contract?*

Genuine curiosity; a return to the exploration.

P: *The pain is getting worse. I want to say bad words about it — F words...*
T: *Are you noticing any emotions in the moment?*

Genuine curiosity.

P: *I felt sad before, but now I feel like I repress my emotions.*
T: *How does it feel in the body when you repress, stuff your emotions? (Turning to class, asking rhetorically) How does it feel for you when you stuff emotions?*

Tending to resonance; keeping curiosity going.

P: *I feel more tension, feel like I am getting squeezed.*
T: *In this moment are you feeling pain in your jaw?*

Returning to the exploration.

P: *Yes. It's there. I Don't Like It!!*
T: *You don't like it. And right now the pain is here. What happens when I say that this is the way it is in this moment?*

Offering the "truth" of the moment.

P: *I say, "That's not right!" (Clenching hands and face, squeezing legs together)*
T: *But the actuality of this moment, Hope, is that this is the way it is.*
P: *I feel resistance to that.*
T: *I can understand that and I see people nodding — they understand too.*

Acknowledging; tending belonging and resonance.

P: *I feel like arguing with it, with you.*
T: *I can understand that you have resistance and emotions that make you want to fight with the pain and to argue with me. But where does that put you in the body, Hope?*

Pointing to the "truth" of the moment.

P: *More pain...*
T: *I am inviting you to make a choice in this moment, to allow yourself to be with the actuality of what is. Opening even one percent more to what is here... the pain, the tightness, including the resistance, which is here as well. (pausing, noting what is happening nonverbally with Hope and the other participants, then, turning to all) Whatever is here for you, it is the actuality of your moment. Noticing if you are resisting the moment, and how that feels, or opening to what is, and how that feels... (long pause, then, to Hope) What is happening?*

P: *I feel less tension in my shoulders, not feeling squeezed. I am aware of the pain in my jaw and I see that there is a tendency for me to rush there, to say, "It's still there."*

T: *So you are able to notice your tendency to rush to the area of pain, and also to notice what you are telling yourself about the pain?*

Acknowledging; allowing her to hear her own statement.

P: *Yes. (slight smile, body more relaxed, more open posture...long pause)*

T: *It takes a lot of courage to turn toward pain, to open to what is not wanted. And I see a lot of heads nodding. Do you see this Hope? Your classmates are acknowledging your courage...*

T: *(to group) Let's just sit now... (after a couple of minutes, to group) What quality or qualities are you noticing in the moment?*

Tending belonging and resonance.

P2: *Strength...*

P3: *Compassion...*

P4: *Encouragement...*

P5: *Sense of understanding...*

T: *How does that feel in the body?*

Demonstrating preference for embodied knowing.

P5: *Peaceful...*

P6: *Not acknowledging what is happening can hurt more than acknowledging it.*

Part III
Towards an "Empty" Curriculum

Chapter 6
Organizing the Intentions of Teaching

In learning to teach mindfulness as a professional, the questions about *what* gets taught and *when* are of equal weight with the questions of *how* the teaching happens. Within the mindfulness-based interventions (MBIs), particularly those that explicitly include meditation practices, many of the answers to *what* and *when* (as well as *how)* have been based on the template curriculum of mindfulness-based stress reduction (MBSR). As described in Chapter 1, many of the MBIs, such as mindfulness-based cognitive therapy (MBCT), mindfulness-based art therapy (MBAT), mindfulness-based relationship enhancement (MBRE), and mindfulness-based relapse prevention (MBRP), assume the basic MBSR curriculum of formal mindfulness practices as an armature for specific didactic material and specially elaborated meditations and experiential explorations for their own target populations. In this way, the pedagogy of mindfulness unfolds relatively consistently from intervention to intervention. The measured success and exciting possibilities of the MBIs, we believe, are attributable in no small part to the MBSR armature — a metastructure of the *what* and *when* of teaching mindfulness.

This metastructure was developed and refined through more than 30 years of reflective teaching. It has been shaped by a range of influences. The long-established approaches in the wisdom traditions worldwide form a background, with the Buddhist tradition contributing the key model in the four ennobling truths and four foundations of mindfulness (see Table 6.1, and Chapter 3 for detailed discussion). This organizing impulse has been reinforced and amplified through the findings of empirical research, study of participant responses, and the personal intuition, fearless experimentation, and powerful authenticity and authority of Jon Kabat-Zinn, Saki Santorelli, and the senior teaching staff at the University of Massachusetts medical school (UMASS) Center for Mindfulness (CFM).

As MBSR has moved outward into the world from its origin, refinement of the curriculum and pedagogy has become an ongoing collaborative activity, not only at the CFM but also among the community of teachers in the MBIs, as they conduct classes around the world. Those in the community of teachers have been using their own authenticity and authority to shape responses to what is arising moment by moment in unique circumstances. Such exploration, critique, and innovation have

D. McCown et al., *Teaching Mindfulness: A Practical Guide*
for Clinicians and Educators, DOI 10.1007/978-0-387-09484-7_6,
© Springer Science+Business Media, LLC 2010

Table 6.1 Towards an "Empty" curriculum: Influences and expressions through eight weeks of MBSR

Four Ennobling Truths (see detailed description in Chapter 3)	Foundations of Mindfulness (see detailed description in Chapter 3)	MBSR Curriculum: Themes and content by week	MBSR Curriculum: Formal home practice assignments by week	Spectrum of Teaching Intentions (listed by intensity of focus in class)
• Fully understanding suffering	• Mindfulness of body	1: There's more right than wrong with you 2: Perception and creative responding	1&2: Body scan meditation (plus sitting meditation with focus on breath)	• Experiencing new possibilities • Discovering embodiment
• Letting go of craving	• Mindfulness of feelings	3: Pleasure and power of presence (pleasant events) 4: Shadow of stress (unpleasant events)	3&4: Alternate the body scan with standing or floor yoga practice (plus sitting meditation with focus on breath)	• Discovering embodiment • Cultivating observation
• Realizing liberation	• Mindfulness of mind states	5: Finding space for responding 6: Working with difficult situations	5&6: Alternate sitting w/ choiceless awareness with yoga; add walking meditation	• Cultivating observation • Moving toward acceptance
• Cultivating the path	• Mindfulness of mental contents	7: Cultivating kindness 8: A new beginning	7&8: Choose the practices you prefer	• Moving toward acceptance • Growing compassion

been encouraged from the start as part of MBSR teacher training. From the beginning, Kabat-Zinn (1996) has presented an openness to change, which is stated explicitly in the training materials used by the CFM:

> We emphasize that there are many different ways to structure and deliver mindfulness-based stress reduction programs. The optimal form of its delivery will depend critically on local factors and on the level of experience and understanding of the people undertaking the teaching. Rather than "clone" or "franchise" one cookie cutter approach, mindfulness ultimately requires effective use of the present moment as the core indicator of the appropriateness of particular choices.

Interestingly, despite the license granted to the community, the changes and elaborations that have taken place have been focused more on the *how* of the pedagogy rather than the *what* and *when* of the curriculum. There are many possible explanations for this reticence to change: perhaps a personal admiration for this paradigm-breaking work; maybe a reverence for the Buddhist underpinnings; maybe a scientific conservatism among clinicians that responds to MBSR's empirical success with "if it ain't broke, don't fix it"; there may also be a practical reserve in wanting to maintain continuity for the sake of continued elaboration of the evidence base. It seems most likely, however, that the metastructure has remained unchanged for decades simply because it has an extremely powerful intuitive logic — it *feels right* to the teachers — many of whom have been able to compare the years-long development of their personal practice of mindfulness with the 8-week MBSR experience. In short, it has an undeniable integrity.

Although the metastructure of MBSR in no way can be considered *proven* as the optimum approach to teaching mindfulness, it is certainly widely accepted, and the empirical measures of its success are impressive. Therefore, it would seem to be a useful exercise for teachers steeped in the curriculum to reflectively and critically examine the MBSR metastructure. Such an undertaking promises to make explicit the intentions that the teacher holds for participants' development of mindfulness across the duration of the curriculum. Because these intentions are implicit in the *what* and *when* of mindfulness experience and practice, it will be useful to review the curriculum and practices session by session.

The MBSR Curriculum

The template MBSR program (Kabat-Zinn, 1990) is an 8-week, nine-session course that is educational, experiential, and patient centered. Participants attend 2½h sessions once a week for eight weeks, with a full-day (7-hours) class between the sixth and seventh sessions. Class time each week is divided among formal meditation practice, presentations by the teacher of certain didactic material, small and large group discussions, and inquiry during group time with individuals into their present-moment experiences. The core formal mindfulness practices taught include a body scan, sitting meditation with concentrative focus on the breath, mindful Hatha yoga, sitting meditation that expands the focus of attention, to choiceless awareness.

Additional meditations introduced or reinforced at the full-day session include walking meditation, a loving kindness meditation, and mountain meditation.

The template program undergoes a transformation based on local population, setting, and teacher factors. For example, the frequency and duration of classes may be altered significantly. Several studies report varied course lengths, of 4–10 weeks (Jain et al, 2007; Rosenzweig et al., 2003; Speca et al., 2000), and shorter class durations, ranging from 1½ to 2 hours (Astin, 1997; Jain et al, 2007; Roth and Calle-Mesa, 2006; Rosenzweig et al., 2003). The changes required to adapt to such timings are made primarily in the amount and kind of didactic material presented, and in the opportunity for group discussions and inquiry, rather than in the presentation and practice of the core meditations. In the examples of programs listed here, the core practices were all presented — and in the template order.

The outline below describes themes, learning focuses, and specific practices typically introduced in each class session of an MBSR course based on the template program. The themes and practices are reinforced and built upon in each succeeding week.

MBSR TEMPLATE COURSE PROGRAM

Session One: Theme: There is more right with you than wrong with you.

Learning focus: Problems can be worked with, and the MBSR program offers the opportunity to do this in a supportive environment. Present-moment awareness of body sensations, thoughts, and emotions is the foundation of this work, because it is only in the present that one can learn, grow, and change. This includes formal didactic presentation on "What is mindfulness?"

Practices Introduced: Awareness of breath, body scan.

Session Two: *Theme: Perception and creative responding.*

Learning focus: How you see things, or don't see them, will determine how you will respond to them. It is not the events themselves but rather how you handle them that influences the effects on your body and mind.

Practice reinforced: Body scan. Practice introduced: Sitting meditation (focus on awareness of breath).

Session Three: Theme: The pleasure and power of being present.

Learning focus: We miss many of our pleasant moments, perhaps by focusing only on the unpleasant ones, such as crisis or pain. Yet it is possible to have pleasant moments even when you are experiencing crisis or pain. Developing deeper understanding and present moment contact with the triangle of awareness: body sensation, thought, and emotion.

Practices Introduced: Mindful yoga (floor yoga). Practices reinforced: Body scan, sitting (breath awareness).

Session Four: Theme: The shadow of stress.

Learning focus: Cultivating mindfulness can reduce the negative physiological and psychological effects of stress reactivity, as well as help develop more effective ways of responding positively and proactively to stressful situations and experiences. Includes formal didactic presentation on stress physiology.

Practices introduced: Mindful yoga (standing postures), sitting meditation (expanding focus from awareness of breath to body sensations and sound). Practices reinforced: Body scan, sitting (breath awareness).

Session Five: Theme: Finding the space for making choices.

Learning focus: Connect mindfulness with perception, appraisal, and choice in the critical moment. Particular attention is paid to observing thoughts as events, and distinguishing events from content — "You are not your thoughts."

Practice introduced: Sitting meditation (expanding awareness to whatever arises in the present moment — "choiceless awareness"). Practices reinforced: Yoga.

Session Six: Theme: Working with difficult situations.

Learning focus: How to maintain your center, recognize habitual patterns of relating, and discern skillful options in stressful interpersonal exchanges. Includes formal didactic presentation and experiential activities to demonstrate communication possibilities in both the verbal and nonverbal realms.

Practice introduced: Walking meditation. Practice reinforced: Sitting (choiceless awareness).

All-day Session: Theme: "Dive in!"

Learning focus: Deepen mindful awareness of experience by formally cultivating mindfulness over an extended period of time, fostering the possibility of greater self-knowledge and insight into the impermanence of pleasant and unpleasant body–mind states.

Practices: The full range of practices from prior sessions are reinforced, and two new practices are introduced — mountain meditation and loving kindness meditation

Session Seven: Theme: Cultivating kindness towards self and others.

Learning focus: Attitudes and practices to help develop a disposition of generosity in formal meditation so that it may arise more readily in our day-to-day life. Continued work with interpersonal communication.

Practices reinforced: Sitting (choiceless awareness), loving kindness.

Session Eight: Theme: "The eighth week is the rest of your life."

Learning focus: How do you keep up the momentum and discipline you've developed over the past seven weeks of mindfulness practice? Presents a range of resources, such as books, recordings, advanced programs, and other opportunities for practice in the community, to support continued practice. Meditation practice and opportunities for sharing with the group close the session and the course.

Practices reinforced: Body scan, mountain meditation, sitting (choiceless awareness), loving kindness.

A Spectrum of Teaching Intentions

Reflections on our encounters with the themes, learning objectives, and practices of the MBSR curriculum through study, teaching, and research have helped to distil a way of describing the metastructure of MBSR as an interrelated set of *teaching intentions*. These are different from *learning objectives*, in that they are meant to be held lightly by the teacher, rather than pressed upon the participants. In this way, the pedagogy of the emergent moment can reflect the integrity of the curriculum's metastructure, while the teacher remains open to outcome. The curriculum becomes a potential space in which contingent content can be co-created — teacher, participant, and class are free to respond to the impulse and intention of the present moment.

The description of an "empty curriculum" presented here seems, in this moment, both useful for practice and generative of critique and innovation. It is presented in a "temporary truth" approach to theorizing, which assumes a mindful stance — maintaining a present-moment focus, avoiding the reification of concepts, and contemplating impermanence. Although the diagram below (Fig. 6.1) confines each teaching intention to an independent bar, the graphic should be imagined instead as a spectrum — for two important reasons. First, consider a rainbow. It is one continuous gradation of hues, only a few of which are available to the human eye. The seven colors we see are a social construction, an overlay of language agreed upon and defined in community. They do not correspond to some inevitable essence or "truth" about the rainbow. In our Western view of the spectrum of colors, the designation "red" is agreed upon in narrower or broader ways, and helps us talk about, say, apples and computer graphics. In the same way, then, the teaching intentions overlay five categories on the total experience of learning mindfulness within the MBIs. Designating "discovering embodiment" as one intention is simply meant to help teachers and participants in exploring and reporting on experiences in which the centrality of the body is called to the foreground of attention. The second reason for seeing the set of intentions as a spectrum is their interrelatedness. Experiences in learning mindfulness are often beyond the limits of language; events and insights emerge from and dissolve into the mystery of not knowing. This suggests it will be best to hold the defined intentions lightly — to be open to the infinite shadings as one intention blends with another, and as unforeseen possibilities show themselves in each new moment of experience or reflection. Finally, it's necessary to remember that this rainbow of intentions appears in context — in a sky of relationship and resonance.

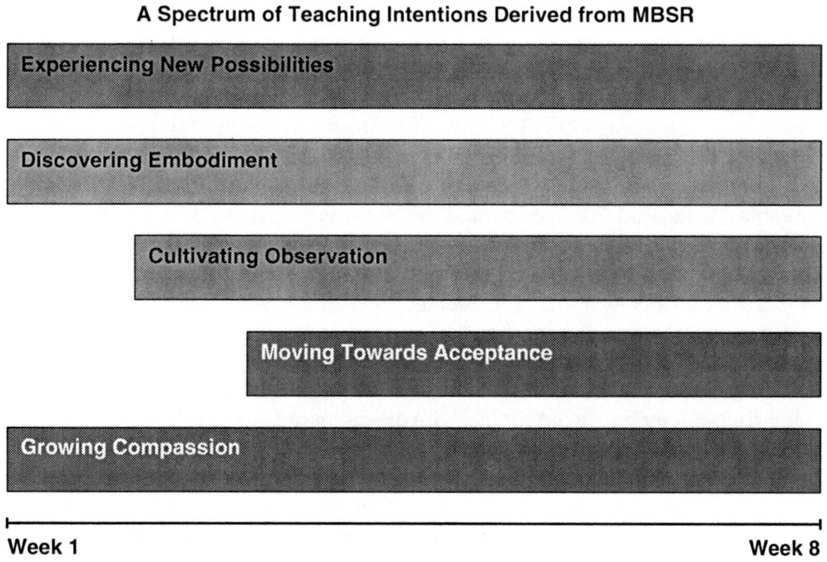

A Spectrum of Teaching Intentions Derived from MBSR

Experiencing New Possibilities

Discovering Embodiment

Cultivating Observation

Moving Towards Acceptance

Growing Compassion

Week 1   Week 8

Fig. 6.1 Both the vertical and horizontal structures of the spectrum of teaching intentions reflect the theoretical underpinnings of the MBSR metastructure. The vertical structure places the unfolding of the course for participants between the experience of new possibilities and the growth of compassion. This suggests the interdependence and simultaneity of the three axioms of mindfulness in the IAA model (intention, attention, and attitude) proposed by Shapiro et al. (2006). The horizontal structure suggests the incremental and experiential nature of the course, in which knowledge is not added to participants, but rather, reflecting the meaning of the Greek root of the verb to educate, is "drawn out" of each participant — gently, in delicate shades that reflect the individual's unique experience in the moment.

PARADOX

The More You Practice, the More You, Well, Practice

In the MBIs that include formal meditation, home practice is considered an integral part of the course. The ideal of compliance to home practice is emphasized to participants when they register, and is actively encouraged by teachers throughout the course. In the CFM's template MBSR program, participants are asked to commit to formal practice, supported by audio recordings that guide the meditations, for about 45 minutes a day. However, what is asked for and what is received can be different. The average practice time reported by participants in the CFM program, depending upon the specific practice, rarely approaches the requested time, ranging from an average of 16–20 minutes per day for sitting meditation and mindful movement, to 31–35 minutes per day for the body scan practice (Carmody and Baer, 2008). In other MBSR programs, shorter durations of formal home practice have been required, ranging from 15 to 35 minutes (Chang et al., 2004; Reibel et al., 2001; Jain, et al, 2007; Rosenzweig, et al., 2003; Roth and Calle-Mesa, 2006), while providing health outcomes consistent with those of the CFM program.

There is no consensus in the research on the relationship between home practice duration or frequency and participant outcomes. Some reports show no significant correlations between formal home practice time and outcomes (Astin, 1997; Carmody et al., 2008; Davidson et al., 2003), while others find correlations between practice time and specific health outcomes (Speca et al., 2000; Carmody and Baer, 2008).

Whether or not researchers find consensus on this question may actually have little relevance to the practice or pedagogy of mindfulness. The question comes from an entirely foreign dimension. Science since Galileo has limited itself to that which is measurable (Whitehead, 2008), and mindfulness researchers are currently working in that paradigm. While clock-time and calendar-time are convenient ways to map the horizontal dimension of *having*, they yield no useful information about the vertical dimension of *being* (Batchelor, 1983; Fromm, 1976; Marcel, 1949). So, *having* a mindfulness practice is reducible to how many days, months, years you've practiced; how often each week or day you practice; and for how many minutes you practice. Yet, *being* mindful is irreducible. You are only fully present in the vertical dimension, where spiritual and esthetic experience is found, and where clock time cannot measure the moments. Surely this is what our practice aims for and where our pedagogy points.

Authentic moments of mindfulness, however and whenever encountered, can be the catalyst for the changes researchers measure over time. The punctuation of the anxious, horizontal having of a life by a vertical moment of being — whether a single moment or an ongoing series — is a powerful discontinuity. It seems appropriate to let a poet speak to the experience and its effects. Rilke describes the inevitability and charge of such a moment of *being* in this esthetic encounter with an *Archaic Torso of Apollo* (Rilke, 1908/Mitchell, 1995):

We cannot know his legendary head
with eyes like ripening fruit. And yet his torso
is still suffused with brilliance from inside,
like a lamp, in which his gaze, now turned to low,

gleams in all its power. Otherwise
the curved breast could not dazzle you so, nor could
a smile run through the placid hips and thighs
to that dark center where procreation flared.

Otherwise this stone would seem defaced
beneath the translucent cascade of the shoulders
and would not glisten like a wild beast's fur:

would not, from all the borders of itself,
burst like a star: for here there is no place
that does not see you. You must change your life.

We know this much: participants who *have* a six-day-a-week, 45-minutes-a-day meditation practice, and participants who simply *are* mindful at some moment, both access the vertical dimension. And both can change their lives.

Defining the Teaching Intentions within the Context of the MBIs

Experiencing New Possibilities

From the first moment of encounter with the curriculum, participants' expectations are subverted. Their habitual worldviews are slightly destabilized. For example, being part of a heterogeneous group that includes people experiencing suffering of very different kinds and levels sends a message that is amplified by the statement often quoted in MBSR: "...as long as you are breathing, there is more right with you than there is wrong, no matter how ill or hopeless you may feel" (Kabat-Zinn, 1990, p. 2). Many participants who have come to closely identify themselves with their conditions are faced with a situation in which their condition is suddenly less interesting — to everyone. This may be frightening or freeing. It is almost certainly new. This sense that taken-for-granted frames of reference are available for reflection and reconsideration runs throughout the entire course. Also, this teaching intention emphasizes the liminal characteristics of the group, thereby contributing to the development of *communitas* (Turner, 1969) and catalyzing resonance.

Discovering Embodiment

Our contemporary culture in the West privileges the cognitive domain over the domains of affect and embodiment. Direct experience, in Hamlet's phrase, is "sicklied o'er with the pale cast of thought." In contrast, beginning with the first class, participants in MBSR are invited to experience whatever body sensations are arising, without judgment. Initial guidance of the body scan practice, and inquiry into participants' responses to that practice, help participants to disembed their immediate experience from their stories *about* the experience, and to separate anticipation or opinion from the present-moment happening. Early emphasis on embodiment helps make more available the interoceptive sensations that catalyze and deepen resonance with others. Across the entire eight weeks, inquiry into experience returns persistently and patiently to the body, steering participants away from the privileged cognitive domain, and leading them from the known to the not-yet-known. In exploring experience, the holistic relationship of the triangle of awareness is instrumental. For example, when a participant is feeling strong emotion, the teacher can invite her to drop the "story" — the thoughts supporting it — and simply be with/in the body sensations of the moment without judgment. Such an exploration of, say, anger, may lead to a discovery that the bodily sensations by themselves are energetic and even pleasurable, which in turn may gently prompt a reframing.

Cultivating Observation

This is the realization of the metamechanism of reperceiving described in the intention, attention, and attitude (IAA) mindfulness model of Shapiro, et al. (2006). Participants very often come to the point where they discover the capacity to detect their own inner experiences. This realization may begin to dawn as early as week two, when the initial challenge of the MBSR approach has settled. Not coincidentally, this is also the week when sitting meditation is first introduced. In the formal practice of both the body scan and sitting meditation in class 2, guidance assists participants in working *with* rather than *against* the "wandering mind." As they notice when and where the mind has wandered, participants begin to discover the observing consciousness that does the noticing, and can use this capacity to open themselves to meet their moment-to-moment experience, or even choose to reframe it.

Moving Towards Acceptance

This is the actualization of the *attitude* of mindfulness, the third of the IAA axioms of Shapiro, et al.'s model (2006). It is a subtle sense of caring that has its roots in nonjudgment, and that flowers into "an affectionate, compassionate quality...a sense of openhearted, friendly presence and interest" (Kabat-Zinn, 2003, p. 145, quoted in Shapiro et al., 2006). Moving towards acceptance is not merely a function of the reduced reactivity of the individual participant, it also is supported by the authentic presence of the teacher and the co-created mindfulness of the group, which can hold the individual in a way that maintains the stance of lowered reactivity in the face of aversive sensations, thoughts, and emotions in the moment.

Growing Compassion

Over the duration of the 8-week MBSR course, compassion reveals itself, at first implicitly and mostly directed towards the self, and later, explicitly and extended towards the other as well as the self. Compassion is implicit in the nonjudging attitude with which formal and informal mindfulness practices are introduced and explored in the early weeks of the course. Later, an explicit practice of loving kindness is introduced — often during a full-day session when participants have cultivated mindfulness for several hours and the group has built intra- and interpersonal resonance that allows and supports approach to such tender, vulnerable emotions. This practice of offering wishes for happiness, safety, well-being, and ease helps many participants link their personal practice to the relational dimension. They discover the potential impact of their individual transformations on their families, social circles, and workplaces; their awareness of political, social, and environmental situations; and on their religious and spiritual lives. Compassion becomes a powerful force for them.

Applying the Teaching Intentions to Shape Curricula and Guide Responses

Thinking through the spectrum may be useful to the professional teaching mindfulness in four different ways. (1) *Adjusting standard content*: Limitations may impinge, of time and/or space, as well as of culture, cognitive capacity, or other participant characteristics, requiring a shift in content that must be shaped through the teacher's authority and reference to the salient intentions. (2) *Guiding inquiry*: Professionals can use this simple scheme in the emergent pedagogical moment to locate a direction for inquiry with class participants. (3) *Improvising one-on-one teaching*: In educational or therapeutic dyads, the intentions can be a flexible tool to engage with a clients' unique, ongoing concerns, allowing the teacher to meet the client where she is at any given moment by selecting from available curricular content or improvising with the material arising in the session to fashion unique content. (4) *Creating unique content*: New MBIs can be generated as the empty curriculum can be filled with concrete content to leverage the practice of mindfulness in working with new populations. The intentions are also valuable in the creation of curricula that follow on from one of the foundational mindfulness-based interventions — so-called "graduate courses" in which past participants can refresh their skills and explore new practices and applications.

The remainder of this chapter offers examples of how the spectrum of teaching intentions can be used in each of the four ways described above. The examples are presented as illustrations of *ways of thinking,* and are not meant as concrete answers or programs. They are simply expressions of the authenticity, authority, and friendship of the authors to specific situations and within certain relationships. In teaching mindfulness as a professional, each teacher's response will be in the moment, for the moment, and will arise more from who she is than from any knowledge she has. In short, these examples are for inspiration not imitation.

Following on, Chapter 7 discusses the philosophical and pedagogical understanding of each intention. Each discussion links the intention to the theoretical and practical concerns of teaching mindfulness as a professional, as presented in Parts I and II. Further, each discussion offers examples of the typical content of the MBSR curriculum, as well as of contingent curricula that may prove useful — annotated scripts are provided for the core MBSR practices that are most associated with each intention, and there are scripts for practices for each intention that may help illuminate how it may be expressed in particular settings or with specific populations. In addition, vignettes of individual and group inquiry are offered to illustrate how inquiry can be used to point participants towards the particular intention.

Example 1: Adjusting Standard Content

We were asked to provide a "field test" of mindfulness for an editor of *Prevention* magazine (Foley, 2006; Reibel and McCown, 2007). The editor wanted to report on a one-time training for a small group of participants with a range of different reasons for investigating mindfulness practice. Conditions reported by group members included anxiety, depression, sleep problems, chronic pain, heart disease, asthma, gastrointestinal disorders, arthritis, and fibromyalgia — with all members reporting multiple conditions. We did not believe that a single session could provide all that we hoped group members could experience and come to understand. So we proposed a more intense alternative — the 8-week MBSR program. Our proposal made sense and was of interest, but the project had significant constraints of geography, participant time, and project finances. Participants were to be drawn from four different Mid-Atlantic States; we had to meet the publication deadline; and the budget required a creative solution to deliver what we believed to be essential opportunities for learning.

Our strategy for adaptation started from the teaching intentions. We designed a course that was launched in a way that allowed heavy initial emphasis on the three intentions of experiencing new possibilities, discovering embodiment, and growing compassion, while building a platform from which the other two intentions of cultivating observation and moving towards acceptance could be explored and expanded over time.

MAPPING OUT THREE LESSON MODULE

1. *A full-day introductory workshop:* Participants came together for 7 h and were given what amounted to an MBSR mini-course. They were introduced to the full range of practices: body scan, sitting meditation with awareness of breath, yoga stretching, sitting meditation opening to choiceless awareness, walking meditation, and loving kindness meditation. In addition, they received what we believe to be the basic didactic presentations: a definition of mindfulness, an exploration of stress physiology, and experiences of the limits of perception.
2. *Six weeks of practice and support:* Participants followed a schedule of formal and informal practices and readings from *Full Catastrophe Living* for each week. At each week's end, the group assembled by teleconference. Time on the phone was spent practicing together, processing participants' experiences, and reviewing insights occasioned by the homework. The group also maintained connection with each other and with the teachers between calls through group and individual emails.
3. *A half-day silent retreat:* Participants traveled and gathered again to renew the sense of interconnection, review the formal meditations, gain a taste of extended practice, learn about resources for continued support, and come to closure.

The Full-day Introductory Workshop

Underlying the workshop's design was the effort to create personal connections and intersubjective resonance in the group, for two reasons. First, this was important so that during home practice during succeeding weeks, each participant, although meditating alone, could draw on their remembered and internalized support of the teachers and the group. Second, it was critical so that intersubjective resonance could be more easily restored in the sparse interpersonal environment of the weekly teleconferences, where the only cues to another's presence are the content of verbal communication and paralinguistic vocal information.

These considerations shaped the presentation of each experience (see sidebar). Given the short amount of face-to-face time available in the overall course design, concentrated exposure to just one teacher would have increased the potential for internalization by participants. However, due to teachers' commitments and schedules, two teachers were necessary. To best facilitate and maintain connections with the teachers, the practices and experiences were led by one or the other, based on the plan for the six weekly teleconferences. Teachers taught the practices for which they would be leading the teleconferences, and CDs of their recording of the practice were provided to the participants for home practice. To facilitate connections among group members during the workshop, opportunities were created for one-to-one sharing. Significant time was spent on introductions. Then, of course, the mindfulness practices catalyzed the possibility of intersubjective resonance in the group. Further, in the quiet after each practice, participants met and spoke first in dyads or triads — with different partners each time — before opening to group processing.

The three intentions of new possibilities, embodiment, and compassion also shaped the design. The three shifted in dominance from moment to moment, yet continually supported and informed each other.

Discovering new possibilities dominated in the introduction and definition modules. In the introduction experience, the question "What brings you here?" was dropped into the meditation again and again. For many, different answers arose each time, introducing the uncertainty and potential for change inherent in mindfulness practices. In the definitions module, participants found their assumptions challenged: stress is more subjective and controllable than it seems, and raisins are very different when encountered one on one.

Embodiment bore the most weight for the day. From practice to practice, the emphasis of guidance and initial inquiry was on body sensation. The order of the practices built on what was experienced: from the interoception of the body scan to proprioception of the yoga sequence of standing and floor postures, and flowing right into the introduction of sitting meditation with awareness of the breath, where the freedom and sensitivity from the prior practices could precipitate a more intimate con-

DESIGN OF THE FULL-DAY INTRODUCTORY WORKSHOP.

9:30 Introduction module
- Self-introduction of teachers
- Experience: Meditation repeating the question, "What brings you here?"
- Self-introduction of participants, in answer to the question

9:50 What is MBSR?
- Fill out precourse research forms

10:20 Definition module
- Stress definition, and segue to:
- Practice: Relaxing sighs
- Mindfulness definition, and segue to:
- Experience: Mindfully eating a raisin
- Practice: Body scan
- Dialog about practice, first in dyads, then as group

11:30 Practice: Yoga (flowing directly into the next practice)

11:50 Practice: Sitting meditation with awareness of breath

12:15 Dialog about both practices, first in dyads (different partner), then as group

12:30 Lunch

nection with the gross and subtle motions and influences of the breath on the body. It is also possible that this emphasis on awareness of sensations in the body — particularly while resonating intra-subjectively — helped to intensify the experience of resonating intersubjectively, and thereby created stronger connections in the group.

Compassion by participants for themselves and each other was a potential right from the introductions. The repeated "What brings you here?" question probed personal motivations, and the sharing of personal stories of suffering and hope made empathic feelings more likely and more available. The definition of mindfulness, of course, contains the attitude of nonjudgment in which compassion is implicit, while the presentation of the definition made it explicit, noting that practicing mindfulness cuts across the grain of our default desires for permanence and certainty, so it requires a little bit of effort and whole lot of gentleness and kindness towards ourselves. Again, the potential for discovery of an unforeseen level of intersubjective resonance in the practices and the subsequent dyads, groups, and teacher-participant exchanges made cultivation of compassion more likely and possi-

	– Eating and resting in silence, together
1:15	Practice: Walking meditation
	– Dialog about practice, first in dyads (another different partner), then as group
1:50	Perception experiments
	– DVD presentation of experiments
	– Dialog about experience; first in triads, then triads reporting in to large group
2:10	Experience: Narrating one's moment-by-moment experience in dyads
	– Group discussion of experience
2:30	Practice: Sitting meditation opening to choiceless awareness
	– Dialog about practice; first in dyads (another different partner), then as group
3:20	Practice: Seated yoga
3:35	Description of and dialog about logistics for the six weeks of teleconferences
3:50	Practice: Loving kindness meditation
4:00	Mindful good byes

ble. Ending the workshop with loving kindness practice brought the intention of compassion and its dual motions towards self and others into the foreground at last.

For the editor, the experience of the day was an encounter with all the "judgments, fantasies, to-do lists, hopes, regrets, crazy stuff out of left field" (Foley, 2006, p. 159). Her take-away illustrates the new possibilities intention at work: "If that kind of chatter went on in my brain all the time, no wonder I often found myself struggling to put one word in front of the other…. And it hit me. This was why I needed to be in the present moment. The perpetual mental struggle to reconcile the past and control the future was futile, not to mention exhausting" (p. 159).

The Six Weeks of Practice

The six weeks of home practice supported by once-a-week, one-hour teleconferences continued the progressive foregrounding of the intentions (see sidebar). The design assumed that the majority of the teaching emphasis could now be placed on the intentions that are bracketed by discovering new possibilities and growing compassion. The experiences of teachers and participants of the teleconferences were rich; voices did, indeed, help to recall the embodied presence of the individuals we had come to know at the workshop. The silences on the telephone seemed natural, companionable, and resonant. And the entire conference felt supportive and refreshing.

Week one reinforced the exploration of embodiment, through exclusive daily formal practice of the body scan and informal practice of mindful eating. The first teleconference practice, reversing the body scan direction, highlighted how quickly habits arise, and what it is like to have a fresh experience — reinforcing the teaching intention of discovering new possibilities. Week two, through the addition of sitting meditation (awareness of breath, AOB) and the seeking and recording of pleasant events arising during each day began also to point towards "cultivating observation." Week three, with a focus on recognizing and reporting on unpleasant events, helped to bring the intention of moving towards acceptance to the fore. This was made more explicit in the teleconference practice at the end of the week to which participants were invited, during a body scan, to bring attention to a place in the body that was calling out in some way — often interpreted as some form of discomfort. Participants were asked to turn towards the discomfort, to "make more space" or "soften" that area, so they could observe with a caring curiosity whatever sensations were arising from moment to moment. In inquiry with the teacher, participants came to see that through curiosity and acceptance their experience changed over time — in different and unpredictable ways. Weeks four and five allowed deeper exploration of this. The focus of practice moved to sitting meditation with choiceless awareness, amplifying and tying together the intentions of embodiment, observation, and acceptance. The week-5 teleconference practice of loving kindness meditation brought compas-

SCHEDULE: HOME PRACTICE AND TELECONFERENCES.

Week one Formal practice: Body scan
Informal practice: Mindful eating
Teleconference practice: Body scan, reversing direction — foot-to-head versus head-to-foot

Week two Formal practice: Alternate body scan and sitting meditation (AOB)
Informal practice: Pleasant events calendar
Teleconference practice: Sitting meditation (AOB)

Week three Formal Practice: Alternate body scan and yoga
Informal Practice: Unpleasant events calendar
Teleconference practice: Body scan, dwelling in a region of the body that "calls out" to you

Week four Formal Practice: Alternate sitting (AOB) and yoga
Informal Practice: Mindful Shower
Teleconference practice: Sitting (choiceless awareness)

Week five Formal Practice: Alternate yoga and sitting (choiceless awareness)
Informal Practice: Mindful walking
Teleconference practice: Loving kindness meditation

Week six Formal Practice: Sitting (choiceless awareness)
Informal Practice: Mindful listening

sion from the background to the foreground, and began to move it towards others. The editor summed up weeks three to five by highlighting the shift underway in her approach to moment-to-moment experience: "I was beginning to think that I'd been wrong to dread being 'in the moment' — that the struggle to avoid pain is what actually prolongs it. Meditation doesn't change what happens to you, but it helps change your response" (Foley, 2006, p. 160). Week six, by spotlighting sitting with choiceless awareness, offered encounters with the full spectrum of teaching intentions, and led into the closing half-day workshop.

The Half-day Silent Retreat

Participants met face to face for the second time on a warm and bright day that allowed the option to hold the retreat outside in a quiet, park-like setting. By design, the full spectrum of teaching intentions came into play. Compassion flowed immediately as participants, several of whom had weathered health crises or family tragedies during the course, came together. The setting, the discipline of silence and refraining from eye-contact, the unbroken flow of one practice into another, all encouraged discovering new possibilities in practice and in the way participants carried themselves. Teachers led the formal practices (see sidebar) with an emphasis on embodiment — inviting participants to come closer and closer to their sensory, proprioceptive, and interoceptive experience of the moment. The embodied being-together after the weeks of voices as the only contact helped to heighten awareness of feelings of intra- and intersubjective resonance. With such feelings as background, observation and acceptance were eased. Further, according to teachers' observations and participants' reports, the practices often brought participants to a deeper sense of stillness, quiet, and well-being. We broke the silence in a Council Circle (Zimmerman and Coyle, 1996), offering a resonant space for individual reflection to grow gently to dialog. The experience closed with food and socializing.

The editor describes the outcomes of the total course: "Over time, my daily meditations helped me regard what was happening in any moment with curiosity and kindness, without the mindless chatter and instant evaluation that used to whip me into a frenzy.... Most of my classmates had similar life-changing experiences" (Foley, 2006, p.160). A look at the outcome data shows that there is little hyperbole in that statement. Of the nine participants who began the program, eight completed. Their experience of change is reflected in the outcomes of the 18-question Brief Symptoms Inventory (BSI-18)

HALF-DAY "CLOSING RETREAT"
1:00 Arrivals and greetings
1:10 Sitting meditation
1:30 Yoga
1:50 Body scan
2:10 Walking meditation
2:25 Mountain meditation
2:40 Group process, council circle format (How have you benefited? What are your intentions to move forward?)
3:20 Loving kindness meditation
3:30 – 4:00 Fill out post-course research forms; goodbyes

(Derogatis, 2000), which provides an overall measure of psychological functioning, called the global severity index (GSI), and subscales measuring depression, anxiety, and somatization (Fig. 6.2). Pre- to post-intervention differences were significant for the group for GSI, depression, and anxiety, though not for somatization. The GSI was reduced by 52%, depression score by 70%, and anxiety score by 55%. Quite a small sample, of course; yet, comparison with the typical outcomes of these variables in standard MBSR courses for medical patients (e.g., Reibel, 2001) reveal comparable if not greater changes.

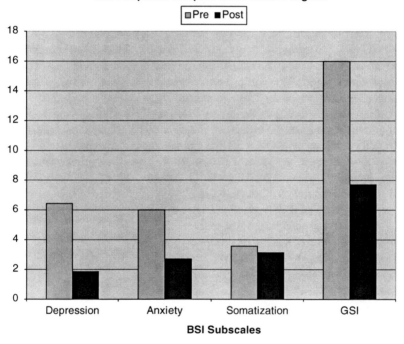

Fig. 6.2 Participants showed significant improvements pre- to post-intervention on three of four measures. Depression symptoms improved 70% ($p<0.05$). Anxiety symptoms improved 55% ($p<0.01$). Somatization showed no significant change. And the global severity index, the measure of overall psychological distress, improved 52% ($p<0.001$) (Reibel and McCown, 2007).

A Very Short Course

An introductory workshop is an often-requested format for presenting the MBIs. The spectrum of intentions can be useful in shaping such presentations, providing structure and ensuring that the teacher presents the work authentically in its breadth, if not in depth.

MBSR for workplace populations is a frequently requested topic. Time for such presentations is often from one to three hours. Our experience (McCown and Reibel, 2008) suggests that it is extremely difficult to work with less than 90 minutes, and that negotiating for additional time past that mark is rewarding in the greater spaciousness allowed in experiential explorations with the group. The empty curriculum suggests a default agenda (see sidebar) that can be shared and promoted for "sales" purposes, yet can be fine-tuned or even entirely improvised as teacher–participant dialog suggests interesting directions. All of the activities and meditation practices mentioned in the following description are described in detail in Chapter 7.

A short workshop can start with experiencing new possibilities — bypassing the expected introductions and walk-through of the agenda. A smaller group with spacious time could begin with an activity during which the teacher asks participants to pause several times to check into internal experiences of body sensation, thought, and mood state. For example, the "trading pinkies" activity, in which rubber balls are exchanged from hand to hand as the group walks at random in the room, can be used to generate some of the feelings encountered in the workplace environment as exchanges are made faster and faster, or formally, or casually, or secretly. A larger group with less time might be brought to new possibilities through a short exploration of a common experience in the moment. Such an exploration is easily improvised on the basis of the teacher's immediate circumstances, as in a guided experience of sitting in the particular room, in a particular kind of chair. A simple practice such as "the soles of the feet," in which a kind curiosity is brought to that area, may also be useful. Introductions and other formalities can then take place inside a dialog based on the shared experience, which provides a multitude of segues into the rest of the workshop and shades into all the other intentions.

A didactic module on stress physiology can help participants discover embodiment, although potentially in a cognitive way. Yet, when followed by a demonstration of the "relaxing sigh" which can help participants to shift from their sympathetic nervous system's fight-or-flight stress reaction to the parasympathetic rest-and-repair response, the points are brought home to the felt sense. Although the relaxing sigh is not a mindfulness practice *per se*, it does increase participants' understanding of the body–mind connection. Further, it suggests that knowing what's happening with you in the

---

A 1.5- TO 3-HOUR INTRODUCTORY BSR WORKSHOP: A DEFAULT AGENDA

1. Beginning with an experience
   - Group dialog and introductions follow
2. Presentation on stress physiology
   - Learning the relaxing sigh for self-regulation
3. Presentation on "What is mindfulness?"
   - Experiencing mindfulness for yourself
4. Break
   - Practicing mindful stretching
5. Exploring the present moment
   - Mindfulness dyads
   - Sitting meditation
6. Dialog and questions
   - Next steps?
7. Close with "unconditional friendliness" meditation

moment, and finding the space in which to make choices may be the start of a new way of being.

New possibilities, embodiment, and observation are all in play even before mindfulness is defined. When the definition is presented, the cognitive understanding should be grounded in experience — such as an eating meditation or a body scan, for example. The definition and the guidance of the experience will necessarily return again and again to nonjudgmental awareness and kind curiosity, which helps to foreground the intentions of acceptance and compassion — particularly self-compassion. Now all intentions are in play.

In a longer workshop, a break might allow participants to leave the room and return to begin an activity of mindful stretching — bringing them back into the body and the moment after any distractions. In a shorter workshop, the activity of stretching can be the break itself. The practice can engage the intentions of embodiment, and participants can come to realize that when they observe their condition in the moment, they have a choice of acceptance, or, if possible and desired, change. The shifts in experience that mindful stretching can prompt lead all the way through the spectrum — from new possibilities onward.

Observation comes to the foreground in exploring the present moment through sitting meditation. The use of "mindfulness dyads" can help many participants grasp the practice of choiceless awareness, of being with/in the experience of each moment as it arises. Each member of the dyad narrates his or her present moment experience to the other, who simply listens mindfully. In processing this, time can be spent exploring not only the capacity for observing but also the experiences of listening mindfully and being deeply heard — usually identified as rare in the workplace setting. The mindfulness dyads, of course, provide a smooth segue into sitting meditation practice — which can begin with the embodiment focus of sensation and breath, before expanding to choiceless awareness. In a longer workshop, this module may be followed by instruction in the 3-minutes breathing space as a take-away practice; in a shorter workshop, the 3-minutes breathing space may form the centerpiece of the experience.

The workshop comes to its logical end with group dialog on next steps, often including invitations to participate in an 8-week MBSR program. A formal sense of closure — and a foregrounding of the intention of growing compassion — comes with the teacher leading a short loving kindness practice. For nonprofit, social service-oriented workplaces, the term loving kindness tends to be well received; in other organizations, a term such as "unconditional friendliness" is often less threatening, and helps participants settle into the practice.

Example 2: Using the Intentions to Guide Inquiry

Even a one-question inquiry is determined by a multitude of influences within the context of a typical MBSR course. The timing within the eight weeks, the practice or exercise from which the opportunity arises, the present-moment disposition of — and the history of inquiry with — the participant, the state of group resonance, and the teacher's tacit understanding of the nonverbal communications of the participant and the group are among the salient factors. The work of weighing all of this information may require a split second or a long pause. In any case, reference to the spectrum of intentions can be defining or confirming — in other words, quite useful.

The inquiry by the teacher in the following exchange was shaped substantially by context, and was confirmed by reference to the intentions. The class is in session 5. The bell has just rung to end a 30-minutes practice of sitting meditation in which the focus of attention has been expanded step by step to choiceless awareness. The group has been quiet and still during practice and now appears to the teacher to be intersubjectively resonant and reticent to break the silence. The teacher allows the silence to continue comfortably, and finally, gently, breaks it.

Teacher: *Any discoveries as we moved from breath to body, to sound, thinking, emotions, and then to whatever was arising?"*

The question makes an opening. It brings specific language into the group by naming the experiences of the practice. And it focuses participants on discovery — surprise, novelty, new possibilities. A participant speaks at last.

Participant: *My leg has been hurting me all morning... the pain had been so intense before we started meditating. But when we were practicing I began to feel the air against my face... and then I started hearing sounds in the room... and then I was aware that the pain was still there — but it didn't grab my attention so much.*

This participant has spoken of her pain in several other class sessions. She has been engaged at the outset by the teacher's statement that not an end to pain, but a different relationship to pain is a possible outcome of the course. At this point, the body scan and yoga practice and the class dialogs about them have helped her to clearly sense and articulate her embodied experience. The teacher realizes that pursuing inquiry from the intention of embodiment — about what she perceived moment by moment — will not take her much further in that. The participant's statement that the pain "didn't grab my attention so much" is different, fresh, an insight. She's noticed some distance from her pain that is not simply a distraction. This is intriguing for her, yet not necessarily comforting, so for the teacher to inquire from the intention of acceptance would be premature. The teacher's choice, then, is bracketed and confirmed — to inquire from the intention of cultivating observation. The question is directed to the participant and the rest of the group, as well.

Teacher: *Is the awareness of pain also in pain?*

The first response from the participant and group is silence. The question has dropped right into the ripening experience of many in the group. The momentum of the curriculum has been gathering in this direction. The participant responds, loudly, enthusiastically, speaking for many:

Participant: *NO! It just knows... It knows!*

Here is alignment of curriculum, teacher intention, and participant experience, that prompted in the group further discoveries and enriching dialog.

Example 3: Improvising One-On-One Teaching

The group effects of the MBIs are powerful, and it is recommended that whenever possible, patients or clients should be referred to groups. However, there are two basic conditions in which one-on-one teaching is a valuable solution: (1) for convenience — participants may not have the structured time that allows regular class attendance, or may have a condition or way of being that precludes group participation; (2) for inclusion with other dyadic work — a structured approach to learning mindfulness may be helpful in counseling, psychotherapy, occupational therapy, performance coaching, and spiritual direction, to name just some applications.

It's helpful to remember in such situations that the dyadic relationship can offer many of the advantages of the group, and several unique advantages as well. Mindfulness in a dyad is a very focused co-creation. Instruction and exploration of the practices can be influenced in the moment by feedback from the participant: verbally, as the teacher can ask questions and receive a spoken answer during practice; and nonverbally as the near space and opportunity for lengthy observation can reveal valuable information. Interpersonal resonance is available for support and exploration, although it may be less stable than in a group, and more dependent on the teacher to catalyze it and sustain it. Shared dialog arising from practice experience is available, provided the teacher is also authentic about how the practice is for her in the moment. What's more, opportunities may arise more regularly than in a group to work mindfully in the moment with specific content that is meaningful to the participant.

When convenience is the dominant force in bringing the teacher–participant dyad together, the spectrum of intentions plays its typical role of generating a structure and allowing responsiveness within it. The typical MBSR course content, for example, can be offered through eight one-hour sessions — making certain that there is sufficient time between sessions to experience the home practice. It may be that the participant contracts formally for an eight-session course. Or it may be that teacher and participant negotiate the time commitment depending on the client's particular needs — in the event that it is helpful to dedicate occasional sessions for working mindfully with personal issues as they arise or for learning beyond the typical curriculum about specific topic areas that capture interest. For example, a participant may wish to spend extra sessions working mindfully with the symptoms of a chronic illness, or a participant may wish to gain an expanded knowledge of mindful communication within their personal relationships or workplace. Whatever the needs, the spectrum of intentions may be useful in planning sessions and assessing progress. In teaching mindfulness as a professional, such planning and assessment is not about expecting a particular outcome, but rather about ensuring that each intention comes to the foreground and allows for the participant's authentic response.

When the teaching of mindfulness is to be included with other dyadic work, from counseling to spiritual direction, the planning and assessment applications of the spectrum come into play. In such situations, the teacher has two basic approaches. She can choose to interrupt the other work for a time, setting aside a block of sessions to introduce and explore a range of mindfulness practices, perhaps even using the curriculum of an MBI. Or she can choose to integrate — or titrate, so to speak — mindfulness practice into the process of sessions as it seems appropriate. The first approach is discontinuous, and requires a certain amount of persuasion on the part of the teacher and a willing commitment on the part of the participant. The major benefit is that it sets formal and informal mindfulness practice up as an existing resource that the teacher–participant dyad can call on as needed in their ongoing work. The second approach is more subtle, calling for less persuasion and less participant commitment, although the result over time may be the same as the first approach. The teacher can suggest using mindfulness practice — formal or informal — to encounter some experience that is arising in the moment, in session. Such a move would bring to the foreground the intention of experiencing new possibilities, and, using the spectrum, it would seem best balanced if the practice also emphasized embodiment. Once mindfulness practice is introduced with some success, the dyad can continue to move through the intentions as opportunity and need present themselves. For example, a woman came into psychotherapy to better cope with neurological problems resulting from chronic Lyme disease, including joint pain and feelings of depersonalization and derealization. Due to the latter, she was reticent to engage in meditative practices. She found that simple body-based practices such as the soles of the feet and the body scan were stabilizing and grounding. Using just those practices, and bringing in the full spectrum of intentions, over time she was able to come to a sense of acceptance — "…that's not who I am, it's just how I feel." In spiritual direction or other dyadic work that explores spiritual practices, the spectrum can be used as a guide for assessment and prescription. A man in spiritual direction exhibited openness, embodiment, the capacity to observe, and a deep compassion for others. Self-compassion and acceptance, however, were significantly less developed. This became clear to him as he was directed to note his attitude and response each time his attention strayed from the breath in a focused sitting meditation. Working with his own reactions in formal meditation, and making loving kindness meditation a regular practice for a period of eight weeks, he began to notice a change in the way he carried himself throughout the day.

Example 4: Creating Unique Content

There are myriad reasons for designing new mindfulness-based courses, for example, to reach underserved populations, to target particular issues or sets of issues, or to help participants who have "graduated" from MBIs to continue to explore the practice of mindfulness. In any of these cases, the spectrum of teaching intentions can be used directly as an armature to develop a curriculum that is congruent with the unfolding of an MBSR course, or the spectrum can be used indirectly as a collection of essential theoretical elements that support the pedagogy and learning of mindfulness, although the emphasis and order may differ because of specific content. The following example has been chosen because it illustrates a broad range of development challenges, and because, as a short course, its components are limited and concise.

The course *Meeting Aggression* was designed as a "graduate" course, to be offered to participants who completed an MBSR course, or who are experienced in mindfulness meditation from some other training. Structure and content were chosen to appeal to men, as men are significantly underrepresented in MBI classes, at roughly 25% (e.g., Baer, 2003; Coelho et al. 2007; McCown et al., 2007). The appeal of the curriculum included an emphasis on physical practices, with the martial-arts-derived practice of Taijichuan (simplified) as a centerpiece, and incorporating readings, films, and discussions featuring the image of the mindful warrior. The language used in promotion paints the picture:

> *In our daily lives it can feel as if we continually meet with aggression — from within and without. This four-week course will explore the habitual physical postures, intellectual positions, and emotional attitudes we assume in such encounters. Are they truly helpful? Or are there more skillful ways to work with aggressive energy? We'll use a range of mindful physical practices from* Taijichuan *to playground games to see what the body-mind reveals to us. We'll deepen our practice of mindfulness meditation to encounter and understand our own aggressive positions and attitudes. And we'll engage in small and large group dialogues to develop both clarity and compassion. A CD of new practices, plus readings from across the contemplative traditions will support personal explorations between classes.*

The 4-week structure (see sidebar) derives from the flow of the spectrum of teaching intentions, in which the intentions build upon each other. Practices, readings, and activities, each bring into the foreground two intentions, which overlap and reinforce the potential learning experiences week to week, culminating in a week-4 review of practices that touches the first four intentions — before the fifth, compassion, is made explicit in a closing that encourages further practice in the times to follow.

Class 1 focuses on experiencing new possibilities and discovering embodiment. The course begins with the activity "chaos and systems," in which each participant is in a circle and each is given a playground ball. Just seeing and holding the ball can be explored for the memories and ideas of aggression towards the self and others that it prompts. As the activity begins, instructions are simple and amusing, bringing the group together lightheartedly. Further on, the instructions move the group to discipline and systemize their actions to accomplish a task, and then to accomplish it faster and faster with greater and greater precision. As participants assume roles and authority, a range of experiences of aggression towards self and other begin to arise and become available for mindful exploration directed by the teacher towards the body — "What are you feeling right now?" Eventually, the exploration is pursued verbally in group dialog and inquiry, and many come to see that the group moved from the ease of being simply present with each other in fun to the anxiety and aggression of doing or the sake of achievement. Also, individuals come to see the strategies, often habitual, that they used to protect their weaknesses — or to exploit them. The insights and material that become available can be referred to throughout the rest of the course. The course theme of meeting aggression is highlighted through the introduction of the 10-posture *Taijichuan* sequence and its layers of seeming contradictions — as a martial art whose moves contain defense and attack simultaneously, as a mindful movement practice of grace and beauty built on a potential for violence. The teacher demonstrates each of the postures, as a volunteer "opponent" experiences in slow motion the powerful forces involved: new possibilities in an embodiment practice, intensified by the sense of contained energy. The practice of *Being Present* is a lying-down meditation that explores through small movements — such as lifting an arm without breaking contact with the floor — the possibilities of aggression towards your own experience. Guidance frames as a form of aggression any sense of wanting your experience to be a certain way rather than simply allowing it to be as it is. Surprises may come from small resistances at the tissue level. (The practice is described and guided in Chapter 7, as are the other practices in this curriculum.) Finally, the weekly reading assignments are subverted through the introduction of a contemplative reading practice. Rather than aggressively reading to have knowledge and gain "truth," participants learn a method that is a *being with*, not a *doing of* the text — an embodied, not a cognitive encounter.

Class 2 shifts the major focus to discovering embodiment and cultivating observation. *Taijichuan* practice expands with more postures in the sequence, and the being present practice is reviewed and elaborated. The new practice of *Being Open* is a 10-minute standing meditation, which for many is a physical challenge. There is much to notice as you hold the body still and vertical for a prolonged period; the challenge then becomes to respect rather than become aggressive towards the moment-by-moment experience — to "look again" at it, which is what the root of the word respect means. Participants are encouraged to remain open, to observe, and to respond with what is needed, without aggression. This is dramatized in a scene from the film *Gettysburg* (Esparza et al., 1993) that sets up the group dialog and the contemplative reading for the week.

MEETING AGGRESSION: A "GRADUATE COURSE"

Class 1: Being and Doing

"All men seek peace first of all with themselves."

... Thomas Merton

Practices in class:
- Ten-posture Tai Chi Chuan (learn 1–3)
- Introduce *Being Present*
- Introduce the practice of contemplative reading

Reading for the week:
- Thomas Merton (1955): "Being and Doing"

Class 2: The Warrior

"The principle that guides the Warrior is showing up and choosing to be present."

... Angeles Arrien

Practices in class:
- Ten-posture Tai Chi Chuan (1–3 & learn 4–6)
- Review *Being Present*
- Introduce *Being Open*

Film clip and dialog on theme:
- *Gettysburg* — choosing to be present

Reading for the week:
- Angeles Arrien (1993): "The Way of the Warrior"

Class 3: The Sage Commander

"Because the sage commander has settled into being who he is, he is no longer constantly comparing himself to others."

... The Denma Translation Group

Practices in class:
- Ten-posture Taijichuan (1–6 & learn 7–10)
- Review *Being Open*
- Introduce *Being for Others*

Film clip and dialog on theme:
- *To Kill a Mockingbird*–not comparing self to others

Reading for the week:
- The Denma Translation Group (2002): Commentary on "The Sage Commander"

MINDFULNESS AT GETTYSBURG

Colonel Joshua Chamberlain, in charge of the 20th Maine Regiment, is brought a group of 120 deserters and told that he can shoot any who refuse to march or fight. Rather than treating them as the other officers had, he shows them respect — looking again — and treats them with care and deference. By appealing to their common humanity, Chamberlain wins their confidence and cooperation; in fact, almost to a man, the soldiers take up arms again to fight beside him. Had they not, it is doubtful that the 20th Maine could have repelled the Confederate attackers at Little Round Top, which was essential to the Union Army victory at Gettysburg. Many participants clearly see and feel the power that Chamberlain's embodied presence and attitude of respect has on the men — both before and during the battle.

Class 4: Hearing the Call of the Other

"The Other does more than suffer, the Other calls out in his suffering... the Other calls out to you."

... Stephen Batchelor

Practices in class:

– Review ten-posture Taijichuan (1–10)
– Review *Being Present*
– Review *Being Open*

Closure:

– Council circle on theme of hearing the call of the other
– Review *Being for Others* practice
– Goodbyes

Reading for the coming week:

– Stephen Batchelor (2004): "Hearing the Call of the Other"

Class 3 moves to a focus on observing and accepting. *Taijichuan* practice completes the entire 10-posture sequence, maintaining the importance of embodiment, and keeping the balance of being and doing, aggression, and non-aggression available for dialog. The being-open practice reviews the idea of observation with discernment — respect. For many during the past week, the practice has raised challenges about when and how to respond to discomfort by moving or sitting, and when to work with acceptance. Inquiry and dialog about this can set up the introduction of the new practice of *Being for Others*, which explores the capacity to be open to suffering — emphasizing the intention of acceptance, of simply being with/ in an experience as it is. This contemplation asks participants to imagine four different scenes of suffering. First, participants imagine a small child that they do not know who has been hurt in some way — nothing grave. Then they imagine themselves as children, hurting, but not too badly, and explore the possibilities for remaining open: then attempting to turn towards and be open to their own suffering in the moment. Finally, they choose someone for whom they wish to practice. The practice with each scene is to model for the person in the scene a way of being with/ in one's experience of the moment, of turning towards and opening to the way it is; each scene ends as the participant imagines placing a hand on the shoulder of the sufferer, with the statement, "I wish you were not suffering."

TO KILL A MOCKINGBIRD

The film clips from *To Kill a Mockingbird* (Pakula and Muligan, 1962) that lead to group dialog show attorney Atticus Finch (Gregory Peck) accepting the request to defend the falsely accused African American Tom Robinson although he knows the pain it will bring to himself and his family; and then his faultless, but futile, performance in the courtroom, where he turns and faces with truth the hatred and prejudice of his fellow townspeople. Finch's capacity to accept — to be with/in each moment as required — does not involve capitulation, and does not negate the futility of his effort, nor any of the pain or consequences for himself, his family and friends, the defendant and his family, or the local African American community. Yet, through his way of being, there is the potential for transformation.

Participants continue to pursue this theme in the contemplative reading of the week, a commentary on Sun Tzu's *Art of War* (Denma Translation Group, 2002), that explicates the core principle of *taking whole*: "True victory is victory over aggression, a victory that respects the enemy's basic humanity and thus renders further conflict unnecessary."

This is the also the victory that St. Joan of Arc was seeking in her ultimate efforts to turn the tide of battle and history with England and France in the fourteenth century: respect and acceptance, creating a segue for the intention of growing compassion.

Class 4 is designed as a retreat — the first hour flows in silence from one practice to another, reinforcing the intentions of embodiment, observing, and acceptance. As the group comes together for dialog, the reading from *Art of War* provides plenty of fodder, suggesting that the practices the group has been doing may help participants meet aggression differently. The practices have predominantly focused on work with aggression coming from inside. Now the issue is about how to meet aggression coming from outside. And the intention of growing compassion rises to the surface at last. In the presence and openness that brought Joshua Chamberlain "true victory" at Gettysburg, and in the openness and acceptance that brought Atticus Finch "true victory" in the courtroom and town of Maycomb, Alabama, compassion is showing. The dialog explores how to bring compassion into the very real situations participants are facing. The dialog closes with the practice of being for others; at the end, everyone stands, and, given permission, pair by pair, they place a hand on the other's shoulder and with eyes open wish them well. With the memory of so many faces, the final weekly reading assignment brings particular poignancy, introducing the idea that the other's face calls out to us, making a compassionate response imperative.

Chapter 7
Fulfilling the Intentions of Teaching

In teaching mindfulness as a professional, using your authenticity, authority, and friendship, each session is fresh and different, like a new wave breaking on the shore. Each progress through a course is unique. Participants and teacher find other ways of saying, demonstrating, learning, understanding — together. Participants and teacher are never the same, course to course, or even session to session, again like the river flowing past the shore. Never the same people again, as they are changing in each moment. There will never be these same sufferings, these same questions, these same jokes or joys — each a challenge to the teacher and the others. And so, there will never be these same responses. Holding this. Exploring that. Sitting with the terrible, the unanswerable, the riotous, and the oh-so-sweet.

It is because of this fluid nature of teaching that the curriculum must be empty. Not so that it can be filled, but that it may be fulfilled.

That is the challenge of this chapter: to offer ways of thinking, organizing, creating, and simply responding that lead to fulfillment. No laws, no rules, no step-by-step instructions can make that happen. Only the teacher and participants, co-creating their experience in the present, can do it. So this chapter, and this book, cannot be a recipe book to follow, to make the same casserole over and over again. (Amazingly, there are cookbooks for both practitioners and clients that purport to offer recipes for integrative experience – but not this one.) It can't be a coloring book, to make the sheep, say, blue, this time. It can't even be "Mad Libs," to generate infinite variations on the same story. Rather, our presentation of the spectrum of teaching intentions here is as a series of elemental motions or gestures that mark the presence of an intention — and its effects. Like watermarks on a riverbank or tide lines on the shore, the following presentations of each teaching intention are tracings of something at once more majestic, delicate, harrowing, and beautiful than could be prescribed or predicted. They are one way, our attempt, to capture the central motion of each intention. Our strategy is to keep descriptions gestural, broad, abstract, so that they can more easily be applied in the co-creation of mindfulness and the curriculum among particular teachers and participants. Each intention is offered through (we hope) a simple description, as well as through other descriptive methods that may help to make it available for reflection and use.

D. McCown et al., *Teaching Mindfulness: A Practical Guide for Clinicians and Educators*, DOI 10.1007/978-0-387-09484-7_7, © Springer Science+Business Media, LLC 2010

There are also graphic treatments that attempt to literally trace the motions. There are verbatim excerpts from inquiries with groups or individual participants that demonstrate how the abstracted motion of an isolated intention can be both near to and far from the actual messy moment of co-creation. And there are stories, poems, and insights from the deeply practiced community of mindfulness-based stress reduction (MBSR) teachers that expand the range of vibrations, hues, tones, and frequencies in which the intentions can be identified or applied. There are also considerations for curriculum development. Finally, in Chapter 8, there are scripts for basic practices that reflect the spectrum of teaching intentions, and in the Appendix there are listings of resources that can help teachers and potential teachers in expanding the possibilities of their ever-changing authenticity, authority, and freedom.

Experiencing New Possibilities

This intention is often the first to be recognized by participants. Mindfulness-based interventions (MBIs) are unlike almost any of the other classes, groups, or individual therapeutic approaches that participants have experienced. The differences can immediately subvert expectations or challenge familiar concepts in a way that engenders an openness to different perspectives and other ways of being. There is a range of these destabilizing factors, which can be ordered in three categories that, we hope, help make the dimensions of this intention a bit more clear. The first, *reordered relationships,* reflects the liminality of the mindfulness-based group; there are no certain roles or identities for participants or even, ultimately, the teacher. The second, *radical redefinitions,* refers to the "content" of the sessions; context, experiences, and languaging all undergo significant shifts of meaning and emphasis. The third, *transformative orientations*, suggests the ways in which mindfulness comes to find its co-constructed definition within the group; the teacher often catalyzes important discoveries in this process.

Reordered Relationships

In the first session, participants are asked to take a second look at their presumed medical and social identities. Particularly in the heterogeneous make up of MBSR groups, a participant's diagnosis ultimately is not sufficient or even useful as a self-definition. The teacher's implicit or explicit statement that, "as long as you're breathing there's more right with you than wrong with you," opens what may be for many a new negotiation of identity. This negotiation can also be evoked in the participant's social identity, as socioeconomic status and educational attainment are revealed to be of little use in meeting the challenges of the curriculum. This intensifies the sense of liminality of the group, which is coming together for purposes of transformation, suggesting development of *communitas*.

Participants may become aware of and open to a more egalitarian, democratic perspective because of two basic characteristics of the work of exploring mindfulness in practice. First, there are no gradients of the ability to be mindful;

everyone in the class can become more aware of and open to their own experience. This equal capacity certainly runs counter to the expectations of Western society, in which a group quickly stratifies by grades or levels. Suddenly, however, differences are not an important way of thinking about people. In fact, any possibility of competition is trumped by the larger vision of the course — it is not about improvement or change, rather it is about becoming more of what one already is. Everyone is therefore working towards the same goal — which is unique for each. Second, as the work of exploring one's experience in the moment begins, words fail — for everyone. It quickly becomes evident that verbal language, which is the main communicative instrument in almost all classes, is a tool that is hard to control. It bucks and slips in the authentic teacher's hand as much as in anyone else's; it is nearly always inadequate to convey the full weight of felt meaning (e.g., Gendlin, 1962). Relationships are indeed reordered — and everyone's in the same boat.

Radical Redefinitions

The course itself is in need of redefinition right from the start. Participants come into the first session with particular expectations, which are shifted or challenged quite early on. In MBSR classes, the central challenge is in the participant's understanding of the term stress reduction. They come in believing that they will be learning to turn off their roiling, racing minds and relax, only to hear that they're actually being asked to turn towards that roiling and racing — and to *welcome* it! Their expectations may be met with other reversals as well. A teacher might state: "You may think you signed up for a once-a-week class supported by homework assignments,

---

MBSR PERSPECTIVES ON EXPERIENCING NEW POSSIBILITIES

The immediate subverting of expectations and destabilizing of familiar concepts can be seen from a number of different perspectives that are more or less acknowledged as influences on the development of the MBSR curriculum and pedagogy (Santorelli, 2004).

The Buddhist perspective is succinctly presented by Daniel Goleman: "In mindfulness, the meditator methodically faces the bare facts of his experience, seeing each event as though occurring for the first time" (1988, p.20). This is made explicit as "beginner's mind," one of the attitudinal foundations of MBSR. As Kabat-Zinn (1990, p. 35) explains, "Too often we let our thinking and our beliefs about what we 'know' prevent us from seeing things as they really are."

Another acknowledged perspective is that of transformative learning, defined by its originator Jack Mezirow (2000, pp. 7–8), as one by which "…we transform our taken-for-granted frames of reference (meaning-perspectives, habits of mind, mind-sets) to make them more inclusive, discriminating, open, emotionally capable of change, and reflective so that they may generate beliefs and opinions that will prove more true or justified to guide action."

A perspective that is highly useful though less pointedly acknowledged is the concept of reframing, most distinctly defined in the family therapy literature by Watzlawick et al. (1974), p. 95), as meaning "to change the conceptual and/or emotional setting or viewpoint in relation to which a situation is experienced and to place it in another frame which fits the 'facts' of the same concrete situation equally well or even better, and thereby changes its entire meaning."

---

but it's helpful to see it as six days of homework supported by a once-a-week class."

The course also can be redefined through its activities — and their order. For example, the first session may begin by dropping participants right into the middle of things. With little preamble, without group introductions, the teacher can begin with an experience — a contemplative practice, a game, a story — that provides opportunity for discovery and reflection. Participants must hold their questions of who's who and what's what in abeyance. They must live for a time with *not knowing*, which is still another opportunity for discovery and reflection. A participant in a college class wrote in his journal: "I was expecting the class to go around in a circle and tell our names and a little about ourselves. As I sat getting myself prepared for what I was going to say, our instructor had us get into groups with a ball. The exercise was excellent. I wasn't nervous anymore and I became comfortable with the students in the class. After the exercise I didn't know what to expect out of the class, but I knew it was gonna be very different than any other class I've taken."

On a more global level, many of the class activities, particularly the formal meditation practices, are beyond the bounds of most participants' everyday experiences. Being asked to lie on the floor for the first body scan suggests that just about anything could happen in the classroom. Yet, all of this is presented as simple and ordinary, nothing special. That is certainly a redefinition.

Transformative Orientations

As the group and teacher begin the co-creation of a definition and experience of mindfulness, spaces often begin to open up for experiencing new possibilities. Those spaces are generated in any number of ways. Very often, they come from one of four orientations.

The first is orientation towards nonjudgment. We say "towards" because it is such a difficult attitude to hold; it can be a stumbling block in defining mindfulness. Nonjudgment may not be one's immediate reaction with/in an experience. It is likely, rather, that nonjudgment is a response that is negotiated, more or less smoothly, in the moment. The teacher meets participants with this kind of nonjudgment, negotiated through inner dialog — or even through rifts and repairs in the group dialog. Participants then begin to understand nonjudgment through their direct experience. And as they understand it, they may come to see the ways in which acceptance and compassion can arise from it.

Second is orientation in the present moment. This is often manifested in the ongoing co-creation of mindfulness as a privileging of immediate experience. Participants are asked to question their sustained narratives as ways of defining *who they are*, and instead to look closely at *how they are* as valuable and valid information. They are thus taking up a perspective that is opposed to the ingrained practices of Western culture and, particularly, of much contemporary discourse in the humanities and the professions, which posits the narrative perspective as normative for psychological and moral well-being. The emerging resistance to the dominance of narrative (e.g., Abbott, 2007; Strawson, 2004) supports the value of an *episodic* or *lyric* perspective on self-understanding, as is implicit in the MBIs, and reflected in the striking use of lyric poetry as a teaching vehicle.

Third is orientation in impermanence. Participants become sensitive to the constant flow of experience; what one treasures and what one fears can both be seen as continually slipping away. Participants find themselves in an environment in which change is the constant, in which it is *expected* that their condition will not be solid and intractable, but rather will be different moment to moment.

Fourth is an orientation of embodiment. This, of course, is a "rainbow gradient overlap" of the next in the spectrum of teaching intentions. Discovering embodiment will be discussed in detail in the next section. It is enough to say here that as participants find that the default question in exploring their experiences is not *What do you think*, but *What do you feel in the body*, they realize they may find answers they never believed possible.

Curricular Considerations

When these orientations are skillfully titrated for the sensitivities of the particular population, the participants will likely neither shut down when their fixed understandings and identities are challenged, nor be lulled into a sense of safety and familiarity that inhibits serious exploration. For example, in a college class, participants have the physical and emotional resources to be pitched without preamble into an experience that may feel like pointless chaos, as in the exercise with playground balls (Practice 1). Or in a patient class in which physical illness and limitations of aging are evident, participants can be guided towards new possibilities through a formal contemplation that confronts them with a question that is repeated again and again (Practice 2).

In the first class of the Center for Mindfulness (CFM) template MBSR curriculum, experiencing new possibilities is explicitly offered in two directed exercises (Santorelli and Kabat-Zinn, 2003). First is the mindful eating of a raisin. Through a guided encounter with one raisin at a time, participants are nudged into "not knowing" and an encounter with the present moment. By exploring the raisin with all the senses, new information challenges familiar ways of perceiving. As one example, when asked to "listen to" the raisin, an unconsidered dimension opens up; participants react with humor and real curiosity. Through such a contemplative approach to an ordinary undertaking, participants find they have challenged their understandings and habitual patterns. A participant in a recent class noted, "I've been eating raisins since I can remember, because I like sweet things and raisins are sweet. Now, I don't think I really like them. They are sweet, but I noticed the texture of the skin and the pulp...I don't find that particularly pleasant." The second exercise is the nine-dot problem, often given as homework after the first class. Try it yourself; the answer is given below. To struggle with the problem, and then to see the "out of the box" solution, can suggest the power of experiencing new possibilities. Coincidentally, Wátzlawick et al. (1974) discussed the nine dots in their work, and the continuing effect of seeing the solution: "Once somebody has explained to us the solution of the nine-dot problem, it is almost impossible to revert to our previous helplessness and especially our original hopelessness about the possibility of a solution" (p. 99). It is this reduction in helplessness and hopelessness that the "experiencing new possibilities" outcome emphasizes. Throughout the eight weeks, and into post-course life, we, as teachers, trust that new possibilities tremble at the edge of participants' experience, and that from week to week the potential for reframing experience moves from a guided offering by the teacher to a personal capacity within the participant.

THE NINE DOTS: A PUZZLE

. . .

. . .

. . .

Instructions: Without lifting the pencil from the paper, draw four lines so that all of the dots are connected with a line passing through them.

Discovering Embodiment

This Western culture in which participants (and teachers!) are embedded creates distance from embodied experience in many ways — perhaps three general views can help define this distancing and suggest how the intention of discovering embodiment can be actualized in a mindfulness-based curriculum.

First, contemporary culture encourages a life lived routinely "in the head," to the virtual exclusion of the body. We privilege cognitive understanding at the expense of the tacit, and language-based knowing at the expense of the inexpressible. This is evident, for example, in the unequal position of the crafts and trades in our educational systems. Even the MBIs have been critiqued for cognitive bias, for conflating thoughts and body sensations, seeing both as cognitive events (Drummond, 2006). As well, consider the overwhelming dominance of the visual and auditory media. Television, radio, the Internet, the graphic environment, and other technologies present to us a description or vision of life, not a direct experience. We spend hours every day in a simulated reality that points toward our heads — the location of eyes and ears, screens and headphones. Experience is "mediated" by technologies, developed under a cultural imperative of individualism, that help isolate us from others, and from our own bodies. It is perhaps easier to stay "in the head" than to sense into the changes in posture, breathing, heart rate, muscle tension, and energy flow that may be brought about by that cop show or even that cell phone call home.

Second, and flowing from our privileging of the visual, is the tendency to conceive of the body as object rather than as subject, as something to be seen from outside rather than as the locus of perceptions of actual lived experience. The question

"Does this suit make me look fat?" is seemingly far more captivating than "What am I feeling as I prepare for this meeting?"

Third, and flowing from body as object, is the focus on the body as a goal or achievement. Wanting to look a certain way, perhaps to be in accord with cultural norms, we subdue the body to the will in drastic and subtle ways. Whether in choosing to be shaped to fit boundaries of beauty by surgical procedures, or in adopting a diet discipline and exercise regimen to achieve a proposed ideal of health, something is left out: the body's own voice and wisdom.

All in all, it is possible that participants in the MBIs may have heard very little from their bodies — aside from the pain, discomfort, and other symptoms they are attempting to turn away from. They literally may be disconnected from enormous portions of their experience — and life. The intention of discovering embodiment helps to make this important link, both to the experience of movement in the outer world, proprioception, and the happenings in the inner world, interoception. By connecting with gravity and the breath, as emblematic of proprioception and interoception, participants can make a beginning of embodiment.

Navigating Towards Embodiment

As we've shown in the previous intention, participants are almost immediately invited to "be with" or "be in" whatever experience is arising in the domain of body sensation, without judgment. The experience of the body scan, the first practice introduced in many MBIs, is a useful example. The teacher's guidance attempts to bring participants to an unmediated experience of their bodies. The guidance provides permission for *any* experience to be present; we begin, say, at the top of the head, calling the participant's attention there, and offering language that names a range of experiences, from variations in temperature, to tingling, itching, pressure, to "nothing at all" — with an emphasis that "nothing at all" is a possible, acceptable experience. Further, participants are helped to parse immediate experience from stories *about* experience, to separate anticipation or opinion from the present-moment happening. Discoveries are very often pre-semantic, later processed in language as, "I feel more connected to myself," or "I know that my back hurts, but I didn't know what that actually feels like until now." Discoveries also may reflect the intersubjective dimension of the mindfulness co-created in the group, as in, "I don't quite understand it, but when I'm here with the group, I feel like my practice is better — I go deeper."

The discoveries brought about through embodiment multiply and deepen over time, as participants learn to navigate the territory of body sensations. To accomplish this, participants may need assistance in locating and approaching such experiences. Teachers can be helpful by finding and creating opportunities within the curriculum to emphasize implicitly and explicitly the essential navigational tools: gravity and the breath. These two can be seen as generating the cardinal points on a compass that assists participants in working beneficially with direct experience in the moment (see Fig. 7.1).

THE NINE DOTS: AN ANSWER

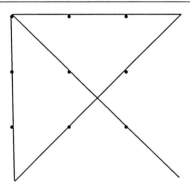

Solution: The "box" shape of the dots suggests that the solution is found inside the confines or boundaries of the dots. It is only through the discovery that the lines can be drawn "outside the box" that solutions become possibilities.

INQUIRY: "RESULTS" OF A BODY SCAN

Working with participants in a first session, immediately after a body scan, many sitting on the floor, turned towards each other. A few questions can point both to new possibilities and embodiment.

Teacher: What are you feeling right now?

An open question dropped into the silence. Expecting brief answers, and getting them.

Participant 1: Relaxed...

P2: At peace...

P3: Sleepy... I didn't know how tired I was until now.

  T: It's good to take the time to find these things out... to see how it really is, not how we need it to be, or want it to be...

Encouraging exploration; acknowledging new possibilities.

  T: How about anxiety... frustration...? Anybody? It's not necessarily all smooth sailing through the body scan...

Acknowledging the range of possible experiences. Giving permission.

P4: I couldn't be still. I kept having to move, and then peeking around to see what everyone else was doing — to see if I was doing it right... if I was OK...

  T: You are very OK... (pause) So you noticed that your body felt uncomfortable?

Reassuring. Nonjudging. Choosing a direction for inquiry that might touch on permissiveness.

P4: Oh, yeah! (laughing)
 T: And you were aware of moving and sneaking a look around?
P4: Sure...
 T: Then I'd say you were doing the practice very precisely, just right. Look at all the things you found out...

Further reassurance. Reframing the experience as about learning and knowing.

P4: I never thought of it that way.
 T: (Directed to everyone) This is a very simple practice, just moving through the body and noticing what is there in the present moment. There's no need to add anything more. And when you find yourself judging and reacting, that's right there in the body in the moment, you can simply notice that too... Everything fits in the practice, everything belongs...

Speaking to the judgments each speaker has implied, without directing comment to anyone.

P5: But I actually didn't feel anything in my legs...
 T: Did you notice judging that?
P5: Well, it just seems wrong...
 T: In this practice, there is no right or wrong... there is just present moment awareness, and yours was that you weren't feeling anything in your legs... the next present moment could be different.

Now a choice point; a reason to return to the practice, to refocus on the body.

 T: Maybe you could check it out right now... In the present moment, what's your experience of your legs?
P5: No, it is... it's different. I can feel them against the floor, their weight... my feet are cold... there's a kind of tingling... OK, yeah, I feel and sometimes I don't.

Exploring With Gravity

Gravity is such an all-pervading force that it is rarely considered or explored under its own name. Rather, it is commonly experienced in its relationship to bodily aliveness (Selver and Brooks, 2007). The body moves against or with it, with differing levels of energy expenditure, differing amounts of *up* negotiating with the constancy of *down*. It is unrelenting. It is inescapable. And it is, in many ways, comforting. Coming to standing from sitting, for example, requires widely varying amounts of *up* energy, from the burst of exertion as you start to rise, to the smaller negotiations as the knees and pelvis come into the more vertical plane, to the infinitely tiny adjustments that bring you into ease of standing — a relationship in which gravity is doing the vast majority of the work in holding you vertical. This relationship and the negotiations around it can be transposed into every posture you assume. Sitting, standing, lying, walking, in each there is an open invitation to feel out your yieldings and resistances as the earth draws you towards itself. The relationship can not only be transposed, but also translated — as the objects that you handle relate to gravity through you. Lifting, holding, carrying, placing, in any activity with whatever is given in the moment — book, tea cup, tire iron, stone — there is much to be learned. In lifting, what is the right amount of up for the tea cup, and how do you know? In placing, what is required to control the down of the cup to the saucer so that it comes to rest without being dropped or pressed?

In all the formal mindfulness practices with participants, then, they can be asked to explore the body's relationship with the constancy of gravity. As they work with its unrelenting nature and their own energies — sometimes triumphantly, sometimes fruitlessly — they can explore struggle, comfort, surrender, refreshment. They can use gravity's "down" and their own "up" to orient themselves, to discover themselves as an embodied presence in this present space. On a finer level, they can use down and up, their own giving and resistance to gravity, to help discern, explore, and even comfort a particular event in the body. This reflects the rainbow gradient relationship to cultivating observation.

In informal mindfulness practices, participants can attend to this orienting relationship — say, in the shower, on the bus seat, carrying a package, or washing the dishes. They can also use it to discern and work with embodied events. Such attention has the capacity to bring them right *here*.

Exploring With the Breath

The breath is equally as pervasive as gravity, but in another mode. It is constant in its inconstancy, flowing steadily, providing a sense of *in* and *out* — the other two cardinal points on the compass. The breath's motion, its cycle, is usually soothingly repetitive, and the supply of air almost always seems vastly greater than the demand. When you turn the attention to the breath, it can create a sense of well-being, a sense of unimpeded flow from moment to moment.

All the points of the compass.
The relationships to gravity and the breath bring out the cardinal points on the compass with which participants can navigate direct experience, but there are an infinite number of other points on the compass rose as well. Every sense, every form of knowing, contributes to what is revealed in everyday language as "finding yourself." The poem below, by David Wagoner (1976), is used in many MBI classes and contexts to describe this process. It is a version of a teaching story from the Native Americans of the Pacific Northwest, where to venture off the path in the old growth forests could be a disorienting experience. Think of these lines as instructions.

Lost
Stand still. The trees ahead and bushes beside you
Are not lost. Wherever you are is called Here,
And you must treat it as a powerful stranger,
Must ask permission to know it and be known.
The forest breathes. Listen. It answers,
I have made this place around you.
If you leave it, you may come back again, saying Here.
No two trees are the same to Raven.
No two branches are the same to Wren.
If what a tree or a bush does is lost on you,
You are surely lost. Stand still. The forest knows
Where you are. You must let it find you.

The cycle of in- and out-breaths creates and keeps a kind of time, marking out the "vertical" time of *now*. Daniel Stern (2004) in attempting to define the present moment, notes its relationship to perceptions, verbal and nonverbal behaviors, relational understandings, and mental operations, attributing an average duration to all these of from three to five seconds. For example, most spoken phrases last about three seconds, five at the outside; a musical phrase is likewise three to four seconds, and a greater than three-second stop suggests an ending; baby talk and nonverbal communications in the mother-infant dyad have been measured at between two and five seconds and turn-taking in adult conversation takes two to three seconds. The breath cycle of in and out takes about three seconds, as well — a present moment.

In all the formal meditation practices, participants can use the breath to explore embodiment. When they bring the body to stillness and quiet, they may find it possible to sense the influence of the breath in surprising places and ways. In a body scan, perhaps the effects of the breath can be felt in the arms and hands, the pelvis, and the feet. A growing sense of the breath being available everywhere allows it to be used in exploration of constant and transient sensations, from pain to pleasure, from head to toe. Through this familiarity, participants can develop an ability to

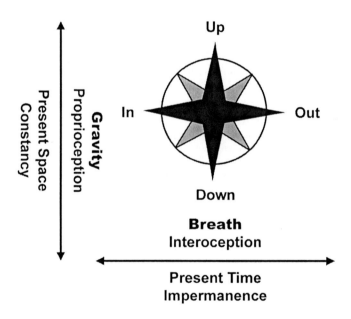

Fig. 7.1 *A compass for navigating direct experience.* This simple instrument can be combined with the triangle of awareness to help participants locate and approach direct experience. Using gravity to center the body in space, to come to a disposition of stillness and constancy. Allowing the breath to center the body in time, in the fluidity and impermanence of the present moment. Located at these coordinates, the participant has a certain physical and psychological freedom to look closely at the flow of sensations, thoughts, and emotions arising now.

"direct" the breath like an instrument to find, touch, surround, and even soothe a particular area. Again reflecting the next intention.

In informal practice, participants can bring attention to the response of the breath to brushing teeth, sitting in a boring meeting, mopping the floor, petting the cat, or lying down to go to sleep. Or, pointedly, to explore and work with specific sensations. In any case, participants can be using the breath to have the experience right *now*.

Curricular Considerations

Gravity and breath, up and down, in and out, meet in the here and now. The teacher can leverage curricular opportunities, or create them, for participants to develop more intimate relationships with gravity and the breath. Through such standard offerings in the MBSR curriculum as the body scan (Practice 3) and mindful Hatha yoga (Practice 4), particularly in the repeated exposure through audio recordings used for home practice, many facets of these relationships emerge over time. The sense of embodiment can be discovered and deepened, creating the conditions for the cultivation of observation as that rainbow gradient begins to show.

INQUIRY: IN THE MIDDLE OF A MINDFUL STRETCH

At the opening of Session 3 of an MBSR course. After several standing stretches, introducing a spinal twist — hands on hips, turning the body from the waist, while keeping the hips in the original plane, to look beside and behind. Asking participants to hold the posture and check in to body sensations. Then asking them to relax the muscles that don't need to be used.

T: What are you noticing right now? Anybody? It might be anything...

> Choosing the moment to ask by noting the perceptible shifts in expressions and postures. Giving plenty of space and time for responses.

P1: Easier...
P2: Not so tiring...
P3: I didn't know I was holding so tight...
P4: I can actually turn a little more now...
P5: My breath is calmer, slower...

T: So you're doing just what the situation requires, no more, no less... that's mindful practice... And it's the same with thought and emotion... Is worry "just the right amount of effort?"

> Offering the new embodied knowing as larger, workable in all the "tensions" participants may experience.

P3: Oh my god, no! (General laughter)

Cultivating Observation

So much happens with new possibilities and embodiment in early sessions that this intention, the third and pivotal one of the five, is often not held explicitly by the teacher or uncovered intuitively by participants until later.

In the flow of the curriculum, participants begin to settle in to home practice and to appreciate the new possibilities that their participation brings. At some point, they begin to tune in to their capacity to notice discrete events — sensations, thoughts, emotions. The attention in the body scan or sitting meditation drifts away, perhaps, into a thought, and they see that it has happened. They often then assume the default position of "I am having this thought," in which the "I" is identified with the thought. This position of self as subject is natural, logical, and extremely limiting. The ingrained and well-worn ways of experiencing that support this self-as-subject help to maintain its limits. The thoughts or events identified with this "I" are judged through prediction, memory, and desire. This cold hospital chair, this dim lighting, this dull ache, these recurring thoughts of death, this pulse of fear, this is my world. My *little* world. There is a sense of constriction, almost a claustrophobic quality to the experience, as graphically suggested in Fig. 7.2. It is such suffering, more often than not, that etches the limits of the little world of "I" in ways that show it clearly.

> **RUMI REFLECTS ON THE UNITY OF AWARENESS.**
>
> With all this explanation of stepping back, observing, and seeing thoughts and sensations as "not me," it is helpful to be reminded by the mystical literature that we are not divided but whole. Across traditions, around the world, there is insistence on the unity of awareness. In poetry, song, or art, this is not an abstract idea, it is a felt meaning. Rumi's meditation in verse (Barks and Moyne, 1997) makes the truth of it available in ways that literally "make sense."
>
> We are the mirror as well as the face in it.
> We are tasting the taste this minute
> of eternity. We are pain
> and what cures pain, both. We are
> the sweet cold water and the jar
> that pours.

The pivot of this intention comes when "I" see the "I" that is suffering, and know that the identification of that "I" with the thought, pain, or emotion is not true. Participants make those statements, such as "I am not this thought," "I am not this pain," I am not this fear." The event is dis-embedded and becomes observable. The second observing "I" is a step away from the first, suggesting an expanded space in which events can be reflected upon. What's more, if this second "I" can see the first, the way is opened for a third to see the second seeing the first — and on back and back, like the ever-receding images created when two mirrors face each other. These observing "I"'s, then, are neither solid nor central. Nor are they separate. Each is simply a temporary, albeit useful, platform for observation within a unity of awareness. Now the constricted "I" is part of a much larger context, and has room for expansion, as suggested in Figs. 7.2 and 7.3.

Identification

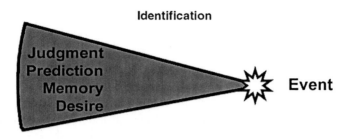

Fig. 7.2 The little "I" observing an event, say, a thought or pain, identifies directly with it: "This is my pain." Judgment based on prediction, memory, and desire intensifies identification, and, in the case of pain, constricts in suffering, as the narrowness of the band suggests. Pleasant and neutral events also have this structure, yet the felt quality of the "pinch" is often less evident — at least for a time.

Observation

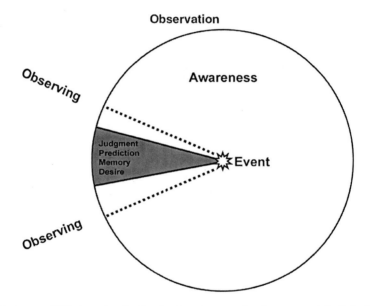

Fig. 7.3 A second "I" observing the first is a larger context for the event and the little "I." It is a context in which awareness expands around the little "I" allowing exploration and offering space in which constriction can find relief. (Note that the graphic convention of the circle makes a boundary where none is implied; awareness is boundless).

Curricular Considerations

The challenges in holding this intention in teaching, particularly after class 1, are to leverage or create opportunities for participants to recognize and cultivate this capacity for expanded observation. Within the template MBSR curriculum, participants may first recognize it while formally practicing or inquiring into experiences of the body scan, Hatha yoga, or awareness of breath practice. This suggests how the intention of cultivating observation shifts and gradates from discovering embodiment in the spectrum of intentions, as participants come to understand that the illimitable expanse of awareness and the life of the body coincide. Constriction and expansion have felt meanings for which gravity and breath provide a vocabulary — heaviness and lightness, effort and ease, depth and shallowness, suspension and flow.

Once observing awareness is available, it is most explicitly cultivated in the template curriculum through the formal expanding awareness practice (Practice 5). The practice allows exploration into discrete domains at first, from breath, to body sensation, to sound, into thought, and then emotion. Then it shifts to choice-less awareness, in which the capacity for observation is cultivated in attending to virtually any event to which the attention is drawn in the ongoing expanse of awareness. A standing meditation such as the one on "being open" (Practice 6) can offer further unexplored perspectives, especially as it works directly with the visual domain and the proprioceptive sense.

Opportunities for inquiry with the group and individual participants are extremely important in cultivating observation for two reasons: first, to be able to point to the vast-ness of awareness, its infinite capacity for expansion; second, to ensure that awareness is understood as a unity, that the observing "I"s are not reified (made into "things") but understood as fluid. If the big inquiry questions about discovering embodiment are "What" questions — "*What* are you noticing?" — the central questions in cultivating observation are "Who" questions — "Who is noticing?" or "Whose thought is it?"

This intention and the next, moving towards acceptance, are intimately related, dif-ficult to disconnect within the rainbow gradient. They are connected in the same way as discovery and exploration — there is an ever-recurring simultaneity of true richness.

INQUIRY: "NOW I SEE"

After an expanding awareness practice, opening up to the movement — the pivots of observation that come early and later, unbidden and worked through.

T: What did you discover in this practice?

Open, permissive, allowing for anything.

P1: I was actually worried about worrying today... Before the meditation, I was worried that I wouldn't be able to meditate, because I was having so many thoughts about something that happened at home before I came to class. I am such a worrier... But during the meditation when you said "Just notice the process of thinking and let thoughts be," I realized that thoughts were there, but — so what! I didn't attempt to push them away, to get rid of them. I realized that they were just going to be there, and I didn't pass judgment on them. I'm going to have worrisome thoughts, but if I don't focus on them or fight with them, they just come and go... and it's OK for them to be there. To me that's really, really a light bulb moment.

Unbidden, within the expanding awareness practice with its intention to cultivate the observing capacity, the pivot happens. Space opens in awareness for whatever is there to be there, be seen and acknowledged, and to shift in its own time.

Later in the same discussion, a participant notices the hard time she's giving herself, the difficulty of clearly observing what's present.

P: I have a lot of trouble identifying what I'm feeling. I know there is a feeling there, and it even feels familiar, but I don't know what it is. And I am struggling to figure out what's happening, what the feeling is. And then I start asking myself how is this meditation really going to help me.

T: What would you call that "how-is-this-meditation-going-to-help-me?"

Offering help with the identification process. Using what's present in the moment.

P: (After silence) I guess it's a thought.

T: It is a thought… and it is also a thought that is leaning into the future. So when you notice this thought arising you can label it with a whisper, "thinking." and come back to your breath or whatever you have chosen to focus on. Also, when you are noticing that you are struggling to try and figure out what's happening you can label that "trying to figure out" or "struggling."

Suggesting labeling as a strategy for clarifying and reducing reactivity towards what may feel like a jumble of events.

T: How do think your body feels when — … Actually, rather than thinking about this, would you like to explore with a direct experience right now? (Looking around the group in nonverbal invitation to others to undertake their own exploration)

Making (and remaking) a choice to move back into practice, to return to the body for help in clarifying experience. Note that as other participants are working along, this return to practice will effect intersubjective resonance, providing a more expansive environment for this inquiry dialog.

P: OK…

T: So, now, taking a moment to check into your body and mind and see what is here now…

P: (Settling into chair in meditation posture; long silence) It's a familiar feeling, like I'm efforting, like I have to figure something out.

T: What does that feel like in the body?

Locating the feeling within the space of the body, where it can be observed.

P: I'm tense… so tight… It's anxiety.

T: When you notice thoughts that tell you that you have to figure something out, label them as thoughts and come back to your breath…

Responding to the effort, the need-to-know of "It's anxiety." Making the thought process observable.

T: (After a long silence) What are you noticing?

Choosing to ask when cued by shifts in posture and breathing.

P: I'm relaxing. This is wonderful. I hadn't really realized what I was doing, trying so hard to figure everything out in my head. And how that makes me so tight and anxious. Now I see. This is wonderful.

Moving Towards Acceptance

If the intention of cultivating observation is the pivot on which the curriculum swings, this intention of moving towards acceptance is the swing itself, using all the momentum available in the teacher and participants. It is the "turning towards the symptoms" at the historical root of the MBIs. It is the being with/in of experience that is the central invitation to participants. It is the transformation through which participants find that they are "big enough" and "have enough space" within them — within awareness — to hold whatever is arising in the moment.

It is not surprising, then, that moving towards acceptance is the bulk of the work of the mindfulness-based group or dyad. It is quite common that more time is devoted to this than to any other single intention. This intention is in many ways the most full and important, while, in curricular terms, it is the most "empty" and imperceptible. Inquiry into participant experience is the primary perceptible activity, bringing an exploratory, unpredictable, and improvised quality to sessions, particularly the later ones.

Exploring in the Space Outside

The environment of mindfulness and the intersubjective resonance co-created by the teacher and participants is the context that allows participants to inquire, explore, and move towards acceptance. The ideal environment for each session reflects an ongoing diminishment of judgment and reduced roles for prediction, memory, and desire in defining peoples' stories. This often prompts participants to say things like "I feel safe here," and "This class is a refuge for me each week," and "I never thought I'd be saying this out loud... ." The environment then is an outer expression of the space of awareness that is the context for

Beauty, gratitude, and an awareness filled with fear.

As sessions proceed, the practice of mindfulness shows itself to participants to be very different from the coping strategy or "way out" of undesirable situations that they may have been wishing for or imagining. As they come to explore the boundlessness of awareness and the movement towards acceptance, they may come to understand that it is not about change, but about freedom — the freedom to simply be with/in the experience of the moment without coping or escaping.

The psychiatrist, spiritual director, and lover of wilderness, Gerald May (2006), recounts a story from a solo camping trip that makes the potential of acceptance obvious. He is deep in bear country, deep in the night. He has secured his camp, put food and other bear attractors in the car. Still, he feels insecure — fearful, in fact. A night of nerves and fitful sleep, and then, a bear:

> The bear is right next to me, its side brushing the tent canvas, its growl deep, resonant, slow. This is no dream and I am terrified and yet I feel a strange calmness over everything, so difficult to describe. It's like some kind of fierce embrace...
>
> For the first time in my life, I am experiencing pure fear. I am completely present in it, in a place beyond all coping because there is nothing to do. I have never before experienced such clean, unadulterated purity of emotion. This fear is naked. It consists, in these slowly passing moments, of my heart pounding, my breath rushing yet fully silent, my body ready for anything, my mind absolutely empty, open, waiting. I *am* fear. It is beautiful. (pp. 31–32)

Fear is running free in the space of awareness, and can be seen for precisely what it is — the cultivating observation. It is an intersubjective version of the fullness of the circle representing awareness in Fig. 7.2 in the last section.

Although direct inquiry with the teacher is the most perceptible form of exploration in each session, it would be unwise to privilege it as the main vehicle for moving towards acceptance. Given the environment of intersubjective and intrasubjective resonance, participants who seem to be simply watching the inquiry into another's experience may actually be doing deeper work. They may be working along and accepting and changing in ways they may never report. They may even be keying in to different facets of the spoken inquiry, as becomes clear in the two selections below from participant reflections from the same class. The first participant was helped to turn towards, locate, and open space for a pain in the lower back through inquiry that catalyzed curiosity with questions about what the sensations felt like, including if they had a size, shape, color, and with suggestions for the use of gravity and the breath. The second was one of several who spoke up after working along.

Participant 1: In class on one particular Tuesday, after the meditation, my back was hurting. You had me close my eyes and focus on the pain and its location. You asked what the sensations of pain felt like — did they have a size, a shape, even a color. At first, I was not getting it. All of a sudden, the shape was oblong and the color was blue. Concentrating on the area, the pain slowly subsided. It was amazing. Even more amazing was that others in the group did it too and had a similar reaction to it.

Participant 2: After the scan when we got up, you asked us a few questions about the body scan. June spoke on how she couldn't get comfortable because her back was in extreme pain. My back was hurting too. You had us do a breathing exercise to focus directly on our back. The pain began to move, it felt like waves in my back. It was weird. I actually saw the pain as a color. It was blue. I was totally amused. It was really cool to actually focus my breathing into my pain and it went away.

Of course, participants are also exploring and inquiring entirely on their own, as the

embodied experience — and how it is — beautiful. The outcome, when the bear leaves and May ventures out of the tent, is exhilaration at the brilliance of the starry night and an overwhelming sense of gratitude:

The real gift of that night was that I had been unable to do anything about my fear of the bear. Lying there in the tent, I could not run away; I could not make the bear go away; I could not reassure myself that things were going to be all right; I could not trick my mind into thinking about something else. There was nothing to be done, and that was the gift. I could only be there in the real situation, being real, being pure fear. (p. 34)

For those of us teaching mindfulness as professionals, May's reflection on his experience points to just how profoundly different from much contemporary practice in the helping professions our work really is:

In my psychiatric practice, how many times did I help patients cope with their feelings, tame the power of their emotions? I no longer believe that was helpful. Even when I assisted people in uncovering long-buried emotions, I seldom encouraged them to savor the life-juice of the feelings themselves...

Instead, for the most part, I helped them cope. I have come to hate that word, because to cope with something you have to separate yourself from it... Wild, untamed emotions are full of life spirit... They don't need to be acted out, but neither do they need to be tamed... They are part of our inner wilderness; they can be just what they are.

Our work is not about separation from experience, but rather about discovering, exploring, and tending to unity.

intersubjective context supports or even catalyzes inner exploration. This unseen activity is a part of the co-created curriculum too, whether or not it ever receives outward expression — or acknowledgment.

Exploring in the Space Inside

There is a movement from macrocosm to microcosm, from the space in which the teacher and participants interact, to the space of awareness perceived in an embodied way by a participant. It is a space that opens to exploration: as observation is cultivated, the space becomes more vast. Thus, to explore awareness *is* to move towards acceptance. Participants are given the suggestion and the opportunity to observe their troubling event — thought or pain, perhaps — within a context that can expand until the view is more tolerable. This is described graphically in Figs. 7.4 and 7.5, which can be seen as continuous with the graphics of cultivating observation.

There are two traditional metaphors that define the expanding action of moving towards acceptance in ways available to the senses. The first considers the event as a wild animal, say, a horse, in a small enclosure. From up close to the fence, the bucking, rearing, galloping are threatening — uncontrollable. Yet if the fences are set back further and further until the horse is in a large meadow, there is a sense of control. In fact, the once threatening actions and energy reveal a rare grace and beauty. The second metaphor takes the event as a handful of salt. Added to a glass of water, the taste is overwhelming. Tossed into the reservoir, it's undetectable. It's just tiny bit of a natural nutrient.

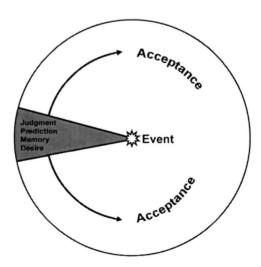

Fig. 7.4 *Moving towards acceptance means expanding awareness.* The motion of this intention is a sweeping opening of the constriction of the little "I" defined by the limiting factors of judgment, prediction, memory, and desire. As the constriction moves into a larger and larger space of awareness, acceptance moves through possibility to actuality.

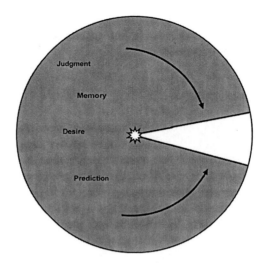

Fig. 7.5 *Expanding awareness allows greater ease*. With the sweeping open of constriction, the space of awareness becomes a wide meadow in which the wild horse of the event — thought, sensation, and emotion — is free to run. In that boundless space its energy, grace, and beauty become clear. Likewise, to use our other metaphor, when the limiting factors are dispersed as a handful of salt in a reservoir, they lose their bitterness. Moving towards acceptance is an expansion of awareness that brings participants greater ease.

Curricular Considerations

The challenge, then, is to find opportunities in each session — and beyond — for participants to bring events into larger and larger contexts. As this intention becomes more salient, curricular material is almost of necessity less structured and planned, more arbitrary and contingent on participants' and teachers' present-moment experiences. Just as the teacher and participants are drawn more and more to co-create mindfulness and intersubjective resonance in the earlier sessions, they are drawn as well to co-create more and more of the curriculum in the later ones. Material is generated both from the participants' experiences and from the teacher's authenticity, authority, and friendship.

Formal practices in session can be used to generate opportunities to move towards acceptance. In a body scan, participants can be invited to be with an area of the body or that is "calling out to them" — language that suggests "unpleasant events" yet leaves room for exploring the pleasant as well. Their curiosity can be catalyzed and they can be guided to explore and to open the awareness around the target area — to step back, to make space, to soften. The same can be done with an expanding awareness practice. Or practices can be designed explicitly to move participants towards acceptance (see Practices 7 and 8). Such practices often result in engaged and resonant inquiry, during which it is often helpful to return to the embodied experience of formal practice again and again.

Moving towards acceptance in informal practice simply becomes life lived with a larger awareness. Participants are invited by their own curiosity and encouraged by their own experiences to identify what in their ongoing experience is asking for acceptance and then moving towards it. Health, work, career, relationships, moment by moment, events come into awareness — which can constrict or open in response.

INQUIRY: CONSTRICTING AND EXPANDING AROUND FEAR

This inquiry did not come out of a practice, but rather before one. It is the sixth session of an MBSR course; participants have spent a week working with the expanding awareness practice. The teacher describes a practice designed to help with understanding choice-less awareness, in which participants narrate in a whisper the flow of their present moment experience to a partner. One participant is visibly upset, and is engaged nonverbally by the teacher.

P: I have a lot of fear... I want to run out of the room... I feel vulnerable.

T: That's what you notice now... a lot of fear and vulnerability... Are you able to be with this on your own right now, just voicing it, or is there something that would be helpful in addition?

Acknowledging. Allowing things to be as they are. Trusting that the participant knows what is needed.

P: I'm not sure. Vulnerability has come up pretty strong.

T: Where do you feel this vulnerability in the body?

Bringing an abstract feeling into view in the body. Giving it limits and definition.

P: My stomach and my back... my back is in pain.

T: If you bring your attention to your stomach or back, what does it feel like?

Making space, distance required to see and answer.

P: I don't really want to say this, but it feels like I am going to throw up.

T: Why wouldn't you want to say this?

Genuine curiosity and nonjudging.

P: I don't want to make other people uncomfortable.

T: So, you don't want to make others uncomfortable, but this is your truth in the moment. (Silence) In this moment, you feel nauseous. As much as you are able, stay with the sensations in your body...

Pointing to the validity of present moment experience. Returning again to embodied experience as observable.

T: (After silence) What are you noticing now?

Permissive, curious. Cued by nonverbal shifts.

P: I'm sad.

T: Something has shifted and you are experiencing emotion, sadness.

Acknowledgement. Staying with the experience.

P: (After silence) I'm noticing that I am picking my finger nails, trying to distract myself I think... I'm going in and out of feeling.

T: So you are going in and out of feeling. Is the nausea still here?

Acknowledging. Returning to observation in the body, a gentle insistence.

P: No, that's gone. I'm just sad. (Long silence) My mind says I can't cope.

T: Do you have thoughts/beliefs that tell you that sadness and coping don't go hand in hand?

Locating, observing thought.

P: Yes, I've always had to be strong and I can't fall apart.

T: Is there another belief that if you allow sadness, you will fall apart and not be able to function?

P: Yes...

T: Allowing ourselves to feel sadness doesn't mean we are not strong, and falling apart does not mean we will not function — falling apart can be a step in regrouping, coming together in a new way, perhaps even stronger and wiser than before.

Offering an opportunity for a shift. Note the use of the plural, drawing in the other participants. Working within intersubjective resonance all this while.

T: (After silence) What are you noticing in the body now?

Gently insistent, returning to the workable space of the body.

P: I feel like crying... I am more comfortable though... It's OK.

There is more space.

T: Do you have a sense of wanting to run out of the room like before?

Bringing perspective.

P: No, but my thoughts are about me being weak... I have lots of judgments about myself, and that's so sad... (Crying quietly; silence) I'm not perfect... (said softly, sincerely).

There is space now for observing, identifying, parsing experience.

T: That sounds more like a kind acknowledgement of being human than a judgment?

Genuinely curious.

P: Maybe a little judgment, but I'm really feeling more kindness right now.

T: (After silence) How does that feel?

A prompt to move from the abstract to the observable.

P: My mind is peaceful. I feel soft, kind of tender. My body is not hurting… My body is not hurting. I'm just noticing my breath.

T: Let's all do that… noticing our breath for a few moments…

Turning the group's attention to individual experience. Offering time and space just to *be* together, with no one at the center.

Growing Compassion

As the bottom gradient band on the spectrum of teaching intentions, growing compassion can be seen as an underscore, an added emphasis to the four intentions above it. All are held with an intention of growing compassion. It is a constant, integrated into the curriculum both implicitly and explicitly. It is evident in the actions and interactions of teacher and participants from the first session to the last. But it does not have the same qualities from first to last. There is a shift that coincides with the pivot of cultivating observation and the subsequent transformation of moving towards acceptance. To fully understand this shift, and to make use of it in fulfilling a mindfulness-based curriculum, it is best to understand the definition of compassion and its two complementary motions as they are proposed here. It is also best to keep in mind that this presentation of compassion is designed as simple and "empty" to optimize flexibility and facility of use in the moment of teaching.

Definition

Compassion here is not precisely identified with *karuna*, the "wish to take away the suffering of others" as described in the four *Brahma Viharas* of Buddhism in Chapter 3, although that wish informs it. Nor is it exactly the emotion-heavy definition from the dictionary, with its cognates of sympathy, sorrow, commiseration, and pity, and its Latin root meaning "suffering with another," although these inform it (Webster's,

---

DO EXPLICIT PRACTICES TO CULTIVATE COMPASSION BELONG IN THE MBIS?

Whether or how compassion-related practices should be integrated into a course devoted to development of mindfulness skills has long been a subject of debate in the MBSR community. Kabat-Zinn (2005) notes that for pedagogical and practical reasons, he was reluctant to include such practices, as they are implicitly embodied in all of the practices and teaching, and as they may confuse participants just learning mindfulness practice by interjecting a sense of *doing*, by "…invoking particular feelings and thoughts and generating desirable states of mind and heart" (p. 286). However, he justifies limited introduction of loving-kindness practice because, "on a deeper level, the instructions only *appear* to be making something happen. Underneath, I have come to feel that they are revealing feelings we actually already have, but which are so buried that they need continual invitation and some exceptional sustaining to touch" (p. 286).

Other MBSR teachers have not found such pedagogical dissonance, or teach in venues that virtually require introduction of compassion practices early on, and thus have developed curriculum adaptations that include loving-kindness and other

1961). And, again, it is informed by, though not identical with the Buddhist-influenced psychological concept of self-compassion (Neff, 2003), with its three basic components: "(1) extending kindness and understanding to oneself rather than harsh self-criticism and judgment; (2) seeing one's experiences as part of the larger human experience rather than as separating and isolating; and (3) holding one's painful thoughts and feelings in balanced awareness rather than over-identifying with them" (p. 224). Compassion in the context of the "empty curriculum" is meant, rather, as a larger, more encompassing, and less emotionally charged term reflecting its relationship to the other four intentions and the co-created relationship of teacher and participants.

compassion-oriented practices from the earliest weeks of the course. They also routinely include such practices as ongoing home practice for participants, supported by audio recordings. To defuse any dissonance of doing versus being, practices can be guided with recurring injunctions such as "noticing how it is with you right now, in the body, emotions, and thoughts," and "knowing that you can offer loving-kindness [for example] with all that you are in this moment — whether you're feeling loving-kindness, or anger, or sadness, or any other way of being." From such a perspective, participants can simultaneously allow their own experience and hold a compassionate intention.

Protestant theologian Tillich (1957, 1963) speaks of *love* in a way that can be recruited to assist in a definition of compassion for mindfulness pedagogy. Tillich states that "Love is the drive towards the reunion of the separated" (1963, p. 134). He sees the driving power towards reunion as essential, the nature of life itself. Aligning with this drive, then, could be seen to be compassionate — suffering with the separated, and wishing and doing whatever is possible to bring about unification and reduce suffering. Transposed into the mindfulness curriculum, this is seen most clearly as a participant is able to observe the little "I" constricted around an event in a larger context, and to accept that event and thereby realize the unity of awareness. Such an action often has the result of reducing the participant's suffering and expanding her capacity to be with/in her experience. Her growing capacity to be with/in whatever is arising also makes her more available, more present, to others in the group — and in the world. Simply through her greater capacity to be present, to turn towards rather than away from her own or another's suffering, she is being compassionate.

Two Motions

At the start of the first session, participants are often suffering from separation from part of themselves; they are constricted in their relationship to the experience of their lives — reflected in discomfort in the body, in thoughts, in emotions. They may attempt to work with this separation and the discomfort it brings through compassion — moving it in one direction or another. Some will find, particularly in the early sessions, that they need the compassion of others, particularly of the teacher. They draw compassion towards them with a kind of centripetal force that moves it inward to help relieve their constriction. Others

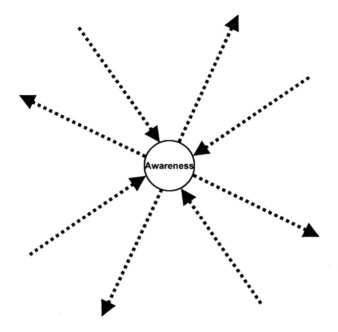

Fig. 7.6 *Centripetal and centrifugal compassion in early sessions.* When awareness is constricted around an event, a participant may find a certain amount of relief by drawing compassion towards herself — often from the teacher. It is also possible that a participant cannot accept compassion into his constricted little "I", and that relief is found instead in offering compassion to others — often approached as "fixing" the other. As suggested by the thin dotted lines, such experiences of centripetal or centrifugal compassion in this constricted context are relatively weak, intermittent, and barely "touch the surface" of suffering.

will find that they have difficulty accepting the compassion of others, and that they find some relief from their constriction in a centrifugal motion as they feel others drawing compassion outward from them. Of course, any combination and degree of the two is possible, including no engagement with compassion at all.

The Shift

Centripetal and centrifugal motions of compassion continue session to session, yet there is a significant change in the quality associated with each motion over time. In the early sessions, the centripetal motion has a focused, needy quality. It draws most significantly on the teacher, whose being in many cases reflects a relatively more open and unified awareness, with a less judgmental view and a more permissive approach. The teacher is thus more present for others than most other participants. At this same time, the centrifugal motion has an anxious quality about it. The need to find relief from separation, from constriction, may manifest in the drive to tell personal stories, to offer advice, in short, to "fix" others. From this perspective, the teacher's more expanded awareness and greater capacity for holding may be frustrating, as it does not fit the classic frame of *helping*.

As sessions go on, and participants are able to observe their constricted little "I" and to open around it, the quality of compassion does indeed change. With an expansion of awareness, a diminishment of the limiting factors, and a motion towards acceptance, participants may be reunified with their own experience. With this shift comes a notable change in the quality of centripetal compassion. Because there is less constriction, there is a greater capacity to receive, and to receive from participants as well as the teacher. What is new is that because awareness has expanded and there has been some reunification of the separated, it is also more possible for participants to draw in compassion from themselves. There is also a corresponding change in the quality of centrifugal compassion, as the constricted little "I" expands, and the other can be seen as less distant, less different, and less threatening. There is a reduced need to prop up the little "I" with stories, to demonstrate competence by giving advice, or to "fix" others. At the same time, the presence and authenticity generated by the reunion of the separated — the participant's less reactive relationship with her own experience — transforms whatever may be offered into something more valuable and nourishing for the other.

Participants who are more unified, whose awareness is expanded, also find compassion drawn from them by others. A professional example comes from the reflections of a participant in a graduate-level mindfulness program in which the final session was a silent three hours of practice — a mini-retreat:

> I had a really cool experience at work. In fact, it was the day after the mini-retreat. That next day, three patients revealed amazing and highly emotional stories to me in the process of their testing. One woman from another country began crying when we spoke of her past in the country she came from. She missed her country; her family is struggling to adjust here... Another woman revealed a story of her disabled sister and her mother's metastatic cancer... Another patient stopped by to show off her baby. She herself has some health problems but looked radiant. She said – oh by the way – she just separated from her husband... Now, patients often share personal stories during their time with me, but on that day the number and depth of emotions they shared was striking. I had to wonder if I was more open and more present after the mini-retreat, such that they were more comfortable expressing themselves to me. Or, was it just coincidence?

This participant felt the pull of the centripetal force of compassion, and, although she does not describe her own responses, there is a sense that one who would notice this experience would respond centrifugally with care.

Of course, the two motions of compassion and this significant shift can be framed and spoken about in many different ways. For example, a description based on intra- and intersubjective resonance, as they develop from session to session and influence the group and individual participants, would be another way to account for the same motions and shifts.

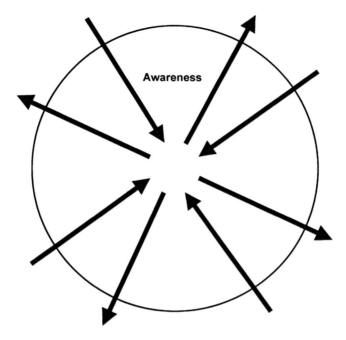

Fig. 7.7 *Changed quality of centripetal and centrifugal compassion in later sessions.* When awareness is expanded so the participant has some freedom to observe her experience, compassion takes on a different quality. Centripetal compassion is drawn less insistently, and can be accepted more fully and consistently. Centrifugal compassion is offered more gently, from a deeper understanding of the common human condition. As the graphics suggest, such compassion is more affecting, stable, and connected to experience in the moment.

Curricular Considerations

Compassion, particularly its centripetal motion, is implicit in the formal and informal mindfulness practices, and in the didactic material introduced in the early sessions of the MBSR template. That is, the teacher's early role makes it salient, particularly through nonjudgment, permissiveness, and authentic empathy. The centrifugal motion in those early weeks is most likely discovered in teacher–participant inquiry, group dialog, and participants' budding intragroup relationships. As curricular focus shifts to the intentions of cultivating observing and moving towards acceptance, the shift begins to take place for many participants, so inquiry and languaging of practice guidance can shift along to explore the possibilities of greater centripetal compassion from within the participant herself and more centrifugal compassion for others in the class and in participant's lives.

In the template MBSR curriculum of the CFM, an explicit practice of loving-kindness is introduced somewhere between weeks five and seven, often during the all-day session. This practice of offering wishes for happiness, safety, well-being, and ease is usually designed to broach the subject of centripetal compassion very permissively, so participants may explore with reduced reactivity. A version of a loving-kindness practice that we use (Practice 9) presents permissively an opportunity to offer intentions of loving-kindness for oneself and for others from whatever emotional space one is in; the practice is not to change one's feelings but to acknowledge them and offer intentions through them and with them — to be completely accepting of one's own experience. The loving-kindness practice is often a link that helps many participants connect their personal practice to the relationships in their domestic and work lives. Further, they discover the potential impact of their individual transformation on family, social circle, workplace, and political, social, and environmental awareness, as well as on their spirituality.

Outside the template MBSR program, many MBSR teachers integrate explicit compassion practice in much earlier sessions. The shift to an expanded awareness and movement towards acceptance may or may not happen earlier for participants, yet this addition would seem to offer additional relief from the constriction of the little "I". It is also common — and popular with participants — for graduate courses to be devoted to compassion practices. A compassion practice that works deliberately with the relationship of expanded awareness — the capacity to remain open — to catalyze acceptance is included in Chapter 8 as well (Practice 10).

INQUIRY: SOME MOTIONS AND MOVEMENTS OF COMPASSION

In the sixth session of a foundation MBSR course, the group is heterogeneous, with helping professionals mixed in with patients. This fact adds poignancy to the dialog.

P: If you were to ask me how I am this morning, I would have said I'm feeling good, even happy. But when you asked us to sit and check in, I noticed how bad I feel.

There is something I am angry about, and every time I sat to meditate this weekend there were lots of feelings that were unpleasant. It was really hard to meditate. What was up was how much was uncomfortable — lots of sadness, and underneath that, fear, and underneath that, despair. That's what's coming up. Anger is the one I struggle with the most. It's really hard to sit with for me. There was a lot of it. I had the awareness of how inward it goes. I was angry at some of the choices I made. Someone was not returning my phone calls and what emerged was feelings of helplessness. But the more I sat with it the more angry I got at myself. It's hard to admit but there is really a lot of self hatred that came up with the helplessness.

It's funny that I was reading about mindful communication this week. I would fucking communicate mindfully with this person, if they would fucking call me. And I would even do it fucking compassionately. (Laughter in class.) But I made four calls and didn't get a reply. The more rage I felt, the more I felt it going inward, toward myself.

T: There's lots of emotions arising for you.

P: Yeah, yeah... It's Awful!

T: It's hard to be with all this...

Acknowledgement. Compassion both drawn centripetally and sent centrifugally.

P: *(Sighing, crying; then, after silence) I'm a therapist and I work with people who self-injure. My God, I really get it now — why someone does that. It's embarrassing to say it, for the first time ever, I really get why someone would cut themselves. I don't want to do it...*

Recognition of authentic compassion.

T: *You can feel that level of pain?*

Recognition of authentic compassion.

P: *(Crying) Yes, wanting to release it (the pain) myself because there is no other release.*

(Crying, then) Just saying it out loud, I'm feeling better.

T: *That was the very question I was going to ask — how are you in this moment?*

P: *I was embarrassed, but it's all really true. It's the truth and I feel better.*

(Crying stopped) I feel calm...

T: *(Silence, looking around the group) Let's take a moment to check in. Anna has been sharing really authentically. Noticing what is coming up for you right now. Seeing if you can simply notice without needing to change anything or do anything.*

Making space for observation.

T: *(After silence) What are you noticing ? What's arising ? Pop-corning out a word or two.*

Offering permission. An opportunity to express, to connect, to acknowledge centripetal and centrifugal compasion.

Group: *Compassion... Empathy... Truth... Tension... Sadness... Being human... Connection...*

T: *Anna, how are you right now? What are you noticing?*

P: *Relief... Gratitude... I'm tired and a bit weary... And in this moment, I'm OK.*

Chapter 8
Practice Scripts and Descriptions

This chapter presents scripts for a range of practices, including the core practices of mindfulness-based stress reduction (MBSR), and practices that approach the teaching intentions from different perspectives. They are specific embodiments of the "emptied" motions or gestures of the teaching intentions, drawn from our own authenticity, authority, and friendship. If Chapter 7 characterized the water marks or tide lines of the intentions, perhaps the practices in this chapter are objects found at those lines — a piece of driftwood, a pretty shell, a polished piece of broken glass. They are that concrete, and that unique. Perhaps their usefulness is found in the way that driftwood might be used by an artist: taken home, looked at reflectively, and then abstracted into a new creation. Take these for inspiration, not imitation. Feel the gestures called out in the margins, don't follow them.

Practices for Experiencing New Possibilities

Practice 1: Playing Attention
Approximate Timing: 15–20 minutes

This activity can provide a common experience that translates easily into a group dialog about mindfulness. There are countless variations possible from the basic gestures of the one-to-one encounters and the attempts at group-relating.

This practice is guided as a meditation — one that gets pretty wild. The description given here is actually just a sample of what can be done. The "object" for the teacher is to improvise instructions that toggle the participants' expectations and experiences between order and chaos, joy and frustration, or whatever else arises in the group or suggests itself to the teacher. Use of inviting language is important, as is the use of bells or some other method of attracting attention in class? chaos.

D. McCown et al., *Teaching Mindfulness: A Practical Guide for Clinicians and Educators*, DOI 10.1007/978-0-387-09484-7_8,

Disrupting the circle of chairs before it has been used, declaring the rule of impermanence. And bringing participants into embodied contact with something possibly pleasurable, and certainly not predicted.

Acknowledging the enormous range of possible experiences, and introducing the triangle of awareness.

Facilitating a flow of varied mind–body states.

Moving participants' attention from outer activity to inner. Exploring again the triangle of awareness.

Begin by clearing as large a space as possible in the room, perhaps moving all the chairs out to the perimeter. Then handing each participant a playground ball — anything from a heavy rubber "four square" game ball to a light vinyl beach ball, to a "pinky" or "Spaldeen," depending on the teacher's own childhood memories, available resources, or the size of the budget.

Guidance at this point is something like: "Noticing what having one of these in your hands does to your experience of your body, your thinking, and your emotions. Maybe this is part of your history...of triumph...or sadness...or embarrassment... Just being aware of how it is."

Then setting the essential ground rules: "This won't necessarily be a quiet experiment, but please try not to talk. Limiting yourself to nonverbal communication. Following the instructions as best you understand them. I'll ring a bell from time to time. When you hear it, simply stop where you are... bringing your attention to what is happening within you... perhaps closing your eyes if that helps and feels comfortable in the moment. When the bell rings again, continuing what you were doing.

Commencing the action by asking participants to walk at random through the room, explaining that, when they make eye contact, they should exchange their ball with the other person's, hand to hand, and then move on. When participants have found a rhythm, modify the instructions every minute or two, by asking them to make the exchange in different ways. For example, "Making the exchange... from a distance ...from up close... in a formal way... in a casual way... in a fancy way... over a tall fence... under the fence... without anyone seeing... one-handed... behind the back..." Remember, this is an improvisation, so key into what is happening in the group, shifting instructions to amplify or oppose ongoing action, speed, mood, or whatever draws your attention and curiosity.

At any time during these shiftings, when participants are in states that you deem interesting to investigate, ring a bell to stop, and have them turn attention to what is happening in the moment: "Coming to quiet and turning your attention to the energy in the room; what is it like right now?... And, if it feels comfortable, closing the eyes and tuning in to the body; how is it with you?... Noticing breathing... possibly the heart rate... aware of thinking — not so much the content, but the speed, density, and quality of thoughts... and attending to emotion — how do you feel right now?"

Ring the bell again and have the participants return to their activity. On one of these returns, perhaps changing the instruction to something like "Making the exchange precisely," to give them an opportunity to experience the potential of greater clarity after pausing and turning inward.

Reordering relationships.

As the activity begins to become routine — or, better, before — ask participants to come together as groups of 6 to 10, depending on the overall count. Perhaps you can improvise an interesting way for this to happen, or maybe you just step in and make an arbitrary division. Ask each group to come into a circle, and have all but one person put down their ball. Begin by asking them to throw the ball to someone in the circle. Whoever receives the ball will say their first name and throw the ball to someone else. As a rhythm develops, you will move from group to group, handing another person a ball from the ground, so that more balls come into play. Ask the group to see how many balls they can get into play. This can become quite chaotic — and fun.

Ring the bell at a chaotic moment. You'll know when. And check in as before; moving from outer to inner experience, using the triangle of awareness. Then, beginning again, ask them to also try to say the name of the person to whom they're throwing. Add more balls as it goes on. Ring the bell, come to quiet, and check in.

May point up the contrast between flowing, embodied experience and experience dominated by thought and judgment.

Then shift again, asking them to use speech and to figure out a pattern through which they can get all the balls into circulation — but they can't simply pass them to the person next to them. As they negotiate, ring the bell, come to quiet, and check in to experience in body, thoughts, and emotion.

Inquiring particularly around *reordered relationships, radical redefinitions,* and *transformative orientations.*

Shift one last time, away from the dominance of thought and judgment. Allow them to pass to the person next to them, so the balls simply flow around the circle. When all are in circulation, ask for variations, such as more speed, greater precision, complete silliness — amplify or oppose whatever draws your attention in the groups. Ring the bell, come to quiet, and check in. Then bring the circle of chairs back together and spend some time in dialog about what people noticed about individual and group experience.

Practice 2: Well Meditation (from the teaching of Saki Santorelli, EdD)
Approximate Timing: 10 minutes

This is a guided contemplation that does not require an introduction to mindfulness. As such, it is useful as an opening experience for initial sessions. The material that becomes available to participants through the repeated asking of a question often touches deep human longings and concerns. In the sharing after the contemplation, relationships are often reordered, as common themes are revealed. There is a sense that the shared human condition is in the foreground, and age, gender, race, diagnosis, professional identity, move to the background.

Giving the permissive option to use imagery or not.	Sitting in a comfortable position. Bringing your attention to your body... Feeling the support beneath you... Noticing your breath wherever you feel it most vividly in the moment, with the air flowing in and out the nostrils... or with the rising and falling of the chest or abdomen... Simply following your breath moment to moment."
Repeating the question.	If imagery is helpful to you, you may want to imagine a deep well... And imagining a pebble beside the well. ... picking up the pebble, feeling it in your hand.... The pebble carries with it a question ... and when you are ready, dropping the pebble into the water with the question that it carries... *"What brings you here?"*... And noticing what answer or answers splash up." Just sitting in silence and listening...
Repeating the question. Potential for radical redefinitions, answers different than they originally "thought."	*"What brings you here to be sitting in this class?"*... Sitting in silence.
	"And now, as the pebble drops deeper into the water, notice if any other answers reveal themselves from a deeper place within in response to this question, *What brings you here?"*
Preparing for introductions and sharing of answers — "as much as you care to."	"And when you're ready, bringing your attention back to the breath...simply noticing the in-breath and the out-breath... and feeling the body sitting here.... And when you're ready, allowing your eyes to open..."

Practices for Discovering Embodiment

Practice 3: Body Scan
Approximate Timing: Introduction, 3 minutes; Practice, 25 minutes

This is a recording script for this core practice of the MBSR curriculum and of many interventions that make use of the MBSR armature for teaching. Within a research paradigm utilizing MBSR as the intervention, the preferred version of this practice begins with the feet and moves upwards to the top of the head. This version begins at the top of the head. However, the practice can be started and finished anywhere, and there are many ways of moving through the body, such as section by section, or first one side then the other, or following a circle or ring around the body that progresses gradually up or down. All are useful at particular moments in teaching, depending upon intention. The intention of this version is to effectively initiate and support "discovering embodiment."

Introduction

This is a recording of a mindful body scan, designed for you to use regularly to help you assume an active and powerful role in your own health and well-being.

It is best to listen to this recording — and to do what it says — while in a comfortable place where you can feel safe, secure, and free from interruption... Looking at this practice time as an opportunity to be both *by* yourself and fully *with* yourself... an opportunity to nourish yourself, to open to and experience the potential of strength and healing within yourself.

A radical redefinition, suggesting a preference for embodiment over cognitive, verbal processes.

Our culture asks us to live so much in our thoughts, in our heads, that we may sometimes forget that the *whole body* feels and knows... that there is a wisdom beyond words... we may have built-in habits that ignore, minimize, or completely shut down the possibility of feeling our own aliveness... Now, the body scan is an opportunity to connect a little more to the body — this marvelous sensing instrument that can bring you closer to yourself, to the world, and to others... this practice is a time for gentle exploration of each *present* moment.

Reinforcing nonjudgment. Offering options.

The opportunity to explore bodily experience can be very helpful... you can begin to notice what feels good, what you withdraw from, when you tense up, and when you can give yourself space... this is a time for simply *being* your experience ... *being* just as you are... without criticizing, judging, wishing, or trying to change the experience in any way... While many people prefer to do the body scan lying on their back on the floor, the body scan can be done in any position, lying or sitting... on the floor, on a bed, or on a chair... what really matters is your presence in the moment.... what really matters is that you are choosing to show up for what's happening *now*.

Body Scan Practice

Lying on your back, with your arms and hands at your sides and legs outstretched ... or with the knees bent and the soles of the feet on the floor, if that is more comfortable ... or sitting in a chair in a relaxed posture... making a choice to allow yourself to be exactly as you are in this moment...

Exploring the breath and its soothing potential.

Coming gently to notice the breath... it's such a constant feature of life that it's easy to ignore... so taking time with it now... actually feeling the sensations as the breath enters the body and leaves the body of its own accord... allowing it to move through its cycle of in-breath and out-breath without controlling... if it feels right to you, attending to the belly, the lower abdomen, noticing that it may be rising and falling with the cycle of the breath... if you care to, placing your hands on your belly... feeling the movement of the breath, the rhythm, the waves of the breath... simply riding the waves of your breath from moment to moment.

Offering a safe haven.

As you listen to this body scan, if at any time sensations in the body become too uncomfortable, or emotions arise that are too difficult, knowing that it is always possible to return to the breath as a safe place, a haven, a retreat for you to rest in, until you are ready to venture again into the body scan... wherever this recording is in its progress.

How far can you feel the breath?

If you've placed your hands on your belly, taking them off now, and moving your attention to the top of your head... noticing that sensations may arise when you bring attention to a particular part...maybe tingling, maybe pressure, maybe a feeling of the breath or the pulse affecting this area... or perhaps there's no sensation — that's OK, that's simply your experience of this moment.

And when you're ready, moving your attention to your forehead... observing any sensations...perhaps furrows of tension, or tingling, or a sense of relaxation... allowing yourself to feel whatever you feel.

Exploring with light and breath.

Now moving your attention from the forehead to the eyes and eyelids... noticing how you're holding them... how much or how little pressure does it take to keep them closed? Experiencing the eyes from the inside, from behind the eyelids... are the eyeballs moving or still? Is there darkness? light? color? How does the breath affect this area?

Moving attention from inside to outside the body.

When it feels right, beginning to pay attention to the cheeks... sensing the bones, the muscles, the skin of the cheeks... noticing the play of air, sensations of coolness or warmth... noting perhaps that some sensations stay for a while, while others pass quickly... and that intensity may change one way or the other as you bring attention to them...

...and attending now to the nose, from the bridge to the edges of the nostrils... perhaps feeling the breath in the nostrils as it enters and leaves... noticing temperature, moisture, sensations on the upper lip, perhaps...

Suggesting interoception of "echoes" of the movement of the jaw.

Moving the attention to the jaw... being aware of tightness or softness... allowing the lower jaw to drop down slightly, and noticing any changes in sensations in the muscles of the face and neck, or in other parts of the body which that small movement may create... and expanding your focus of attention to include the mouth and lips... inside the mouth, the tongue against the teeth, against the roof of the mouth... if you care to, breathing in through the nose and out through the lips... allowing the air to play on its way out... observing the sensations of dampness, dryness, warmth, or coolness...

Moving away from concepts, towards direct experience.

And expanding the attention to encompass the entire face... not a picture of your face in your mind, but really feeling the sensations in the area that we call the face.... What's there for you? ...aware of any thoughts and emotions as well... and if thoughts or emotions arise allowing them simply to come into awareness and pass, like clouds in the sky...

Shifting the attention to your neck... noticing how it is right now in the big muscles in the back of the neck, from the base of the skull to the shoulders... the throat... aware perhaps of the play of air or touch of clothing... being present in this experience...

The breath for navigation.

Moving now to the shoulders, checking into their condition in this moment, any tightness or softness, recognizing that this is the condition *now*... accepting it, knowing that it does not need to be some other way... and knowing also that conditions change... noticing if there is a sense of the breath in the shoulders... how much of the body does breathing affect?

Allowing the attention to travel to the upper and mid back... sensing the muscles, tight or loose... aware perhaps of sensations of the weight of the body here... pressure against the floor or chair back, feelings of the texture of clothing...noting how the breath moves in this area...

Gravity for navigation, and for presence in unpleasant or pleasant moments.

Bringing attention to the lower back, to the sense of contact or lack of contact with the floor or chair, the sense of yielding to gravity or resisting, any tightness or softness... noticing any tendency to move away from or towards any sensations or thoughts, feelings, judgments that may arise... remembering that this is simply how it is in the lower back at this moment...

Moving away from concepts and language.

And experiencing the whole back now, from the shoulders to the base of the spine... aware of the subtle and not so subtle motions of the back as you breathe... dwelling in the sensations of the back, not watching from your head... just knowing what the back knows....

Gravity and breath.

Shifting to the arms... to the upper arms and forearms... aware of the pull of gravity, the weight of the arms... feeling the muscles and joints, the touch and texture of clothing... and expanding the attention to include the wrists and hands... sensations of warmth, or coolness, tingling, moisture, or dryness... how does the breath affect the arms and hands? Is it possible to feel the pulse here? Just being with what's here now...

Exploring interoceptive possibilities.

And moving, as you're ready, to the chest... aware of the lungs and heart in this space... maybe sensing inside, as the lungs fill and empty... perhaps noticing the heartbeat, the rhythm of the heart and the breath together... being present to these sensations of life... and feeling the surface, the touch of clothing, any sense of movement...

Making possibilities of interoception explicit.

Now extending attention into the abdomen, the belly, feeling inside first... this place where we have our gut feelings — there really are nerves here that sense and know — feeling into the motion of the diaphragm, the sense of the breath in the belly...

Gravity and the breath to stay oriented in a potentially uncomfortable physical and psychological experience.

When it seems right, moving attention to the pelvic region, from hip to hip... aware of the effects of gravity, the weight of the lower body ... the buttocks pressed into the floor or chair, sensation in the hip joints... the groin, the genitals... the lower abdomen... tuning in to the sense of the breath, of the pulse here.. how far do they reach? And noticing thoughts and feelings that may arise... aware of judgments, and, as it's possible for you, letting them go...

Shifting the focus into the upper legs — the thighs... aware of gravity's work, the pressing against the floor or chair, the feel of clothing against the skin, and moving in...

Aliveness.

the quality of the muscles, tight or loose…is it possible to feel the bone running through?

… and extending the attention now to the lower legs, the calves and shins… noticing points of contact or lack of contact with the floor or chair, aware of gravity, aware as well that the legs are alive — how does the breath affect them? How about the pulse — is there a sense of the blood flowing?

When you're ready, exploring onward… to the feet… feeling where they are, the floor, perhaps a sense of temperature… warmth or coolness… a sense of the breath and heartbeat perhaps?

Comfort of gravity and the breath.

Now expanding the attention to include the entire body from the soles of the feet to the top of the head… being present to the totality of the experience of sitting or lying here in this moment… perhaps feeling the breath — how it has been a constant companion, how it brings the whole body together…as does the pulse, the heart beat…. feeling the sense of gravity, the sense of being held gently, closely, without fail… dwelling in what the body feels… in what it *knows*…

In the last moments of this body scan, congratulating yourself for spending the time and energy to nourish yourself this way… for continuing to make choices to live a more healthy, satisfying life… and knowing that you can carry this awareness of your body's deep wisdom beyond this practice session and into each moment of the day, wherever you may find yourself.

Practice 4: Floor Yoga (Script for Recording)
Approximate Timings: Introduction, 2 minutes; Practice, 25 minutes

A recording script for the mindful Hatha yoga presented in the MBSR curriculum. While many movement practices are easily presented as mindfulness practice, Hatha yoga is, in our experience, easily accessible for fulfilling the intention of discovering embodiment. Participants make connections to their bodies quickly and in many cases joyfully. Central to the presentation of the practice is the permissiveness with which it is presented. It is offered for the purpose of exploring the body in motion, without expectations of meeting some objective standard or improving one's "performance" or abilities, as participants may first assume from their cursory exposure to Hatha yoga in the popular culture.

Introduction

Activating the schema
of the triangle of
awareness.

This program of gentle yoga stretching is an invitation to enter more deeply into the life of the body… to experience the mind and body as one, as a unity… to bring them together, as the meaning of the word yoga — to yoke or join — suggests. And as with all mindfulness practices, this yoga is about paying attention, moment to moment, to the sensations, thoughts, and feelings that arise in your awareness…

Permissiveness.

The movements in this program are designed to be done on the floor, where a yoga mat or a blanket may make you comfortable… If you are unable to get down on the floor, you may wish to use a bed — preferably one with a firm mattress…

Offering alternatives.

As you go through this program, entering into the experience of the body as deeply as you can, and without judging… this is not about performing, about doing the movements in some ideal way for some critical audience… Rather, it's about doing them to help connect more closely to, and better understand, the body… So, not forcing any movement, rather, relaxing into it… not taking on any part of the program that seems inappropriate for you, instead, using your knowledge of your own body and its limits to guide you and to override the instructions, adapting the movements in a way that works for you… or skipping them entirely and perhaps imagining yourself doing the movements, feeling them in stillness, which is a valuable practice in itself…

Floor Yoga Practice

Let's begin in rest pose…lying on the back… allowing as much of the body to contact the ground as you are able, from head to heels… If you have any problems with the lower back, bending the knees instead, and placing the soles of the feet on the ground as if standing… aligning the shoulders, hips, and feet, so that the spine is straight… if you care to, gently lifting the head, tucking the chin in slightly and setting the head back down…noticing the sense of a straight spine from the base of the head all the way down to the pelvis… legs a bit apart, feet falling slightly outward… arms lying alongside the body, and if it's comfortable, turning the hands to face palm up…

Orienting with gravity and breath.

Noticing how the ground accepts you, how gravity works so you don't have to... and bringing your attention to the sensations of the breath in the body... aware of sensations of rising and falling, expanding and contracting, on in-breath and out-breath... and with each breath, allowing the ground to receive more of your weight... working less, trusting and accepting more...

Breathing in and out... and when you're ready, breathing in, lifting the arms gently and allowing them to travel in an arc upwards to vertical — noticing the sensations as they move through the air — and then allowing them to descend to rest on the floor outstretched above the head...

...pointing your fingers towards the wall behind you and, at the same time, pressing the heels in the opposite direction... stretching the entire body... relaxing the stretch and breathing out, allowing your arms to travel back through the arc — slowly; aware of the sensations of movement — without anticipating their return to the floor; allowing an element of freshness of experience as they come to rest again at your side... and as you lie still now noticing how you feel in your body after having completed one mindful stretch...

Once again, breathing in and allowing the arms to travel through an arc... feeling the changes in effort as gravity pulls and assists... until the arms come to rest on the floor above the head... and pointing the fingers in one direction and the heels in another, feeling the stretch wherever it can be noticed in the body... noticing any thoughts or feelings that may enter awareness, and as much as possible, allowing them to simply come and go like clouds in the sky...keeping attention centered on the sensations of the body...

Now releasing the right side of the body from the stretch while maintaining it in the left side... noticing the stretch in the left side... and noticing the sensations in the right side as well...

And releasing the left side and stretching the right side, noticing the sensations in both the right and left... then, breathing out, allowing the arms to return through their arc to rest by your side...

Refocusing on embodiment.

Aware of how you feel, lying in rest pose again... aware of thoughts and emotions, and as much as possible letting them go as you focus on bodily sensations right now... in this moment...

Exploring relationship with gravity and breath.

Moving the arms out from the sides to rest outstretched as a "T"... and if the knees are not already bent, bending the knees and bringing the soles of the feet to rest on the floor ... aware of the sensations in the body in this position, aware of breathing... and on an out-breath contracting the lower abdomen and moving the lower back down towards the ground, lifting the tailbone slightly and making as much contact with the back to the ground as is comfortable... feeling this stretch... and on the in-breath, then, relaxing the abdominal muscles and pressing the tailbone down to raise the lower back, noticing the sensations associated with this arch... On an out-breath, again contracting the abdomen and lifting the tailbone... and on the in-breath releasing the abdomen and pressing the tailbone down... and in your own time, following your breath, rocking the pelvis... noticing thoughts and feelings arising and allowing them to pass as clouds in the sky as you focus on the sensations in the body...

Pausing... aware now of stillness and sensation... ... Then drawing the knees up towards the chest and embracing them with the arms... interlacing the fingers, perhaps... breathing like this... and on an out-breath, seeing if you can draw the knees a bit closer to the chest... finding the limit where you are comfortable, and not passing it ... then beginning with small movements, rocking gently from side to side, massaging the back... how much effort does it take to get started?... When does gravity take hold and begin to pull the body too far? ....aware of the sensations in the back... and if it's comfortable for you, bringing the head towards the knees; again not passing your limit of comfort... learning to accept the limitations of the moment, and knowing that limits change one way and another from moment to moment *and* over longer periods of time... lowering the head to the ground... and coming to stillness...

Discerning essential from added effort. Then letting go of the right leg and extending it along the ground, while continuing to hold the left knee to the chest... stretching the right heel towards the wall and at the same time drawing the left leg closer... ... noticing how much of the body is involved in this stretch... investigating the face perhaps... is there tension generated there? And investigating the need for that tension... how does the stretch in the right leg feel without it? Is it possible to work with just the legs and arms in this posture? ...then releasing the left leg and allowing it to stretch out along the floor, while simultaneously bringing the right leg up towards the chest and embracing it with the arms...

extending, stretching the left leg... what tension and looseness is required? And, when you're ready, releasing the right leg, placing it back next to the left.... Aware of the sensations in the resting body...

In your own time now, rolling over onto your belly and coming to hands and knees, with the back parallel to the ceiling — like a table... ...then moving the knees outward a bit and the feet inwards, perhaps with the big toes touching... and lowering your buttocks back and down into this open triangle... the head and trunk moving downwards as you do this, and the arms can be outstretched with the forehead touching the ground between, or if it is more comfortable, you can fold the hands on top of the other, and rest the forehead there...this is child's pose, a rest pose for when we are working in this orientation on the ground... adjusting your body for comfort and rest... breathing into this pose and experiencing the sensations in the body in this moment...

Pressing down with the hands and raising the buttocks to return to hands and knees, like a table... as you breathe in, arching the back so the abdomen moves towards the ground, and lifting the head up, looking up and out in front of you... breathing in and out in this cow pose... and on an out-breath contracting the abdomen and moving into cat pose, by arching the back towards the ceiling and drawing the head down in between the arms...And moving back into cow pose, relaxing the abdomen and arching the back, so the abdomen moves toward the ground, and bringing the head up to look outward... And when you are ready, moving back into cat pose, abdomen contracted, back arching toward the ceiling, and head to chest. Moving back and forth now, at your own pace, between cat and cow, following your breathing... If you need to rest at any point, in this or the next set of movements, feel free return to child's pose...

Exploring the relationship to gravity; framing experience with sensations of breath and pulse.

...Coming back to a table position, aware of sensations — the breath and the heartbeat, perhaps... how far can you feel them in the body?... Now, while focusing your visual attention on a point ahead of you to steady yourself, releasing the weight from the right knee and extending the right leg out behind you, holding it out parallel to the ground, with the toe pointing back... then, shifting weight to the right hand, lifting the left arm to shoulder height, parallel with the ground, pointing it forward, the fingers pointing forward, and balancing... noticing what is required to achieve this... what tiny motions? what shifts and adjustments? Feeling free to touch down as often as needed to remain steady —

relatively! (said with humor) — and now drawing the arm and leg in under you to resume the table pose... ...now shifting weight to the right knee and lifting and stretching the left leg back while at the same time weighting the left hand and stretching out the right arm... stretching... holding... adjusting... aware of the whole body's involvement at this moment... now drawing the arm and leg back and coming to stillness...noticing the breath and perhaps the heartbeat in this moment, perhaps a sense of warmth from exertion...

Then coming down to the ground and resting on your belly... aware of your relationship with gravity and the breath... aware of sensations, thoughts, feelings in this moment... letting thoughts and feelings go by without following, without attaching to them...

And in your own time, rolling over onto your back... Bending the knees and bringing the soles of the feet to the floor as if standing, with the feet close together... bringing the arms out in a "T" position... and letting both knees very slowly fall over to the right... letting gravity work... keeping the shoulders on the ground, and turning the head look out to the left... looking out over the left arm and hand... sensing this spinal twist throughout the body... how far does your awareness extend?... and bringing the knees slowly back to center... and allowing them to fall slowly to the left, while turning the head to face right, to look out over the right arm and hand... at your own pace, doing a few of these spinal twists... aware of the sensations along the back, and throughout the body... and bringing the knees to center and to stillness... and on an out-breath, extending the legs along the ground...

Assuming rest pose... and resting now, at the end of this session... if it feels right, acknowledging the effort, the care, and the caring-for-yourself that you bring to this practice...

Practices for Cultivating Observation

Practice 5: Expanding Awareness
Approximate Timing: Introduction, 2 minutes; Practice, 30 minutes

This is a recording script for this core practice of MBSR. This is perhaps the practice that allows the fullest expression of the spectrum of teaching intentions. As the central practice for most professionals teaching mindfulness, guidance of it may very well go through the most constant change and refinement — as the teacher discovers or is drawn to investigate the innumerable facets of the practice.

Introduction

Acknowledging the inevitability of judgment.

In your formal practice of sitting meditation, you are taking a seat right in the middle of your life. You are intentionally bringing yourself into a direct and intimate relationship with the present moment and what is arising in it for you — as much as possible without judging.

Possibilities of transcending the little "I".

In this recording, you have the opportunity to expand your attention to explore body sensations, sounds, thoughts, emotions, and, when you are ready, to open to all of these — to the full range of events within and without as they move and change, appear and disappear in awareness. You are taking time to become more familiar— moment by moment — with who you *are*, beyond all the wanting and having and doing...

Encouraging willingness to be present to whatever arises.

In a sense, this practice is a perfect expression of your own unique presence in the world... So it is helpful to come to this practice with a sense of kindness and care for yourself ... and to bring a dignity and nobility that befits your special status to the time, place, and posture of your sitting practice... Setting aside a regular time, when you won't be interrupted... In a quiet and comfortable place that can nurture your practice... And sitting, whether on a chair or cushion, with an attitude of confidence and stability — not leaning into or moving away from anything, simply present with and open to what is happening now...

Expanding Awareness Practice

Orienting with gravity.

Sitting in an upright position with your back straight and yet relaxed. Dignified... Embodying confidence... Feeling the floor or chair or cushion beneath you, supporting you. Feeling gravity holding you, the earth receiving you. Finding a point of balance where gravity is holding you comfortably upright, without strain. Allowing the body to become still...

Orienting with the breath.

And bringing your attention now to the sense of the body breathing, the breath entering and leaving the body...

Bringing curiosity and freshness to this moment... and noticing where you feel the sensation of breath most vividly now... and centering your attention there...

Emphasizing impermanence.

Simply breathing in and out... noticing that there is a beginning, middle, and end of an in-breath and a beginning, middle, and end of an out-breath... (long pause).

Watching the entirety of an in-breath from the beginning to the end.

Noticing the moment, the space, or pause, when it shifts to become an out breath... and then noticing the out-breath from its beginning to its shift as it becomes an in-breath... (long pause).

Realizing that no matter how many times the attention leaves the breath, awareness of that does arise, and there is an opportunity to choose and to bring the attention back... to this in-breath and or this out-breath, now... (long pause).

Allowing the breath to be at the center of your attention and allowing any thoughts to come and go like clouds in the sky... (long pause).

If the attention has wandered from the breath, gently but firmly escorting it back, making the breath the center, the focus of attention again... (long pause).

And now, when you are ready, expanding your attention beyond the breath to include also the entire body, sitting... Becoming aware of sensation in the body... Perhaps sensations of contact with the chair or cushion... Perhaps the touch of clothes on your body, or how your hands feel in the moment. Sensations of temperature. Being present with any sensations as they arise...

Emphasizing impermanence.

Noticing how sensations sometimes stay for just a short while, and how other times they linger... Noticing how they change in intensity, shift, and pass away as new sensations arise... like the breath, they have a beginning, middle, and end... (long pause).

Staying in touch with sensations in the body as you sit... If the attention wanders, noticing and making a choice to bring it back with care and kindness to the awareness of the body and the breath... (long pause).

Options and permission to explore experience. Recalling impermanence.

If sensations arise in the body that are very intense, making it difficult to focus on the body or the breath, there are two ways to be with this. You may choose to change your posture mindfully, attending to the sensations of movement as you shift... *Or* you may choose to direct attention right into the intensity of the sensation itself...

Exploring it with a gentle curiosity... Noticing nuances of sensation... perhaps thoughts and judgments... Perhaps resistance or bracing... and, as much as possible, stepping back to observe, to open space in awareness, perhaps to soften... and attending to duration — noticing that sensations change, that they have beginning, middle, and end... (Long pause).

Observing sound.

Now, allowing your attention to shift from the breath and the body to the sense of hearing... Not seeking sound, rather receiving whatever is available... from within the body and from the environment near and far... becoming particularly aware of hearing... Noticing how the awareness receives sounds without effort... (long pause).

Recalling impermanence. Encouraging spacious observation.

Being aware of how sounds have a beginning, middle, and end... How some are very short and some are long... How they are varied and textured... How there is space between sounds... Noticing how the mind labels sounds, has opinions about sounds, likes and dislikes certain sounds... Noticing any desire to move away from some sounds and towards others... as much as possible making space in which sounds can be experienced as they are... (long pause).

Observing thought.

And when you are ready, allowing attention to shift from hearing, and letting it expand this time into thinking — the realm of thought... seeing thoughts not as distractions but rather bringing your awareness to the thinking process itself...

Recalling impermanence. Defining foreground and background to help expand the space of awareness.

Noticing how thoughts arise, stay briefly, or for a more extended period, and then dissolve... beginning, middle, end... So, not getting lost in the content of the thoughts... allowing thought to be in the foreground of awareness with sound, body sensations, and breath in the background... (long pause).

Expanding awareness to observe body sensations.

Noticing thoughts... they may be about anything — about sleep, obligations, the past, the future... If you get carried away in the current of thinking, coming back to observing thoughts as separate elements that come and go... Thoughts moving through an open and spacious mind... (long pause).

Noticing also that emotions arise in the body and mind... Perhaps frustration, or restlessness, or peacefulness, or sadness, or joy, or fear.

Observing emotion. Often more accessible when framed as mood state.

Now bringing attention to emotion... to the mood state... What is here for you right now?... Noticing where in the body certain emotions seem to live... (long pause)...

Exploring emotion... Noticing how what is here may be wanted, or unwanted.... How there may be a tendency to cling to emotion judged as pleasant... and to struggle with others judged negatively — like sadness or fear... (long pause).

Recalling impermanence. Encouraging an embodied observation that may lead to insight into the relationship of thought and feeling.

Noticing whatever emotions arise in the moment... knowing that they have a beginning, middle, and end... perhaps simply observing them in the body — letting go of supporting thoughts or stories... (long pause).

Offering the permissive option to disengage from distressing exploration.

If at any time emotions or sensations become too uncomfortable, remember that you can always return to the breath... finding a safe harbor focused there until you're ready to venture out again... (long pause).

Moving into choiceless awareness.

Moving now, if you care to, into a choiceless awareness... Not choosing to bring your attention to anything in particular... Simply sitting here, fully aware of whatever is presenting itself to you in each moment ...

If sound arises, allowing sound to be the center of attention... If body sensation arises, letting that be the center of your attention... Until the next arising, which may be another body sensation... or a thought about the body sensation... or an emotion... (long pause).

At one moment, the breath may predominate, and then, perhaps, sound might be most prominent... Simply dwelling with an open awareness, attending to whatever arises... (long pause).

Observing whatever presents itself to you in the moment... Being spacious with whatever arises... (long pause).

Cultivating the capacity for observation.

Sitting in stillness with whatever comes and goes... (pause)... Being present with it all... (pause)... Being here now... (pause)... Open to the totality of your experience... (pause)... Being fully human... (long pause)

Returning to the orientation of gravity and breath.

Now returning the attention to the body as you sit... Feeling the breath coming and going... Staying fully present with body and breath... (long pause).

And as this meditation session comes to a close, realizing that by practicing mindfulness you are intentionally deepening your ability to be fully present in your daily life...

If it feels right, perhaps congratulating yourself for having taken this time and energy to nourish and care for yourself... Remembering that practicing in this way helps create access to a wider, deeper, more open way of being in your life, in which you can see more clearly and make more conscious choices for health, well-being and freedom...

Practices for Moving Towards Acceptance

Practice 7: Being Present
Approximate Timing: Introduction – 2 minutes; Practice – 15 minutes

A recording script for a practice that supports the "graduate-level" mindfulness course Meeting Aggression, *described in Chapter 6. Although the script specifically mentions aggression, the central motions or gestures of the practice may be explored within any context, providing a deliberately body-centered practice that makes the possibility refrain. Further, with its allowing of motion,* Being Present *may have distinct appeal to certain populations — where connecting to movement may strengthen the capacity for focus.*

Introduction

To begin to work with aggression, we need to understand it from inside. This meditation on being present is an opportunity for you to observe the natural interplay of nonaggression and aggression toward your own experience. To see how simply allowing yourself to be as you are in the present moment reveals your true strength and character, and to see, as well, how wanting your experience to be different in this moment exiles you from the power of the present.

Perhaps read nonacceptance and acceptance for nonaggression and aggression. In this meditation you may, very likely, experience a full spectrum of nonaggression and aggression. Keep in mind, though, that your experience is just that — yours. It will be different from others', and different in each session.

This meditation is a lying-down meditation that requires no special place, time, objects, or conditions. It's simple, just you, and the floor, and your senses. You can also feel free to adapt this practice to your own style and circumstances — try it at your desk, on the couch, or in bed. It is possible to be present anywhere, anytime.

Being Present Practice

Beginning by lying down on your back... allowing your arms to lie along your sides, your legs to stretch out fully, or if your back requires, bending the knees and putting the soles of the feet on the floor...

Presence as acceptance of the fullness of the moment.

Noticing if a sense of "doing" this meditation, a sense of working to be present, is arising... realizing that we cannot have presence as our *goal*, we cannot *try* to be present. Goals and striving carry us off... into a fictional future, while just *being* connects us to the reality of the present...

Orienting with gravity and breath.

Bringing your attention to the sensations of the body... in the contact with the surface on which you are lying, in the contact with other parts of your body... and in contact with the motions of the breath...

Permission.

As much as possible, letting sensation and your natural breathing guide you into simple presence... Maintaining gentle, nonjudgmental awareness moment after moment.... Allowing whatever small or large movements happen... spontaneously... to shift you from doing... to being...

At times, in this meditation, you may enter into a sense of rest or quiet... Or it may be that your experience is of tension, discomfort, frustration... leading to a wanting of change, a desire for transformation...

So... noticing when you are pulled out of the present moment and into the wish for some "better" experience... There are roots of aggression in this... this striving to hold on to a pleasant state that is changing ... this fighting to change the experience you don't want in the moment...

Expanding awareness to allow acceptance.

Seeing if it's possible to simply be present in this arising of aggression... Seeing if your presence, your being, is large enough to accommodate it, to hold it without acting on it... just letting be...

Permissive option to use an image for understanding.

Taking a larger view... Maybe an image helps to make this idea clear; if not just let it go: A wild bull in a cage is frightened and frightening, but if we open the cage into a wide pasture, moving the fences way back, both the bull and our perception may change... (Pause).

Attending to the head and neck, where so much "doing" takes place...and where the power of habit so often overrides the experience of the present moment...

How does the head really wish to be held by the floor in this moment? So, lifting the back of the head just slightly, perhaps the hair doesn't even clear the floor...Then allowing it to return slowly, feeling out what is needed... How is it that the head and neck feel present and alive...

Accommodate — from the Latin "to make fit.

There is no right or wrong here, no success or failure, there is just exploring being... noticing when judgment or wanting arise, and, as much as possible, allowing your presence to accommodate whatever you feel... (Pause).

Sensing into the arms and shoulders... are they at rest or are they working — holding themselves on the floor?

Raising both arms from the floor, again, slightly... Can you raise them without breaking contact with the floor?

Accommodating trying.

And slowly allowing them to find rest.... Is there struggle or striving? Knowing that rest is not that typical image of relaxation... a collapse of the arms like when you let go of a puppet's strings... Perhaps seeing rest as FULL presence...The arms are alive... they have muscle tone... blood and energy flowing through them, a marvelous capacity for sensation... So how is it that they can relate to the floor without aggression? Noticing wanting them to be a certain way... noticing trying, if that is what is arising... and making room for that in the moment... present with all your experience.... (Pause).

Acknowledging the real and the alive. Acceptance as ongoing negotiation.

Bringing the attention to the legs, however you are holding them... How can they come into full presence? Lifting the right leg... perhaps a few inches... perhaps it doesn't leave the floor.... Tuning-in to the sense of lifting.... Noticing the aliveness, the freshness, and power of the tension, in the moment.... And allowing the leg to come back to the floor, into presence... expressed, perhaps, as rest.... Remembering that rest is presence, not collapse... not the wilting of a plant, but the fullness of a flower seeking the light... (Pause).

Lifting the left leg... sensing its aliveness, and maintaining contact with that aliveness as it seeks presence, rest, on the floor... Being present in ease... present in struggle... present to the interplay of nonaggression and aggression... (Pause).

Being present in bending the knees — if they're not already bent — and bringing the soles of the feet to the floor as if standing. Attending to the sensations of the lower back in this moment... noticing thought and feeling, any wanting, any interplay of nonaggression and aggression.... And lifting the pelvis slightly... present in this movement.... Noticing how far throughout the body this motion has an effect... present in all of it.... Then allowing the pelvis to come down to the floor... the back to come into greater contact... into presence... perhaps into the freshness and aliveness of rest... (Long pause).

Coming to a sense now of the entire body, lying here, present in sensory experience, present as well in thoughts and emotions...

Remembering that presence is not striving to overcome tension or boredom or fear or sleepiness, it is simply allowing tension or boredom or fear or sleepiness to be your experience without wanting it to be different in this moment... (Long pause)

Allowing, accommodating, accepting.

Are you present in your experience of this moment?... Is this a moment of nonaggression... or aggression? Allowing whatever is arising to be included in your field of being... your presence... (Pause).

As this formal meditation practice ends, carrying a sense of presence, a sense of the power of just being into the doing of you life... moment by moment...

Practice 8: Saying "Yes"
Approximate Timing: 10 minutes

This is adapted from a practice used by the psychotherapist and Buddhist teacher Tara Brach. Although the presentation here is as a short practice, the basic gestures of sitting with No and Yes can be used in many teaching moments — to lead into a longer practice, perhaps of expanding awareness, or to work directly with a particular issue during inquiry with a participant.

Sitting in a comfortable position and bringing your attention to your body... Feeling the support beneath you.... Noticing your breath wherever you feel it most vividly in the moment....

Simply following your breath, moment to moment... As you sit, noticing what is arising in the triangle of awareness — body sensations... feelings or mood state... and thoughts...

Experiencing NO in the triangle of awareness.

To experience first hand what happens when we resist rather than accept our experience, begin by saying "NO" to whatever is arising... If it is a sensation in the body, unpleasant or pleasant, mentally directing a stream of "NO" toward the sensation and noticing what happens to the sensation as you say "NO." If it is a feeling of sadness, or fear, or joy, saying "NO" to the feelings. Let the word "NO" carry the energy of negating, rejecting, pushing away what you are experiencing. Noticing what this resistance feels like. How does it feel in your body? What happens to breathing... heart rate... muscle tension... as you are saying "NO" to your experience? What is life like as you live moment to moment with the thoughts and feelings of "NO" — resisting what is?

Reorienting with gravity and breath.

Now opening your eyes if they are closed and taking a few full deep breaths, and relaxing the body by softening muscles in your face, perhaps letting your draw drop down slightly and allowing the shoulders to drop a bit. When you are ready, following your breath once again. Simply breathing in and out with awareness....

Spaciousness, openness, acceptance. YES in the triangle of awareness.

Noticing what is arising, perhaps body sensations, or feelings or mood states, or thoughts. Simply allowing whatever arises to be in awareness. If a body sensation is arising, whether it is pleasant or unpleasant, directing a stream of the word YES to the experience. Allowing the word YES to carry an openness toward whatever is arising. Letting the sensations, feelings, thoughts float in a larger field of yes. Yes to pleasant, yes to unpleasant, yes to pain, and yes to wanting pain to go away. Saying yes to even resistance if it arises. Noticing your experience as you say YES. How does Yes feel in the body? Is there more spaciousness, openness in the mind? What happens to pleasantness or unpleasantness when you say YES? What happens to your heart as you say YES? What is life like as you open to it moment by moment and say YES?

Sitting for a few more minutes and gently saying YES to your experience as it unfolds.... (Long pause)... And when you are ready, opening your eyes.

Practices for Growing Compassion

Practice 9: Loving Kindness
Approximate Timing: Introduction – 2 minutes; Practice – 15 minutes

A recording script. This practice is offered within the template MBSR curriculum, although it is not emphasized or given as home practice, while in other manifestations of the MBSR curriculum it is given a more core role. The version presented here frames it as a mindfulness practice; knowing and accepting what is arising in the triangle of awareness while holding the intention of loving kindness.

Introduction

The intention of loving kindness runs throughout our formal mindfulness practices...This meditation calls our attention to it specifically... in loving kindness meditation you are setting an intention to nurture the quality of loving kindness that already exists within... while being with whatever is present in the senses, thought, or emotions, without judgment ...

By practicing loving kindness meditation you are becoming more familiar with this quality, so that it is easier to recognize when it arises spontaneously in your practice, so that it is more available to you in daily life. The practice of loving kindness meditation is — just as is mindfulness — a life-long commitment... and an investment of time and energy that delivers immeasurable value....

Permission to change and adapt the practice.

This meditation involves repeating a set of phrases that point to the innate quality of loving kindness... The phrases in this recording are some of many possible phrases that can be used. If any part of the approach or of the four central phrases do not suit you, please feel free to make any changes that make it more friendly and appealing to you... The intention of the practice is to cultivate loving kindness — for yourself and for others...

Loving Kindness Practice

Orienting with gravity and breath.

Taking your usual posture for meditation... feeling your body where it makes contact with the support beneath you, and settling in... perhaps centering yourself by making the breath the focus of your attention...

Feeling the breath moving and the body sitting...

Beginning with an other, as self-directed loving kindness is a challenge for many participants.

And when you are ready, bringing to mind someone that it is easy to feel loving kindness towards... someone from the past or present, perhaps a child, or a pet... an easy, simple relationship may be best...

Allowing yourself to hold them in your awareness ... perhaps seeing them in your mind's eye or perhaps feeling a sense of them in your heart... can you feel a sense of loving kindness towards them?

As you hold them in your awareness, beginning to send wishes of loving kindness to them.... Silently repeating these phrases ...

May you be peaceful and happy
May you be safe from harm
May you be as healthy and strong as you can be
May you live with ease of well-being...

Now turning toward the self, with permission to feel however you feel.

When you're ready, allowing the image or felt sense of your chosen one to fade ... and seeing how it is for you to be the one who receives loving kindness... resting here in your own kind regard, sending yourself these well wishes ... allowing yourself to take in these phrases ... to say them silently for yourself ...

> May I be peaceful and happy
> May I be safe from all inner and outer harm
> May I be as healthy and strong as I can be
> May I live with ease of well-being...

Maybe it seems artificial and stilted to say such things to yourself, for yourself... maybe you're not feeling loving kindness in this moment — and that's OK — whatever you're feeling, you can hold the intention of loving kindness... offering it from wherever you are... however you are now....

So practicing once more... noticing how you may be drawn towards this practice or drawn away from it...

> May I be peaceful and happy
> May I be safe from harm
> May I be as healthy and strong as I can be
> May I live with ease of well-being...

And now exploring the experience of moving loving kindness outward again, bringing to your heart and mind someone to whom you would like to send loving kindness ... and with the same intention you have been directing towards yourself, offering these wishes...

> May you be peaceful and happy
> May you be safe from harm
> May you be as healthy and strong as you can be
> May you live with ease of well-being... (Long pause).

Holding them in your awareness and sending loving kindness with these phrases... or phrases of your own...

> May you be peaceful and happy
> May you be safe from harm
> May you be as healthy and strong as you can be
> May youlive with ease of well-being... (Long pause).

Reinforcing permissiveness. Being mindful of the quality or qualities that are arising in the moment, and letting go of judgment... You may or may not be feeling loving kindness... and that's simply how it is right now — remembering that the heart has its seasons, and feelings cannot be forced... giving yourself permission to be just as you are...

Just as you are, you can continue to hold the intention of loving kindness ... so now, expanding your awareness to include others....intending peace and well being for those you know well...

And those you know less well...
Those you love...
And those you love less...

And perhaps going a step further and intending peace and well being for everyone...

May everyone be peaceful and happy
May everyone be safe from harm
May everybody be as healthy and strong as they can be
May we all live with ease of well-being... (Long pause).

Aware of how it is with you right now...noticing what is arising as you offer these wishes...

May everyone be peaceful and happy
May everyone be safe from harm
May everybody be as healthy and strong as they can be
May we all live with ease of well-being... (Long pause).

And when you're ready, bringing your attention back to the breath moving in the body... Sensing the body sitting here, breathing, in this moment... noticing thoughts and feelings, and allowing yourself to be exactly as you are — which in and of itself is an act of loving kindness.

Practice 10: Being for Others
Approximate Timing: Introduction – 2 minutes; Practice – 15 minutes

A recording script from the Meeting Aggression *course outlined in Chapter 6. This is adapted from the practice of the Buddhist teacher Charles Genoud. The approach is to work with presence, openness, and acceptance as the motion of compassion. The practice is aligned with the practice and pedagogy of mindfulness in its insistence on observing and opening to whatever is arising during the practice.*

Introduction

Emphasizing safety and permission in working with potentially distressing material.

This meditation on being for others brings the sense of presence and openness into the interpersonal and ethical realm. It is a practice to develop the capacity to be with suffering — to offer our openness and thereby our compassion — our feeling-along-with or feeling-for another. It is important to understand this as *practice* — we are working slowly and gently to build our capacity. Noticing any tendency you may have to wish to work with deep suffering or suffering that may be very challenging to you, then stepping back and remembering that this is practice, and we start small, start easy, and build up.

Remembering also that we may have habits of thought and feeling that see compassion as based on sacrifice. This is not a notion that is useful in this practice — sacrifice limits our compassion to what we are willing to sacrifice. Rather, this practice sees compassion as a willingness to face the other — to remain open to the other's suffering — the only limit then to compassion is the limit to openness.

You may wish to use this as a main practice for a time, or you may be moved to take a part of it and add it into your core practice of sitting meditation.

Practice

Orienting with gravity and breath.

Coming into sitting posture...

Becoming aware of the body in this moment... its relationship to gravity... Is it possible to allow gravity to hold you up? Can you find that place of balance and comfort? Can you allow the little adjustments the body requires, so you're not holding a posture, just responding to sitting... (Long pause).

And attending to the breath... just allowing the mind to rest lightly on in-breath and out-breath... If it flits away, no muss or fuss, just noticing and coming back... (Long pause).

And opening to presence... to what there is in this moment... being with and in the full experience... not adding anything, not taking anything away... (Long pause)

Offering an orientation — three parts.
A small child.

There are three objects of focus in this meditation:

First, imagine a small child who is unhappy — perhaps you have a picture in your mind, perhaps it is a felt sense — not choosing suffering that is too deep or terrible, as that may bring up a lot of fear or discomfort, and make the practice difficult.... (Long pause).

Noticing closing and opening.

Seeing if it is possible to look into the face of the child, and to be open to the sadness... if it feels right, imagining putting your hand on the child's shoulder ... noticing if you are remaining open or closing up... being gentle with yourself as you do this meditation… closing when you are closing, opening when it is possible for you… learning what is possible, learning what it is like to be there — present and open — for another… (Long pause).

Letting that image or sense fade… And coming back to the breath and body in the present moment… (Long pause).

Participant herself as a child.

Imagining or sensing *yourself* as a child, in a moment of sadness or hurt — again, not choosing something too extreme, this is PRACTICE, not a challenge… See or feel the face,… open to the sadness or hurt… perhaps reaching out and placing your hand on the child's shoulder, compassionately, tenderly … (Long pause).

Noticing when you are open, when you are closing… being a model for the child… knowing that as you open there is less suffering, and if the child can open there will be less suffering as well… (Long pause).

Working with this sense of openness and its capacity to reduce suffering, to bring, in some way, healing to the other… (Long pause).

And letting the image fade and coming back to the breath and the body in this moment… (Long pause).

Participant herself, now.

If you're ready, feeling yourself NOW… Seeing if it's possible to open to our own difficulties in this moment… Again, remembering to approach this with gentleness — this is practice for help and healing, not for endurance or suffering — not for sacrifice but for ease of wellbeing…. (Long pause).

Seeing when and how it is possible to be open to yourself… imagining placing a hand on the shoulder of the you that's before you… experiencing the healing power of openness… (Long pause).

And letting that image fade and coming back to the breath and the body…. (Long pause).

And as this meditation ends, knowing that you can use this practice to build your capacity to open to others, and that you can include others in your practice — imagining them and being open for them in their humanness, their suffering…

Appendix

Resources for Personal and Curriculum Development

The following lists offer potential resources for learning more for your own development as a practitioner, for enhancing your teaching, and for formulating new approaches and practices to refine, change, and create curricula anew. Combined with this book's own bibliography, there is a wide range of material given here to bring into your teaching. We hope you'll find what draws you, taste things that may seem strange, and find what works for you and the participants with whom you co-create.

Books on Clinical Applications of Mindfulness

Baer, R. A. (Ed.). (2006). *Mindfulness-based treatment approaches: Clinician's guide to evidence base and applications.* San Diego, CA: Elsevier Academic Press.

Brach, T. (2003). *Radical acceptance: Embracing your life with the heart of a Buddha.* New York: Bantam Dell.

Brantley, J. (2003). *Calming your anxious mind: How mindfulness and compassion can free you from anxiety, fear and panic.* Oakland, CA: New Harbinger.

Cole, J. D., & Lades-Gaskin, C. (2007). *Mindfulness-centered therapies: An integrative approach.* Seattle, WA: Silver Birch Press.

Didonna, F. (2009). *Clinical handbook of mindfulness.* New York: Springer.

Fishman, B. M. (2002). *Emotional healing through mindfulness meditation.* Rochester, VT: Inner Traditions.

Germer, C. K., Siegel, R. D., & Fulton, P. R. (Eds.). (2005). *Mindfulness and psychotherapy.* New York: Guilford Press.

Goleman, D. (2003). *Destructive emotions: A scientific dialogue with the Dalai Lama.* New York: Bantam Dell.

Hayes, S. C., Follette, V. M., & Linehan, M. M. (Eds.). (2004). *Mindfulness and acceptance: Expanding the cognitive-behavioral tradition.* New York: Guilford Press.

Kabat-Zinn, J. (2005). *Full catastrophe living: Using the wisdom of your body and mind to face stress, pain, and illness: Fifteenth anniversary edition*. New York: Bantam Dell.

McBee, L. (2008). *Mindfulness-based elder care: A CAM model for frail elders and their caregivers*. New York: Springer.

Miller, A. L., Rathus, J. H., & Linehan, M. M. (2007). *Dialectical behavior therapy with suicidal adolescents*. New York: Guilford Press.

Orsillo, S. M., & Roemer, L. (Eds.). (2005). *Acceptance and mindfulness-based approaches to anxiety*. New York: Springer.

Rosenbaum, E. (2005). *Here for now: Living well with cancer through mindfulness*. Hardwick, MA: Satya House.

Santorelli, S. (1999). *Heal thy self: Lessons on mindfulness in medicine*. New York: Random House.

Segal, Z. V., Williams, J. M. G., & Teasdale, J. D. (2002). *Mindfulness-based cognitive therapy for depression: A new approach to preventing relapse*. New York: Guilford Press.

Siegel, D. J. (2007). *The mindful brain: Reflection and attunement in the cultivation of well-being*. New York: Norton.

Williams, M., Teasdale, J., Segal, Z., & Kabat-Zinn, J. (2007). *The mindful way through depression: Freeing yourself from chronic unhappiness*. New York: Guilford Press.

Research Articles

An extensive bibliography including ongoing updates of research articles can be found on the website of the Mindful Awareness Research Center at UCLA http://marc.ucla.edu/workfiles/pdfs/MARC_biblio_0808.pdf

Deepening Personal Practice – and Guiding Others

Boorstein, S. (1995). *It's easier than you think*. San Francisco: Harper.

Boorstein, S. (1996). *Don't just do something, sit there*. New York: Harper.

Boorstein, S. (2002). *Pay attention, for goodness sake*. New York: Ballantine.

Carroll, M. (2004). *Awake at work*. Boston: Shambhala Publications.

Chodron, P. (1991). *The wisdom of no escape and the path of loving kindness*. Boston: Shambhala Publications.

Chodron, P. (2002). *The places that scare you*. Boston: Shambhala Publications.

Coleman, M. (2006). *Awake in the wild: Mindfulness in nature as a path to self-discovery*. Novato, CA: New World Library.

Epstein, M. (1995). *Thoughts without a thinker: Psychotherapy from a Buddhist perspective*. New York: Basic Books.

Epstein, M. (2007). *Psychotherapy without the self: A Buddhist perspective*. New Haven: Yale University.

Goldstein, J. (1976). *The experience of insight*. Boston: Shambhala Publications.

Goldstein, J., & Kornfield J. (2001). *Seeking the heart of wisdom: The path of insight meditation*. Boston, MA: Shambhala Publications.

Gunaratana, B. H. (2002). *Mindfulness in plain English*. Somerville, MA: Wisdom Publications.

Hanh, T. N. (1976). *The miracle of mindfulness: A manual for meditation*. Boston: Beacon.

Hanh, T. N. (1991). *Peace is every step*. New York: Bantam.

Hanh, T. N. (1994). *The blooming of a lotus: Guided meditation exercises for healing and transformation*. Boston: Beacon.

Kabat-Zinn, J. (1994). *Wherever you go there you are*. New York: Hyperion.

Kabat-Zinn, J. (2005). *Coming to our senses: Healing ourselves and the world through mindfulness*. New York: Hyperion.

Kabat-Zinn, J., & Kabat-Zinn, M. (1997). *Everyday blessings: The inner work of mindful parenting*. New York: Hyperion.

Kornfield, J. (1993). *A path with heart*. New York: Bantam Books.

Kornfield, J. (2008). *A wise heart: A guide to the universal teachings of Buddhist psychology*. New York: Bantam.

Langer, E. (1989). *Mindfulness*. Cambridge, MA: Perseus Books.

Levine, S. (1979). *A gradual awakening*. New York: Anchor/Doubleday.

Levine, S. (1991). *Guided meditations, explorations and healings*. New York: Anchor/Doubleday.

McLeod, K. (2001). *Wake up to your life*. New York: HarperCollins.

Nairn, R. (1999). *Diamond mind: A psychology of meditation*. Boston: Shambhala Publications.

Nepo, M. (2000). *The book of awakening*. Berkeley, CA: Conari Press.

Rosenberg, L. (2004). *Breath by breath*. Boston: Shambhala Publications.

Salzberg, S. (1995). *Lovingkindness: The revolutionary art of happiness*. Boston: Shambhala Publications.

Weiss, A. (2005). *Beginning mindfulness: Learning the way of awareness*. Novata, CA: New World Library.

Welwood, J. (2000). *Toward a psychology of awakening: Buddhism, psychotherapy, and the path of personal and spiritual transformation*. Boston: Shambhala Publications.

Whitmayer, C. (1994). *Mindfulness and meaningful work*. Berkeley: Parallax Press.

Mindfulness in World Spiritual Traditions

Judaism

Boorstein, S. (1997). *That's funny you don't look Buddhist: On being a faithful Jew and a passionate Buddhist*. New York: Harper Collins.

Cooper, D. (1999). *The heart of stillness: A complete guide to learning the art of meditation*. Woodstock, VT: Skylight Paths.

Cooper, D. (1999). *Silence, simplicity and solitude: A complete guide to spiritual retreat.* Woodstock, VT: Skylight Paths.

Cooper, D. (2000). *Three gates to meditation practice: A personal journey into Sufism, Buddhism and Judaism.* Woodstock, VT: Skylight Paths.

Fischer, N. (2003). *The Buddhist path to truly growing up.* New York: Harper Collins.

Fischer, N. (2003). *Opening to you: Zen-inspired translations of the psalms.* New York: Penguin Putnam.

Fischer, N. (2008). *Sailing home: Using the wisdom of Homer's odyssey to navigate life's perils and pitfalls.* New York: Simon and Shuster.

Lew, A. (2005). *Be still and get going: A Jewish meditation practice for real life.* New York: Time Warner.

Lew, A., & Jaffe, S. (2001). *One god clapping: The spiritual path of a Zen Rabbi.* Woodstock, VT: Jewish Lights Publishing.

Slater, J. P. (2004). *Mindful Jewish living: Compassionate practice.* New York: Aviv Press.

Sufism

Barks, C., & Moyne, J. (1997). *The essential Rumi.* Edison, NJ: Castle Books.

Helminiski, K. (1992). *Living presence: Sufi way to mindfulness and the unfolding of the essential self.* New York: Tarcher/Putnam.

Christianity

Bourgeault, C. (2001). *Mystical hope: Trusting in the mercy of god.* Cambridge, MA: Cowley.

Bourgeault, C. (2004). *Centering prayer and inner awakening.* Cambridge, MA: Cowley.

Dougherty, R. M. (1995). *Group spiritual direction: Community for discernment.* Mahwah, NJ: Paulist Press.

Jones, A. (1982). *Exploring spiritual direction.* New York: Seabury.

Keating, T. (1999). *The human condition: Contemplation and transformation.* New York: Paulist Press.

Keating, T. (1999). *Invitation to love: The way of Christian contemplation.* New York: Continuum.

May, G. (1982). *Will and spirit: A contemplative psychology.* New York: HarperCollins.

May, G. (2004). *The dark night of the soul.* New York: HarperSanFrancisco.

May, G. (2006). *The wisdom of wilderness.* New York: HarperSanFrancisco.

Merton, T. (1955). *No man is an island.* New York: Harcourt Brace Jovanovich.

Merton, T. (1960). *Spiritual direction and meditation.* Collegeville, MN: Liturgical Press.

Merton, T. (1962). *New seeds of contemplation*. Norfolk, CT: New Directions.
Merton, T. (1967). *Mystics and Zen masters*. New York: Farrar, Strauss and Giroux.
Merton, T. (1968). *Zen and the birds of appetite*. New York: New Directions.
Merton, T. (1969). *Contemplative prayer*. New York: Herder and Herder.
Pennington, M. B. (1980). *Centering prayer: Renewing an ancient Christian prayer tradition*. New York: Image Books.
Rohr, R. (1999). *Everything belongs: The gift of contemplative prayer*. New York: Crossroad.

Buddhism

Analayo. (2003). *Satipatthana: The direct path to realization*. Cambridge, UK: Windhorse.
Batchelor, S. (1983). *Alone with others: An existential approach to Buddhism*. New York: Grove Press.
Batchelor, S. (1994). *The awakening of the West*. Berkeley, CA: Parallax.
Batchelor, S. (1997). *Buddhism without beliefs: A contemporary guide to awakening*. New York: Riverhead Books.
Gethin, R. (1998). *The foundations of Buddhism*. Oxford: New York.
Narada, M. (1980). *The Buddha and his teachings*. Singapore: Singapore Buddhist Meditation Centre.
Nyanaponika, T. (1965). *The heart of Buddhist meditation*. Boston: Weiser Books.
Suzuki, S. (1970). *Zen mind, beginner's mind*. New York: Weatherhill.
Trungpa, C. (1973). *Cutting through spiritual materialism*. Berkeley, CA: Shambhala.

Audiovisual Resources: CDs

Jon Kabat-Zinn's Mindfulness Meditation Practices

www.mindfulnesstapes.com or contact the University of Mass. Bookstore at 508-856-3213.

1. Series 1: 45 min meditations including Body Scan, Sitting Meditation, Floor Yoga & Standing Yoga. This Series is designed to accompany the book *Full Catastrophe Living*. 4 CD set for $30.00; 2 tapes for $20.00.
2. Series 2: 10, 20, 30 min meditations including Mountain & Lake Meditations. This series is designed to accompany the book *Wherever You Go There You Are*. 4 CD set for $30.00; 2 tapes for $35.00.
3. Series 3: 10–45 min meditations, Bodyscape, Breathscape, Soundscape, Mindscape, Walking Meditation & Loving Kindness. This series is designed to accompany the book *Coming to Our Senses*. 4 CD set for $30.00

Saki Santorelli: Mindfulness Meditation Practice CDs/Tapes

Five Tapes – $35.00/set + $4.00 shipping & handling.
15–20 min meditations including Loving Kindness for the Body, Opening Your Heart to Life, Awareness of Breathing, Cultivating Compassion. These CDs/tapes are designed to accompany the book *Heal Thy Self.*
To order write to/make check payable to:
Guest-House Tapes
P.O. Box 1050
Belchertown, MA. 01007

Bob Stahl: Mindful Healing CDs

This Mindful Healing Series gives practical, educational tools to access the deep inner resources of healing. Specific CDs focus on back pain, chronic pain, neck and shoulder pain, insomnia and sleep challenges, heart disease, high blood pressure, opening to change, forgiveness and loving kindness, headaches and migraines, anxiety and panic.
http://www.mindfulnessprograms.com/mindful-healing-series.html

Dharma Seed Tape Library

Box 66
Wendel Depot, MA. 01308
www.dharmaseed.org
Guided mindfulness meditation tapes/CDs and teacher's presentations on fundamental principles of practice.
To listen to tapes online – www.dharmastream.com

Sounds True Audio

735 Walnut Street
Boulder. CO. 80302
www.Soundstrue.com
A variety of guided meditation tapes/CDs and presentations by meditation teachers.
Also DVDs (Mindful Movements- Thich Nhat Hanh)

Parallax Press

P.O. Box 7355
Berkeley, CA. 94707
1-800-863-5290
www.parallax.org
Books and tapes of Thich Nhat Hanh

Pariyatti

Doing Time, Doing Vipassana-Video- Documentary on dramatic changes brought about when inmates at one of India's largest prison are introduced to Vipassana.

Changing form Inside-Video – Documentary on changes brought about in an American prison when inmates are introduced to Vipassana.

http://www.pariyatti.org/Bookstore

Professional Training in MBSR

Oasis: An International Learning Center – Center For Mindfulness Worcester, Massachusetts

Comprehensive training in teaching MBSR is available through the Center for Mindfulness in Medicine, Health Care, and Society at the University of Massachusetts. The program includes two foundation courses, two advanced offerings, and a review for certification.

Foundation courses:

- Mindfulness-based stress reduction in mind–body medicine: A 7-day residential training retreat
- Practicum in mindfulness-based stress reduction: Living inside participant-practitioner perspectives-10 week program

Advanced offerings:

- Teacher development intensive: An advanced mindfulness-based stress reduction teacher training/retreat- 9 days
- Supervision in mindfulness-based stress reduction
- MBSR teacher certification review

For more information: http://www.umassmed.edu/cfm/oasis

Other Training Opportunities in Medical Settings

Jefferson-Myrna Brind Center of Integrative Medicine – Stress Reduction Program, Philadelphia, PA

Offers three programs for which the Oasis MBSR in Mind–Body Medicine Retreat is a prerequisite.

- Practicum in mindfulness-based stress reduction (10 week program)
- Internship in teaching MBSR
- Supervision in teaching MBSR

    For more information: http://www.jeffersonhospital.org/cim

El Camino Hospital Mindfulness Stress Reduction Program, Mountain View, CA

Offers a 10 week practicum in mindfulness-based stress reduction that is certified by the Center for Mindfulness at the University of Massachusetts Medical School as partial fulfillment of requirements for MBSR teacher certification.
For more information: http://www.mindfulnessprograms.com/teacher-training.html

Duke Integrative Medicine, Durham, NC

Mindfulness Training for Professionals
    The training involves two- 4 day sessions and includes the full 8 week MBSR program and core skills for presenting and teaching mindfulness. *Note: completion of the training does not meet established standards for teaching MBSR.*
    For more information http://www.dukeintegrativemedicine.org/educational/mindfulness_training.aspx

Academic Education in Teaching Mindfulness-Based Interventions

Centre for Mindfulness Research and Practice, School of Psychology, Bangor University, UK

Offers a range of degree, diploma, and certificate programs:

- MSc/MA in Mindfulness-Based Approaches
    - Postgraduate Diploma in Mindfulness-Based Approaches
    - Postgraduate Certificate in Mindfulness-Based Approaches
- MSc/MA in Teaching Mindfulness-Based Courses
    - Postgraduate Diploma in Teaching Mindfulness-Based Courses
- Postgraduate Certificate in Teaching Mindfulness-Based Courses
- Postgraduate Certificate in Advanced Mindfulness-Based Teaching Practice

For more information: http://www.bangor.ac.uk/imscar/mindfulness

Postgraduate Master of Studies in MBCT at Oxford University

This new 2 year part-time course offers experienced clinicians from a range of professional backgrounds a unique opportunity to develop in depth specialist knowledge and skills in Mindfulness-Based Cognitive Therapy (MBCT).

The course is offered by the Oxford Mindfulness Centre at the Oxford University Department of Psychiatry, in collaboration with the Oxford University Department for Continuing Education, and will lead to an award of a Master of Studies by the University of Oxford.

For more information http://www.oxfordmindfulness.org

Institute for Mindfulness-Based Approaches (IMA)

Bedburg, Germany

Professional Training Programs in MBSR and MBCT

IMA has been offering MBSR teacher-training programs since 2002. It introduced an MBCT training program in 2007. The Institute's faculty includes some of Europe's most senior mindfulness-based approaches teachers and researchers, as well as guest teachers from the U.S.A.

In addition to offering trainings in Germany, Austria, and Switzerland, the Institute is responding to requests from the other European countries to introduce its highly successful compact yet extensive training program. The Professional Training Programs take place throughout a 12–14 month period. During this period, participants meet seven times for 4-day sessions each.

For more information www.institute-for-mindfulness.eu

MBSR Institute Freiburg (Germany)

The MBSR Institute Frieberg offers a residential 29-day teacher training program over a one-year period for healthcare and allied professionals who also have a solid foundation in mindfulness meditation. The program includes three major components: 1) Development of teaching skills in MBSR, 2) in-depth background knowledge of the psychological, philosophical and scientific foundations of MBSR and mindfulness, and 3) personal experience and self-exploration within the context of meditative practice and its transmission to others. The overriding guiding vision is that learning to teach MBSR be treated as a mindfulness practice in itself and that attitudinal qualities cultivated by mindfulness be embodied in the training program. The Director of the program is Ulrike Kesper-Grossman M.A. and the Co-Director is Paul Grossman, Ph.D.

For more information www.mbsr-institut-freiburg.de

Professional Training in MBCT

Mindfulness-Based Cognitive Therapy: A 5-Day Professional Training for the Prevention of Depression Relapse offered through Omega Institute

www.eomega.org

Mindfulness-Based Cognitive Therapy: A 5-Day Professional Training for the Prevention of Depression Relapse offered through the University of California, San Diego

Zindel Segal, Steve Hickman
http://health.ucsd.edu/specialties/psych/mindfulness/training

Advanced Teaching and Study Programs in MBCT

For more information contact:
Susan Woods www.slwoods.com
Char Wilkins www.amindfulpath.com
Ferris Urbanowski www.ferrisurb.org

Training Programs in Mindfulness-Based Childbirth and Parenting

Nancy Bardacke
Trainings for perinatal and mental health professionals, birthing, postpartum and infant care professionals or anyone interested in the health and well-being of pregnant and birthing families, infants, children and parents.

11-Week Professional Development and
Training Program in Mindfulness-Based Childbirth and Parenting
Mindful Birthing, Mindful Living
A 6-Day Retreat and Training for
Perinatal Health Professionals
For more information www.mindfulbirthing.org

Mindfulness- Based Eating Awareness Training (MB-EAT)

Jean Kristeller and Char Wilkins
A 5 day workshop/retreat has been offered to healthcare professionals. The highly
experiential training emphasizes the foundational nature of mindfulness practice and
the practical application of it in helping people change their relationship to eating,
including working with overeating, binge eating and weight management in general.
    For more information www.amindfulpath.com

Certificate Program in Mindfulness and Psychotherapy

Institute for Meditation and Psychotherapy and Barre Center for Buddhist Studies
    Newton Center, Massachusetts
    This nine-month program, which consists of a 5 day-long residential program, a
3 day-long residential meditation retreat and weekly classes in the Boston area,
comprehensively explores the integration of mindfulness and psychotherapy. With
the guidance of approximately 20 faculty comprised of specialists in their areas,
participants examine the application of mindfulness to a wide range of clinical
populations and conditions, compare and contrast Western and Buddhist perspectives on health and healing, and practice meditation together.
    For more information: www.meditationandpsychotherapy.org

Training Programs in Teaching Mindfulness to Children

Susan Kaiser-Greenland
www.innerkids.org

ACT Training

Steven Hayes
Association for Contextual Behavioral Science
www.contextualpsychology.org

DBT Training

Marsha Linehan
Behavioral Tech Research Inc.
www.behavioraltech.org

Resources for Personal Retreats

Insight Meditation Centers

For a more complete listing of insight Centers visit Insight Meditation Society's
link http://dharma.org/ims/mr_links.html

East Coast

Connecticut
Insight Meditation Community of New Haven
New Haven, Connecticut
Phone: (203) 624-1998
www.newhavenweb.com/insight

Massachusetts
Cambridge Insight Meditation Center -
331 Broadway
Cambridge, MA 02139
Phone: (617) 441-9038
www.cimc.info

Insight Meditation Society
1230 Pleasant Street, Barre, MA 01005, Phone: (978) 355-4378
www.dharma.org

New York
New York Insight Meditation Center
28 West 27th Street, 10th Floor
New York, NY 10001
Phone: (212) 213-4802
www.nyimc.org

Philadelphia
Philadelphia Meditation Center
8 East Eagle Road
Havertown, PA 19083
Phone: (610) 853-8200
www.philadelphiameditation.org

Washington, DC
The Insight Meditation Community of Washington (IMCW)
P.O. Box 212
Garrett Park, MD, 20896
Phone: (202) 986-2922
www.imcw.org

Florida
Gainesville Vipassana Center
5811 NW 31st Terrace
Gainesville, Florida 32653
Phone: (352) 337-9993
http://www.floridavipassana.org

West Coast

California
Insight LA – Los Angeles
2633 Lincoln Blvd. #206
Santa Monica, CA 90405-2005
Phone: (310) 774-3325
www.insightla.org

Insight Meditation Center
108 Birch Street
Redwood City, California 94062
Phone: (650) 599-3456
www.insightmeditationcenter.org

San Francisco Insight Meditation Community
P.O. Box 475536
San Francisco, CA 94147-5536
Phone: (415) 994-5951
www.sfinsight.org

Spirit Rock Meditation Center
PO Box 169,
Woodacre, CA 94973
Phone: (415) 488-0164
www.spiritrock.org

Washington
Seattle Insight Meditation Society
P.O. Box 95817
Seattle, WA 98145-2817
Phone: (206) 366-2111
www.seattleinsight.org

Mid-States

Mid America Dharma
455 E. 80th Terrace
Kansas City, MO 64131, Phone: (314) 644-1926
www.midamericadharma.org

Hawaii

Vipassana Metta on Maui
PO Box 1188
Kula, HI 96790
Phone: (808) 573-3450
www.vipassanametta.org

Canada

True North Insight
4137 Oxford Avenue, Montreal, Quebec, Canada H4A 2Y5, Phone: (514) 488-7484
http://www.truenorthinsight.org

England

Gaia House
West Ogwell, Newton Abbot
Devon, TQ12 6EN
+44(0)1626 333613
http://www.gaiahouse.co.uk

Ireland

Insight Meditation Dublin
Ballyback Co.
Dublin, Ireland
http://www.insightmeditationdublin.com

Netherlands

Stichting Inzichts Meditatie
List of centers and groups:
http://www.simsara.nl/central.html#buiten

Switzerland

Meditationszentrum Beatenberg Waldegg
CH-3803 Beatenberg Schweiz
Phone. ++41 (0)33 841 21 31
info@karuna.ch

References

Chapter 1

Allen, N. B., Blashki, G., & Gullone, E. (2006). Mindfulness-based psychotherapies: A review of conceptual foundations, empirical evidence and practical considerations. *Australian and New Zealand Journal of Psychiatry, 40*(4), 285–294.

Beutler, L. E., Malik, M. L., Alimohamed, S., Harwood, T. M., Talebbi, H., Noble, S., et al. (2004). Therapist variables. In M. J. Lambert (Ed.), *Bergin and Garfield's handbook of psychotherapy and behavior change* (pp. 227–306). New York: Wiley.

Blow, A., Sprenkle, D., & Davis, S. (2007). Is who delivers the treatment more important than the treatment itself? The role of the therapist in common factors. *Journal of Marital and Family Therapy, 33*(3), 298–317.

Carmody, J., & Baer, R. A. (2008). Relationships between mindfulness practice and levels of mindfulness, medical and psychological symptoms and well-being in a mindfulness-based stress reduction program. *Journal of Behavioral Medicine, 31*, 23–33.

Carson, J. W., Carson, K. M., Gil, K. M., & Baucom, D. H. (2004). Mindfulness-based relationship enhancement. *Behavior Therapy, 35*, 471–494.

Cozolino, L. (2006). *The neuroscience of human relationships.* New York: Norton.

Davidson, R. J., Kabat-Zinn, J., Schumaker, J., Rosenkranz, M., Muller, D., Santorelli, S., et al. (2003). Alterations in brain and immune function produced by mindfulness meditation. *Psychosomatic Medicine, 65*, 564–570.

Dimidjian, S., & Linehan, M. M. (2003). Defining an agenda for future research on the clinical application of mindfulness practice. *Clinical Psychology: Science and Practice, 10*(2), 166–171.

Dryden, W., & Still, A. (2006). Historical aspects of mindfulness and self-acceptance in psychotherapy. *Journal of Rational-Emotive & Cognitive Behavior Therapy, 24*(1), 3–28.

Freud, S. (1912). Recommendations to physicians practicing psycho-analysis. In J. Strachey (Ed.). (1958). *The standard edition of the complete psychological works of Sigmund Freud, Volume XII (1911–1913).* London: Hogarth Press.

Freud, S. (1930). Civilization and its discontents. In J. Strachey (Ed.). (1961). *The standard edition of the complete psychological works of Sigmund Freud, Volume XXI (1927–1931).* London: Hogarth Press.

Gallese, V., Fadiga, L., Fogassi, L., & Rizzolatti, G. (1996). Action recognition in the premotor cortex. *Brain, 119*, 593–609.

Goleman, D. (2003, February 4). Cajole your brain to lean to the left. *New York Times.*

Grepmair, L., Mitterlehener, F., Loew, T., Bachler, E., Rother, W., & Nickel, M. (2007). Promoting mindfulness in psychotherapists in training influences the treatment results of their patients: A randomized, double-blind, controlled study. *Psychotherapy and Psychosomatics, 76*, 332–338.

Hayes, S. C., & Strosahl, K. D. (Eds.). (2004). *A practical guide to acceptance and commitment therapy*. New York: Springer.

Hayes, S. C., Strosahl, K., & Wilson, K. G. (1999). *Acceptance and commitment therapy*. New York: Guilford.

Iacoboni, M. (2008). *Mirroring people: The new science of how we connect with others*. New York: Farrar, Straus and Giroux.

Jain, S., Shapiro, S., Swanick, S., Roesch, S., Mills, P., Bell, I., et al. (2007). A randomized controlled trial of mindfulness meditation versus relaxation training: Effects on distress, positive states of mind, rumination, and distraction. *Annals of Behavioral Medicine, 3*, 11–21.

Kabat-Zinn, J. (1996). Mindfulness meditation: What it is, what it isn't, and its role in health care and medicine. In Y. Haruki, Y. Ishii, & M. Suzuki (Eds.), *Comparative and psychological study on meditation*. Netherlands: Eburon.

Kalb, C. (2003, November 10). Faith & healing. *Newsweek*.

Kristeller, J. L., & Hallett, C. B. (1999). An exploratory study of a meditation-based intervention for binge eating disorder. *Journal of Health Psychology, 4*, 357–363.

Lebow, J. (2006). *Research for the psychotherapist: From science to practice*. New York: Routledge.

Linehan, M. M. (1993a). *Cognitive-behavioral treatment of borderline personality disorder*. New York: Guilford.

Linehan, M. M. (1993b). *Skills training manual for treating borderline personality disorder*. New York: Guilford.

Linehan, M. M. (2008). Keynote address. *6th Annual Conference: Integrating Mindfulness-Based Interventions into Medicine, Health Care, and Society*, Worcester, MA, April 10–12.

Lyons-Ruth, K., & BCPSG. (1998). Implicit relational knowing: Its role in development and psychoanalytic treatment. *Infant Mental Health Journal, 19*(3), 282–289.

Martin, J. (1997). Mindfulness: A proposed common factor. *Journal of Psychotherapy Integration, 7*(4), 291–312.

McCown, D., & Wiley, S. (2008). Emergent issues in MBSR research and pedagogy: Integrity, fidelity, and how do we decide? *6th Annual Conference: Integrating Mindfulness-Based Interventions into Medicine, Health Care, and Society*, Worcester, MA, April 10–12.

Meckel, D. J., & Moore, R. L. (1992). *Self and liberation: The Jung/Buddhism dialogue*. New York: Paulist Press.

Monti, D. A., Peterson, C., Kunkel, E. J., Hauck, W. W., Pequignot, E., Rhodes, L., et al. (2006). A randomized, controlled trial of mindfulness-based art therapy (MBAT) for women with cancer. *Psychooncology, 15*(5), 363–373.

Rawlinson, A. (1997). *The Book of Enlightened Masters*. Chicago: Open Court.

Rizzolatti, G. (2008). *Mirrors in the brain: How our minds share actions and emotions*. New York: Oxford University Press.

Robins, C., Schmidt, H., & Linehan, M. (2004). Dialectical behavior therapy: Synthesizing radical acceptance with skillful means. In S. C. Hayes, V. M. Follette, & M. M. Linehan (Eds.), *Mindfulness and acceptance: Expanding the cognitive behavioral tradition* (pp. 30–44). New York: Guilford.

Salmon, P. G., Santorelli, S. F., & Kabat-Zinn, J. (1998). Intervention elements promoting adherence to mindfulness-based stress reduction programs in the clinical behavioral medicine setting. In S. A. Shumaker, E. B. Schron, J. K. Okene, & W. L. Bee (Eds.), *Handbook of health behavior change* (2nd ed., pp. 239–268). New York: Springer.

Santorelli, S. (2001a). *Mindfulness-based stress reduction: Qualifications and recommended guidelines for providers*. Worcester, MA: Center for Mindfulness in Medicine, Health Care & Society.

Santorelli, S. (2001b). Interview with Saki Santorelli, Stress Reduction Clinic, Massachusetts Memorial Medical Center. In L. Freedman (Ed.), *Best practices in alternative and complementary medicine*. Frederick, MD: Aspen.

Segal, Z. V., Williams, J. M. G., & Teasdale, J. D. (2002). *Mindfulness-based cognitive therapy for depression: A new approach to preventing relapse*. New York: Guilford.

Siegel, D. J. (1999). *The developing mind: Toward a neurobiology of interpersonal experience.* New York: Guilford.

Stein, J. (2003, August 4). Just say OM. *Time.*

Stern, D. (2004). *The present moment in psychotherapy and everyday life.* New York: Norton.

Strosahl, K. D., Hayes, S. C., Wilson, K. G., & Gifford, E. V. (2004). An ACT primer: Core therapy processes, intervention strategies, and therapist competencies. In S. C. Hayes & K. D. Strosahl (Eds.), *A practical guide to acceptance and commitment therapy.* New York: Springer.

Wallin, D. (2007). *Attachment in psychotherapy.* New York: Guilford.

Wampold, B. E. (2001). *The great psychotherapy debate: Models, methods, and findings.* Mahwah, NJ: Erlbaum.

Welch, S., Rizvi, S., & Dimidjian, S. (2006). Mindfulness in dialectical behavior therapy (DBT) for borderline personality disorder. In R. A. Baer (Ed.), *Mindfulness-based treatment approaches: Clinician's guide to evidence base and applications* (pp. 117–139). San Diego, CA: Elsevier Academic Press.

Chapter 2

Baer, R. (2006). *Mindfulness-based treatment approaches: Clinician's guide to evidence base and applications.* Boston: Elsevier Academic Press.

Barks, C. (1995). *The essential Rumi.* San Francisco, CA: Harper.

Batchelor, S. (1994). *The awakening of the west.* Berkeley, CA: Parallax.

Bell, S. (2002). Scandals in emerging Western Buddhism. In C. S. Prebish & M. Baumann (Eds.), *Westward dharma: Buddhism beyond Asia.* Berkeley, CA: University of California Press.

Benson, H. (1975). *The relaxation response.* New York: Morrow.

Bevis, W. W. (1988). *Mind of winter: Wallace Stevens, meditation, and literature.* Pittsburgh, PA: University of Pittsburgh Press.

Brooks, V. W. (1936). *The flowering of New England, 1815–1865.* New York: E. P. Dutton & Co.

Brooks, V. W. (1962). *Fenollosa and his circle, with other essays in biography.* New York: Dutton.

Cage, J. (1966). *Silence: Lectures and writings.* Cambridge, MA: The MIT Press.

Carrington, P. (1998/1975). *The book of meditation: The complete guide to modern meditation.* Boston: Element. (Rev. ed. of: *Freedom in meditation.* East Millstone, NJ: Pace Educational Systems, 1975).

Clark, T. (1980). *The great Naropa poetry wars.* Santa Barbara, CA: Cadmus Editions.

Coleman, W. (2001). *The new Buddhism: The western transformation of an ancient tradition.* Oxford: New York.

Cupitt, D. (1999). *The new religion of life in everyday speech.* London: SCM Press.

Didonna, F. (2009). *Clinical handbook of mindfulness* (p. 523). New York: Springer.

Downing, M. (2001). *Shoes outside the door: Desire, devotion, and excess at San Francisco Zen Center.* Washington, DC: Counterpoint.

Dryden, W., & Still, A. (2006). Historical aspects of mindfulness and self-acceptance in psychotherapy. *Journal of Rational-Emotive & Cognitive-Behavior Therapy, 24*(1), 3–28.

Duckworth, W. (1999). *Talking music: Conversations with John Cage, Philip Glass, Laurie Anderson, and five generations of American experimental composers.* Cambridge, MA: Da Capo Press.

Fields, R. (1991). The changing of the guard: Western Buddhism in the eighties. *Tricycle: The Buddhist Review, 1*(2), 43–49.

Fromm, E., Suzuki, D.T., & DeMartino, R. (1960/1970). *Zen Buddhism & psychoanalysis.* New York: Harper & Row.

Fronsdal, G. (2002). Virtues without rules: Ethics in the insight meditation movement. In C. S. Prebish & M. Baumann (Eds.), *Westward dharma: Buddhism beyond Asia*. Berkeley, CA: University of California Press.

Furlong, M. (1986). *Genuine fake: A biography of Alan Watts*. London: Heinemann.

Hayes, S. C., Follette, V. M., & Linehan, M. M. (2004). *Mindfulness and acceptance: Expanding the cognitive-behavioral tradition*. New York: Guilford.

Hayward, J. (2008). *Warrior-king of Shambhala: Remembering Chogyam Trungpa*. Boston: Wisdom.

Hodder, A. D. (1993). "Ex Oriente Lux": Thoreau's ecstasies and the Hindu texts. *The Harvard Theological Review, 86*(4), 403–438.

Johnston, H. (1988). The marketing social movement: A case study of the rapid growth of TM. In J. T. Richardson (Ed.), *Money and power in the new religions*. Lewiston, NY: The Edwin Mellen Press.

Kantner, P. (1967). Won't you try/Saturday afternoon [Recorded by Jefferson Airplane]. On *After bathing at Baxter's* [LP]. New York: RCA Victor.

Mahesh Yogi, M. (1968/1963). *Transcendental meditation*. New York: New American Library.

McMahan, D. L. (2002). Repackaging Zen for the West. In C. S. Prebish & M. Baumann (Eds.), *Westward dharma: Buddhism beyond Asia*. Berkeley, CA: University of California Press.

Merton, T. (1968). *Zen and the birds of appetite*. New York: New Directions.

Metcalf, F. A. (2002). The encounter of Buddhism and psychology. In C. S. Prebish & M. Baumann (Eds.), *Westward dharma: Buddhism beyond Asia*. Berkeley, CA: University of California Press.

Morita, S. (1998; Japanese publication 1928). *Morita therapy and the true nature of anxiety based disorders (Shinkeishitsu)*; translated by Akihisa Kondo; edited by Peg LeVine. Albany, NY: State University of New York Press.

Mott, M. (1984). *The seven mountains of Thomas Merton*. Boston: Houghton Mifflin.

Mukpo, D. J. (2006). *Dragon thunder: My life with Chogyam Trungpa*. Boston: Shambhala.

Nattier, J. (1998). Who is a Buddhist? Charting the landscape of Buddhist America. In C. S. Prebish & K. K. Tanaka (Eds.), *The faces of Buddhism in America*. Berkeley, CA: University of California Press.

Pennington, M. B. (1980). *Centering prayer: Renewing an ancient Christian prayer tradition*. New York: Image Books.

Polanyi, M. (1966). *The tacit dimension*. Garden City, NY: Doubleday.

Obadia, L. (2002). Buddha in the promised land: Outlines of the Buddhist settlement in Israel. In C. S. Prebish & M. Baumann (Eds.), *Westward dharma: Buddhism beyond Asia* (pp. 177–190). Berkeley, CA: University of California Press.

Prebish, C. S. (1999). *Luminous passage: The practice and study of Buddhism in America*. Berkeley, CA: University of California Press.

Prebish, C. S., & Baumann, M. (Eds.). (2002). *Westward dharma: Buddhism beyond Asia*. Berkeley, CA: University of California Press.

Queen, C. S. (2002). Engaged Buddhism: Agnosticism, interdependence, globalization. In C. S. Prebish & M. Baumann (Eds.), *Westward dharma: Buddhism beyond Asia*. Berkeley, CA: University of California Press.

Reynolds, D. K. (1980). *The quiet therapies: Japanese pathways to personal growth*. Honolulu: University of Hawaii Press.

Reynolds, D. K. (1993). *Plunging through the clouds: Constructive living currents*. Albany, NY: State University of New York Press.

Rohr, R. (1999). *Everything belongs: The gift of contemplative prayer*. New York: Crossroad.

Sanders, E. (1977). The Party: A chronological perspective on a confrontation at a Buddhist seminary.

Schwartz, T. (1995). *What really matters: Searching for wisdom in America*. New York: Bantam.

Seager, R. H. (2002). American Buddhism in the making. In C. S. Prebish & M. Baumann (Eds.), *Westward dharma: Buddhism beyond Asia*. Berkeley, CA: University of California Press.

Seeman, W., Nidich, S., & Banta, T. (1972). Influence of transcendental meditation on a measure of self-actualization. *Journal of Counseling Psychology, 19*, 184–187.
Stevens, W. (1971). *The palm at the end of the mind; selected poems and a play.* New York: Knopf.
Suzuki, D. T. (1957). *Mysticism: Christian and Buddhist.* New York: Harper & Brothers.
Suzuki, S. (1970). *Zen mind, beginner's mind.* New York: Weatherhill.
Trungpa, C. (1973). *Cutting through spiritual materialism.* Berkeley, CA: Shambhala.
Tweed, T. (1992). *The American encounter with Buddhism, 1844–1912: Victorian culture and the limits of dissent.* Bloomington: Indiana University Press.
Vanier, J. (2005). *Befriending the stranger.* Grand Rapids, MI: William B. Eerdmans.
Versluis, A. (1993). *American transcendentalism and Asian religions.* New York: Oxford University Press.
Wallace, R. K. (1970). Physiological effects of transcendental meditation. *Science, 167*, 1751–1754.
Watts, A. (1951). *The wisdom of insecurity.* New York: Pantheon.
Watts, A. (1960). *This is it: And other essays on Zen and spiritual experience.* New York: Pantheon.
Watts, A. (1961). *Psychotherapy east and west.* New York: Pantheon.
Watts, A. (1962). *Joyous cosmology: Adventures in the chemistry of consciousness.* New York: Pantheon.
Watts, A. (1972). *In my own way, an autobiography.* New York: Vintage.
Wuthnow, R. (1998). *After heaven: Spirituality in America since the 1950s.* Berkeley, CA: University of California Press.

Chapter 3

Adler, H. (1998). Vicissitudes of Fechnerian psychophysics in America. In R. Rieber & K. Salinger (Eds.), *Psychology: Theoretical–historical perspectives.* Washington, DC: American Psychological Association.
Agazarian, Y. M. (1997). *Systems centered therapy for groups.* New York: Guilford.
Allen, N. B., Blashki, G., & Gullone, E. (2006). Mindfulness-based psychotherapies: A review of conceptual foundations, empirical evidence and practical considerations. *Australian and New Zealand Journal of Psychiatry, 40*(4), 285–294.
Analayo. (2003). *Satipatthana: The direct path to realization.* Cambridge, UK: Windhorse.
Auden, W. H. (1970). *A certain world: A commonplace book.* New York: Viking Press.
Baer, R. (2003). Mindfulness training as a clinical intervention: A conceptual and empirical review. *Clinical Psychology: Science and Practice, 10*(2), 125–148.
Baer, R., Smith, G. T., Hopkins, J., Krietemeyer, J., & Toney, L. (2006). Using self-report assessment methods to explore facets of mindfulness. *Assessment, 13*, 27–45.
Bakhtin, M. (1984). *Problems of Dostoevsky's poetics.* Minneapolis, MN: University of Minnesota Press.
Batchelor, S. (1997). *Buddhism without beliefs: A contemporary guide to awakening.* New York: Riverhead Books.
Batchelor, S. (2004). Handouts and personal notes from retreat, *The path to the deathless,* held at Barre Center for Buddhist Studies, September 12–17, Barre, VT.
Beels, C. (2001). *A different story: The rise of narrative in psychotherapy.* Phoenix: Zeig, Tucker & Theisen.
Beels, C. (2007). Psychotherapy as a rite of passage. *Family Process, 46*(4), 421–436.
Birrell, P. (2006). An ethic of possibility: Relationship, risk and presence. *Ethics & Behavior, 16*(2), 95–115.
Bishop, S. (2002). What do we really know about mindfulness-based stress reduction? *Psychosomatic Medicine, 64*, 71–84.

Bishop, S., Lau, M., Shapiro, S., Carlson, L., Anderson, N., Carmody, J., et al. (2004). Mindfulness: A proposed operational definition. *Clinical Psychology: Science and Practice, 11*(3), 230–241.

Block, S., & Crouch, E. (1985). *Therapeutic factors in group psychotherapy.* New York: Oxford University Press.

Brody, L. R., & Park, S. H. (2004). Narratives, mindfulness, and the implicit audience. *Clinical Psychology: Science and Practice, 11*(2), 147–154.

Brown, K., & Ryan, R. (2004). Perils and promise in defining and measuring mindfulness: Observations from experience. *Clinical Psychology: Science and Practice, 11*(3), 242–248.

Buber, M. (1947). *Between man and man.* New York: The Macmillan Company.

Burlingame, G., Fuhriman, A., & Johnson, J. (2002). Cohesion in group psychotherapy. In J. Norcross (Ed.), *Psychotherapy relationships that work: Therapist contributions and responsiveness to patients.* New York: Oxford University Press.

Carr, L., Iacoboni, M., Dubeau, M.-C., Mazziotta, J., & Lenzi, G. (2003). Neural mechanisms of empathy in humans: A relay from neural systems for imitation to limbic areas. *Proceedings of the National Academy of Sciences, 100*, 5497–5502.

Claxton, G. (2006). Mindfulness, learning and the brain. *Journal of Rational-Emotive & Cognitive-Behavior Therapy, 23*(4), 301–314.

Cozolino, L. (2006). *The neuroscience of human relationships.* New York: Norton.

Creswell, J. D., Way, B. M., Eisenberger, N. I., & Lieberman, M. D. (2007). Neural correlates of dispositional mindfulness during affect labeling. *Psychosomatic Medicine, 69*, 560–565.

Cullen, M. (2008). On mindfulness. In Dalai Lama & P. Ekman (2008). *Emotional awareness: Overcoming the obstacles to psychological balance and compassion.* New York: Henry Holt.

Cupitt, D. (1999). *The new religion of life in everyday speech.* London: SCM Press.

Danto, A. C. (1993). The shape of artistic pasts: East and west. In P. Cook (Ed.), *Philosophical imagination and cultural memory.* Durham, NC: Duke University.

Davidson, R. (2000). Affective style, psychopathology, and resilience: Brain mechanisms and plasticity. *American Psychologist, 55*, 1196–1214.

Davidson, R., Kabat-Zinn, J., Schumacher, J., Rosenkranz, M., Muller, D., & Santorelli, S. (2003). Alterations in brain and immune function produced by mindfulness meditation. *Psychosomatic Medicine, 65*(4), 564–570.

Davidson, R., Schwartz, G., & Rothman, L. (1976). Attentional style and the regulation of mode-specific attention: An electroencephalographic study. *Journal of Abnormal Psychology, 8*(6), 611–621.

de Bary, W. (1969). *The Buddhist tradition in India, China, and Japan.* New York: Modern Library.

Deikman, A. (1966). De-automatization and the mystic experience. *Psychiatry, 29*, 324–338.

Deikman, A. (1982). *The observing self: Mysticism and psychotherapy.* Boston: Beacon Press.

Dryden, W., & Still, A. (2006). Historical aspects of mindfulness and self-acceptance in psychotherapy. *Journal of Rational-Emotive & Cognitive-Behavior Therapy, 24*(1), 3–28.

Foucault, M. (1972). *Archeology of knowledge.* New York: Pantheon.

Foucault, M. (1981). The order of discourse. In R. Young & R. Young (Eds.), *Untying the text.* Boston: Routledge & Kegan Paul.

Gallese, V. (2003). The manifold nature of interpersonal relations: The quest for a common mechanism. *Philosophical Transactions of the Royal Society of London, 358*, 517–528.

Gallese, V. (2006). Intentional attunement: A neurophysiological perspective on social cognition and its disruption in autism. *Brain Research, 1079*, 15–24.

Gallese, V., Fadiga, L., Fogassi, L., & Rizzolatti, G. (1996). Action recognition in the premotor cortex. *Brain, 119*, 593–609.

Gallese, V., & Goldman, A. (1998). Mirror neurons and the simulation theory of mindreading. *Trends in Cognitive Sciences, 2*(12), 493–501.

Gantt, E. (1994). Truth, freedom and responsibility in the dialogues of psychotherapy. *Journal of Theoretical and Philosophical Psychology, 14*(2), 146–158.

Gantt, S., & Agazarian, Y. (2005). *SCT in action.* New York: iUniverse.

Gergen, K. (1999). *An invitation to social construction.* Thousand Oaks, CA: Sage.

Gergen, K., & Hosking, D. (2006). If you meet social construction along the road: A dialogue with Buddhism. In M. Kwee, K. Gergen, & F. Koshikawa (Eds.), *Horizons in Buddhist psychology*. Chagrin Falls, OH: Taos Institute Publications.

Gethin, R. (1998). *The foundations of Buddhism*. Oxford: New York.

Goddard, D. (1938). *A Buddhist bible*. Thetford, VT: Dwight Goddard.

Goleman, D. (1995). *Emotional intelligence*. New York: Bantam.

Grossman, P. (2008). On measuring mindfulness in psychosomatic and psychological research. *Journal of Psychosomatic Research, 64*, 405–408.

Hayes, A., & Feldman, G. (2004). Clarifying the construct of mindfulness in the context of emotion regulation and the process of change in therapy. *Clinical Psychology: Science and Practice, 11*(3), 255–262.

Hayes, S., & Shenk, C. (2004). Operationalizing mindfulness without unnecessary attachments. *Clinical Psychology: Science and Practice, 11*(3), 249–254.

Hayes, S. C., & Wilson, K. G. (2003). Mindfulness: Method and process. *Clinical Psychology: Science and Practice, 10*, 161–165.

Hölzel, B. K., Carmody, J., Evans, K. C., Hoge, E. A., Dusek, J. A., Morgan, L., et al. (2009). Stress reduction correlates with structural changes in the amygdala. *Social Cognitive and Affective Neuroscience*, Sep 23 [Epub ahead of print].

Horvath, A., & Bedi, R. (2002). The alliance. In J. Norcross (Ed.), *Psychotherapy relationships that work: Therapist contributions and responsiveness to patients*. New York: Oxford University Press.

Imel, Z., Baldwin, S., Bonus, K., & MacCoon, D. (2008). Beyond the individual: Group effects in mindfulness-based stress reduction. *Psychotherapy Research, 18*(6), 735–742.

Isanon, A. (2001). *Spirituality and the autism spectrum*. London: Jessica Kingsley.

Ivanovski, B., & Malhi, G. S. (2007). The psychological and neurophysiological concomitants of mindfulness forms of meditation. *Acta Neuropsychiatrica, 19*, 76–91.

Kabat-Zinn, J. (1994). *Wherever you go, there you are*. New York: Hyperion.

Kabat-Zinn, J. (1996). Mindfulness meditation: What it is, what it isn't, and its role in health care and medicine. In Y. Haruki, Y. Ishii, & M. Suzuki (Eds.), *Comparative and psychological study on meditation*. Netherlands: Eburon.

Kasamatsu, A., & Hirai, T. (1973). An electroencephalographic study of the Zen meditation (Zazen). In D. H. Shapiro & R. N. Walsh (Eds.), *Meditation, classic and contemporary perspectives*. New York: Aldine.

Ladden, L. (2007). Mindfulness meditation and systems-centered practice. *Systems-Centered News, 15*(1), 8–11.

Langer, E. J. (1989). *Mindfulness*. Reading, MA: Addison-Wesley.

Langer, E. J. (1997). *Mindful learning*. Reading, MA: Addison-Wesley.

Lazar, S. W., Kerr, C. E., Wasserman, R. H., Gray, J. R., Greve, D. N., Treadway, M. T., et al. (2005). Meditation experience is associated with increased cortical thickness. *Neuroreport, 16*(17), 1893–1897.

Lieberman, M. D., Eisenberger, N. I., Crockett, M. J., Tom, S. M., Pfeifer, J. H., & Way, B. M. (2007). Rutting feelings into words: Affect labeling disrupts amygdala activity in response to affective stimuli. *Psychological Science, 18*(5), 421–427.

Linden, W. (1973). Practicing of meditation by school children and their levels of field dependence, test anxiety, and reading achievement. *Journal of Consulting and Clinical Psychology, 41*(1), 139–143.

Martin, J. (1997). Mindfulness: A proposed common factor. *Journal of Psychotherapy Integration, 7*(4), 291–312.

McCown, D. (2004). The problems of passionate chess: Helping business strategists change the rules of the game through applied meditation. In S. Gopalkrishnan (Ed.), *Organizational wisdom: Proceedings of the Eastern Academy of Management 41st annual meeting*.

Mills, S. (1997). *Discourse*. New York: Routlege.

Narada, M. (1980). *The Buddha and his teachings*. Singapore: Singapore Buddhist Meditation Centre.

Nyanaponika, T. (1965). *The heart of Buddhist meditation*. Boston: Weiser Books.

Pelletier, K. (1974). Influence of transcendental meditation upon autokinetic perception. In D. H. Shapiro & R. N. Walsh (Eds.), *Meditation, classic and contemporary perspectives*. New York: Aldine.

Porges, S. W. (1995). Orienting in a defensive world: Mammalian modifications of our evolutionary heritage. A polyvagal theory. *Psychophysiology, 32*, 301–318.

Porges, S. W. (2001). The polyvagal theory: Phylogenetic substrates of a social nervous system. *International Journal of Psychophysiology, 42*, 123–146.

Porges, S. W. (2003). Social engagement and attachment: A phylogenetic perspective. *Annals of the New York Academy of Sciences, 1008*, 31–47.

Porges, S. W. (2004). Neuroception: A subconscious system for detecting threats and safety. *Zero to Three: Bulletin of the National Center for Infant Clinical Programs, 24*(5), 19–24.

Porges, S. W. (2006). The polyvagal perspective. *Biological Psychology, 74*, 116–143.

Porges, S. W. (2009). The polyvagal theory: New insights into adaptive reactions of the autonomic nervous system. *Cleveland Clinic Journal of Medicine, 76*(Supplement 2), S86–S90.

Rogers, C. (1961). *On becoming a person; a therapist's view of psychotherapy*. Boston: Houghton Mifflin.

Rothwell, N. (2006). The different facets of mindfulness. *Journal of Rational-Emotive & Cognitive-Behavior Therapy, 24*, 79–86.

Safran, J. D., & Segal, Z. (1990). *Interpersonal process in cognitive therapy*. New York: Basic Books.

Schwartz, G. (1975). Biofeedback, self-regulation, and the patterning of physiological processes. *American Scientist, 63*, 314–324.

Schwartz, S. (1986). *Classic studies in psychology*. Palo Alto, CA: Mayfield.

Shapiro, S., Carlson, L., Astin, J., & Freedman, B. (2006). Mechanisms of mindfulness. *Journal of Clinical Psychology, 62*(3), 373–386.

Shapiro, D. H., & Walsh, R. N. (1984). *Meditation, classic and contemporary perspectives*. New York: Aldine.

Siegel, D. (2007). *The mindful brain*. New York: W.W. Norton.

Siegel, D. (2009). Personal correspondence with D. McCown, November 25.

Stern, D. (2004). *The present moment in psychotherapy and everyday life*. New York: Norton.

Thompson, L., Thompson, M., & Reid, A. (2009). Functional neuroanatomy and the rationale for using EEG biofeedback for clients with Asperger's syndrome. *Applied Psychophysiology & Biofeedback*. doi:10.1007/s10484-009-9095-0.

Tronick, E. (2003). "Of course all relationships are unique": How co-creative processes generate unique mother-infant and patient-therapist relationships and change other relationships. *Psychological Inquiry, 23*(3), 473–491.

Tronick, E. (2007). *The neurobehavioral and social-emotional development of infants and children*. New York: W.W. Norton.

Tronick, E., & Members of the Boston Change Process Study Group. (1998). Dyadically expanded states of consciousness and the process of therapeutic change. *Infant Mental Health Journal, 19*(3), 290–299.

Turner, V. L. (1969). *The ritual process*. Chicago: Aldine.

Watson, G. (1998). *The resonance of emptiness: A Buddhist inspiration for a contemporary psychotherapy*. Delhi: Motilal Banarsidas.

Yalom, I. (1985). *The theory and practice of group psychotherapy*. New York: Basic Books.

Chapter 4

Batchelor, S. (1997). *Buddhism without beliefs*. New York: Riverhead Books.

Boorstein, S. (1996). *Don't just do something, sit there: A mindfulness retreat with Sylvia Boorstein*. San Francisco: HarperSanFrancisco.

Bly, R. (1971). *Kabir: The fish in the sea is not thirsty, versions by Robert Bly*. San Francisco: Rainbow Bridge.

Brach, T. (2003). *Radical acceptance: Embracing your life with the heart of a Buddha*. New York: Bantam.

Center for Mindfulness in Medicine, Health Care & Society. (2007). *Oasis: An international learning center. Professional trainings in mindfulness based stress reduction and other mindfulness-based approaches and interventions*. Worcester, MA: Center for Mindfulness in Medicine, Health Care & Society.

Fowler, J. (1981). *Stages of faith: The psychology of human development and the quest for meaning*. New York: HarperCollins.

Kabat-Zinn, J. (1999). Indra's net at work: The mainstreaming of dharma practice in society. In G. Watson, S. Batchelor, & G. Claxton (Eds.), *The psychology of awakening: Buddhism, science and our day-to-day lives*. London: Rider.

Kabat-Zinn, J. (2003). Mindfulness-based interventions in context: Past, present, and future. *Clinical Psychology: Science and Practice, 10*(2), 144–154.

Kornfield, J. (1993). *A path with heart: A guide through the perils and promises of spiritual life*. New York: Bantam Books.

Landy, D. (1977). *Culture, disease, and healing: Studies in medical anthropology*. New York: Macmillan.

Neufelder, J., & Coelho, M. (1982). *Writings on spiritual direction by great Christian masters*. New York: The Seabury Press.

Santorelli, S. (2001). *Mindfulness-based stress reduction: Qualifications and recommended guidelines for providers*. Worcester, MA: Center for Mindfulness in Medicine, Health Care & Society. unpaginated.

Chapter 5

Baer, R., & Krietemeyer, J. (2003). Overview of mindfulness- and acceptance-based treatment approaches. In R. Baer (2006). Mindfulness-based treatment approaches: Clinician's guide to evidence base and applications (pp. 3–27). San Diego, CA: Elsevier Academic Press.

Batchelor, S. (1997). *Buddhism without beliefs*. New York: Riverhead Books.

Berry, W. (1998). *A timbered choir: The Sabbath poems 1979-1997*. New York: Counterpoint.

Carse, J. (1986). *Finite and infinite games*. New York: Ballantine Books.

Homiletic. (2009). In Merriam-Webster online dictionary. Retrieved January 18, 2009, from http://www.merriam-webster.com/dictionary/homiletic.

Homily. (2009). In Merriam-Webster online dictionary. Retrieved January 18, 2009, from http://www.merriam-webster.com/dictionary/homily.

Kabat-Zinn, J. (2004). The uses of language and images in guiding meditation practices in MBSR. Audio Recording from 2nd Annual Conference sponsored by the Center for Mindfulness in Medicine, Health Care and Society at the University of Massachusetts Medical School. March 26, 2004.

Linklater, K. (1976). *Freeing the natural voice*. New York: Drama Book Specialists.

Littlewood, W. C., & Roche, M. A. (2004). *Waking up: The work of Charlotte Selver*. Bloomington, IN: Author House.

McCown, D., Reibel, D., & Malcoun, E. (2007). Psychological type and participation in mindfulness-based stress reduction programs. Presentation at 5th Annual Conference: Integrating Mindfulness-Based Interventions into Medicine, Health Care, and Society, Worcester, MA, March 29–April 1.

Mezirow, J. (2000). Learning to think like an adult: Core concepts of transformation theory. In J. Mezirow et al. (Eds.), *Learning as transformation*. San Francisco: Jossey-Bass.

Neihardt, J. G. (1961). *Black Elk speaks: Being the life story of a holy man of the Oglala Sioux*. Lincoln, NB: University of Nebraska Press.

Rodenburg, P. (2000). *The actor speaks: Voice and the performer*. New York: St. Martin's.

Santorelli, S. (2001). Mindfulness-based stress reduction (MBSR): Standards of practice. Worcester, MA: Center for Mindfulness in Medicine, Health Care & Society, (unpaginated).

Santorelli, S. (2004). Three points to consider when teaching mindfulness-based stress reduction. Personal notes provided by Santorelli at Post-Conference Instructional Institute, *2nd Annual Conference sponsored by the Center for Mindfulness in Medicine, Health Care and Society*, Worcester, MA. March 27, 2004.

Segal, Z. V., Williams, J. M. G., & Teasdale, J. D. (2002). *Mindfulness-based cognitive therapy for depression: A new approach to preventing relapse*. New York: Guilford Press.

Singh, N. N., Wahler, R. G., Adkins, A. D., & Myers, R. E. (2003). Soles of the feet: A mindfulness-based self-control intervention for aggression by an individual with mild mental retardation and mental illness. *Research in Developmental Disabilities, 24*, 158–169.

Speads, C. (1992). *Ways to better breathing*. Rochester, VT: Healing Arts Press.

Steward. (2009). In Merriam-Webster online dictionary. Retrieved January 10, 2009, from http://www.merriam-webster.com/dictionary/steward.

Stewardship. (2009). In Merriam-Webster online dictionary. Retrieved January 9, 2009, from http://www.merriam-webster.com/dictionary/stewardship.

Tronick, E. (2003). "Of course all relationships are unique": How co-creative processes generate unique mother-infant and patient-therapist relationships and change other relationships. *Psychological Inquiry, 23*(3), 473–491.

Tronick, E. (2007). *The neurobehavioral and social-emotional development of infants and children*. New York: W.W. Norton.

Zimmerman, J., & Coyle, V. (1996). *The way of council*. Las Vegas, NV: Bramble Books.

Chapter 6

Arrien, A. (1993). *The four-fold way*. San Francisco: HarperSanFrancisco.

Astin, J. (1997). Stress reduction through mindfulness meditation: Effects on psychological symptomatology, sense of control, and spiritual experience. *Psychotherapy and Psychosomatics, 66*, 97–106.

Baer, R. (2003). Mindfulness training as a clinical intervention: A conceptual and empirical review. *Clinical Psychology: Science and Practice, 10*(2), 125–148.

Batchelor, S. (1983). *Alone with others: An existential approach to Buddhism*. New York: Grove Press.

Batchelor, S. (2004). Hearing the call of the other. *Parabola, 29*(4), 52–58.

Carmody, J., & Baer, R. A. (2008). Relationships between mindfulness practice and levels of mindfulness, medical and psychological symptoms and well-being in a mindfulness-based stress reduction program. *Journal of Behavioral Medicine, 31*, 23–33.

Carmody, J., Reed, G., Kristeller, J., & Merriam, P. (2008). Mindfulness, spirituality, and health-related symptoms. *Journal of Psychosomatic Research, 64*, 393–403.

Chang, V. Y., Palesh, O., Caldwell, R., Glasgow, N., Abramson, M., Luskin, F., et al. (2004). The effects of a mindfulness-based stress reduction program on stress, mindfulness self-efficacy, and positive states of mind. *Stress and Health: Journal of the International Society for the Investigation of Stress, 20*, 141–147.

Coelho, H. F., Canter, P. H., & Edzard, E. (2007). Mindfulness-based cognitive therapy: Evaluating current evidence and informing future research. *Journal of Consulting and Clinical Psychology, 75*, 1000–1005.

Davidson, R. J., Kabat-Zinn, J., Schumaker, J., Rosenkranz, M., Muller, D., Santorelli, S., et al. (2003). Alterations in brain and immune function produced by mindfulness meditation. *Psychosomatic Medicine, 65*, 564–570.

Denma Translation Group. (2002). *Sun Tzu, the art of war.* Boston: Shambhala.

Derogatis, L. R. (2000). *BSI-18: Administration, scoring, and procedures manual.* Minneapolis, MN: National Computer Systems.

Esparza, M., Katz, R. (Producers), & Maxwell, R. (Director). (1993). *Gettysburg.* [Film]. New Line Cinema.

Foley, D. (2006). Find calm in the chaos. *Prevention, 58*(11), 158–161.

Fromm, E. (1976). *To have or to be?* New York: Harper & Row.

Jain, S., Shapiro, S., Swanick, S., Roesch, S., Mills, P., Bell, I., et al. (2007). A randomized controlled trial of mindfulness meditation versus relaxation training: Effects on distress, positive states of mind, rumination, and distraction. *Annals of Behavioral Medicine, 3,* 11–21.

Kabat-Zinn, J. (1990). *Full catastrophe living: Using the wisdom of your body and mind to face stress, pain, and illness.* New York: Delta.

Kabat-Zinn, J. (1996). Mindfulness meditation: What it is, what it isn't, and its role in health care and medicine. In Y. Haruki, Y. Ishii, & M. Suzuki (Eds.), *Comparative and psychological study on meditation.* Netherlands: Eburon.

Kabat-Zinn, J. (2003). Mindfulness-based interventions in context: Past, present, and future. *Clinical Psychology: Science and Practice, 10*(2), 144–154.

Marcel, G. (1949). *Being and having: An existentialist diary.* Westminster: Dacre Press.

McCown, D., & Reibel, D. (2008). Bringing MBSR to the workplace: One institution's experience in marketing, sales, and delivery. *6th Annual Conference: Integrating Mindfulness-Based Interventions into Medicine, Health Care, and Society,* Worcester, MA, April 10–12.

McCown, D., Reibel, D., & Malcoun, E. (2007). Psychological type and participation in mindfulness-based stress reduction programs. *5th Annual Conference: Integrating Mindfulness-Based Interventions into Medicine, Health Care, and Society,* Worcester, MA, March 29–April 1.

Merton, T. (1955). *No man is an island.* New York: Harcourt Brace Jovanovich.

Mitchell, S. (1995). *Ahead of all parting: Selected poetry and prose of Rainer Maria Rilke.* New York: Modern Library.

Pakula, A. (Producer), & Muligan, R. (Director). (1962). *To kill a mockingbird.* [Film]. United Artists.

Reibel, D. K., Greeson, J. M., Brainard, G. C., & Rosenzweig, S. (2001). Mindfulness-based stress reduction and health related quality of life in a heterogeneous patient population. *General Hospital Psychiatry, 23,* 183–192.

Reibel, D., & McCown, D. (2007). Continuity and change: Adapting the MBSR curriculum and delivery methods. *5th Annual Conference: Integrating Mindfulness-Based Interventions into Medicine, Health Care, and Society,* Worcester, MA, March 29–April 1.

Rosenzweig, S., Reibel, D., Greeson, J., Brainard, G., & Hojat, M. (2003). Mindfulness-based stress reduction lowers psychological distress in medical students. *Teaching and Learning in Medicine, 15*(2), 88–92.

Roth, B., & Calle-Mesa, L. (2006). Mindfulness-based stress reduction with Spanish- and English speaking inner-city medical patients. In R. A. Baer (Ed.), *Mindfulness-based treatment approaches: Clinician's guide to evidence base and applications.* Boston: Elsevier Academic Press.

Shapiro, S., Carlson, L., Astin, J., & Freedman, B. (2006). Mechanisms of mindfulness. *Journal of Clinical Psychology, 62*(3), 373–386.

Speca, M., Carlson, L. E., Goodey, E., & Angen, M. (2000). A randomized, wait-list controlled clinical trial: The effect of a mindfulness meditation-based stress reduction program on mood and symptoms of stress in cancer outpatients. *Psychosomatic Medicine, 62,* 613–622.

Turner, V. (1969). *The ritual process.* Chicago: Aldine.

Whitehead, C. (2008). You do an empirical experiment and you get an empirical result. What can any anthropologist tell me that could change that? *Journal of Consciousness Studies, 15*(10–11), 7–41.

Zimmerman, J., & Coyle, V. (1996). *The way of council.* Las Vegas: Bramble Books.

Chapter 7

Abbott, A. (2007). Against narrative: A preface to lyrical sociology. *Sociological Theory, 25*(1), 67–99.

Barks, C., & Moyne, J. (1997). *The Essential Rumi*. Edison, New Jersey: Castle Books.

Compassion. (n.d.). *Webster's Revised Unabridged Dictionary*. Retrieved January 2, 2009, from http://dictionary.reference.com/browse/compassion.

Debord, G. (1994). *The society of the spectacle*. New York: Zone Books.

Drummond, M. S. (2006). Conceptualizing the efficacy of mindfulness of body sensations in the mindfulness-based interventions. *Constructivism in the Human Sciences, 11*(1), 2–29.

Gendlin, E. T. (1962). *Experiencing and the creation of meaning; a philosophical and psychological approach to the subjective*. New York: Free Press of Glencoe.

Goleman, D. (1977/1988). *The meditative mind: The varieties of meditative experience*. Los Angeles: J.P. Tarcher; New York: Distributed by St. Martin's Press. Updated ed. of *The varieties of the meditative experience*.

Kabat-Zinn, J. (1990). *Full catastrophe living: Using the wisdom of your body and mind to face stress, pain, and illness*. New York: Delta.

Kabat-Zinn, J. (2005). *Coming to our senses: Healing ourselves and the world through mindfulness*. New York: Hyperion.

May, G. (2006). *The wisdom of wilderness*. New York: HarperSanFrancisco.

Mezirow, J. (2000). Learning to think like an adult: Core concepts of transformation theory. In J. Mezirow et al. (Eds.), *Learning as transformation*. San Francisco: Jossey-Bass.

Neff, K. (2003). The development and validation of a scale to measure self-compassion. *Self and Identity, 2*, 223–250.

Santorelli, S. (2004). Three points to consider when teaching mindfulness-based stress reduction. Personal notes provided by Santorelli at Post-Conference Instructional Institute, *2nd Annual Conference sponsored by the Center for Mindfulness in Medicine, Health Care and Society*, Worcester, MA. March 27, 2004.

Santorelli, S., & Kabat-Zinn, J. (2003). *MBSR curriculum guide and supporting materials: Guidelines for presenting this work*. Worcester, MA: Center for Mindfulness in Medicine, Health Care & Society, (unpaginated).

Selver, C., & Brooks, C. V. W. (2007). *Reclaiming vitality and presence: Sensory awareness as a practice for life*. Berkeley: North Atlantic Books.

Stern, D. (2004). *The present moment in psychotherapy and everyday life*. New York: Norton.

Strawson, G. (2004). Against narrativity. *Ratio (new series), 117*(4), 428–452.

Tillich, P. (1957). *Love, power and justice*. London: Oxford University Press.

Tillich, P. (1963). *Systematic theology, Vol. 3*. Chicago: University of Chicago.

Wagoner, D. (1976). *Collected poems (1956–1976)*. Bloomington: Indiana University Press.

Wátzlawick, P., Weakland, J. H., & Fisch, R. (1974). *Change; principles of problem formation and problem resolution*. New York: Norton.

Index

LaVergne, TN USA
12 March 2010
175740LV00001B/51/P